Thoughts on the Clinical Diagnosis and Treatment of Infectious Diseases

www.royalcollins.com

Thoughts on the Clinical Diagnosis and Treatment of Infectious Diseases

Editor-in-Chief
Li Lanjuan

RC

Books Beyond Boundaries

ROYAL COLLINS

Thoughts on the Clinical Diagnosis and Treatment of Infectious Diseases

Editor-in-Chief: Li Lanjuan

First published in 2024 by Royal Collins Publishing Group Inc.
Groupe Publication Royal Collins Inc.
BKM Royalcollins Publishers Private Limited

Headquarters: 550-555 boul. René-Lévesque O Montréal (Québec) H2Z1B1 Canada
India office: 805 Hemkunt House, 8th Floor, Rajendra Place, New Delhi 110 008

ISBN: 978-1-4878-1165-5

To find out more about our publications, please visit www.royalcollins.com.

EDITORIAL BOARD

CONTENTS

For current medical education in China (including five-year and long-term courses), the early classroom teaching stage is mainly designed to instill basic knowledge and thinking methods, while the clinical practice stage requires the cultivation of students' thinking ability and creativity in clinical diagnosis and treatment. The most pressing questions are how can we combine basic medicine with clinical practice, and how can we observe the nature of disease through clinical manifestations? Basic medical knowledge must be integrated into clinical practice, where it can be used to explain clinical phenomena. This is the only way that misdiagnosis and missed diagnosis can be avoided in clinical practice, that clinical experience can be accumulated, and that meticulous thinking about clinical diagnosis and treatment can be established. However, among the medical books that are extant in China, few can guide students or junior physicians to develop their thinking around active clinical diagnosis and treatment.

Thoughts on the Clinical Diagnosis and Treatment of Infectious Diseases is one of a series of books on clinical diagnosis and treatment published by the People's Medical Publishing House, and aims to help senior medical students, clinical postgraduates, residents, and attending physicians to improve their clinical thinking ability. It focuses on common and frequently-occurring clinical cases in infectious departments, both typical and atypical, and both complex and simple. It explains how the authors chose consultation methods, physical examinations, and laboratory-based or special examinations depending on patients' symptoms, so as to make a correct diagnosis and propose a reasonable treatment plan. In this way, it helps to encourage precise and systematic thinking on the diagnosis and treatment of infectious diseases. After a diagnosis and treatment plan is established, the accuracy of the original diagnosis and treatment plan (and whether it needs to be modified) can be determined by observing changes to patients' symptoms, signs, and auxiliary examination reports. Meanwhile, readers are guided to link clinical manifestations with basic medical knowledge in the process of diagnostic thinking and treatment. Most of the cases also provide follow-up results and clinical progress of their specific disease.

The book covers 47 common infectious diseases across a total of 65 cases. The authors are experts who have been engaged in clinical practice and teaching about infectious diseases for many years, and most are well-known experts in this field in China. They are familiar with medical students as well as the thinking around clinical diagnosis and treatment, and understand the basic knowledge and skills that should be mastered by residents and attending physicians in infectious disease departments. Therefore, in writing this book, they combine clinical thinking, deep medical knowledge, and extensive clinical experience, and explain complex theories in simple, practical terms. As a result, the text will have important reference value for young physicians in infection departments around the country.

The contributors are clinicians from 21 well-known hospitals in China, such as the First Affiliated Hospital, Zhejiang University School of Medicine. Professor Si Chongwen, Professor Ma Yilin, and Professor Xu Daozhen (the pioneers of infectious disease departments) have offered many valuable insights about case collection as well as the writing and proofreading of articles, for which I express my heartfelt thanks.

The content of this book was finalized after many discussions and revisions. Due to the large number of participating units and varying writing styles, there are inevitably some errors. Please feel free to inform us, so that we can revise the text for future reprints.

Li Lanjuan
Hangzhou, May 2010

Infectious diseases refer to communicable diseases that can cause epidemics in the normal human population, and are caused by various pathogenic microorganisms. Infectious diseases have accompanied the development of human civilization. Epidemics have claimed countless lives, and have also seriously affected economic and social development. At present, the global situation of infectious disease prevention and treatment is still very serious. In the 1996 World Health Report, the Director-General of the WHO warned: "We are on the verge of a global infectious disease crisis. No country can be safe from it or rest easy." The struggle of human against infectious diseases will remain a long-term process.

I. The current status of infectious diseases in China

Since the founding of the People's Republic of China, great achievements have been made in the prevention and treatment of infectious diseases under the guidance of the health policy of prevention first, and the combination of prevention and treatment. Like other countries around the world, China has eradicated smallpox, and the incidence of many infectious diseases, such as poliomyelitis, measles, diphtheria, pertussis, and neonatal tetanus, has dropped significantly. Human plague has been controlled.

At present, the general status of infectious diseases in China is as follows: Firstly, the prevention and treatment of viral hepatitis are still rudimentary, while hepatitis B, hepatitis C, and related diseases are still common. Over the next few decades, patients infected with viral hepatitis will continue to be important targets for treatment. Secondly, some infectious diseases that have been controlled in the past have been revived and made a comeback, such as tuberculosis, schistosomiasis, brucellosis, malaria, and syphilis. Thirdly, new infectious diseases have been discovered, such as AIDS, severe acute respiratory syndrome (SARS), highly pathogenic avian influenza, enterohemorrhagic Escherichia coli O_{157}:H_7, O_{139} cholera, Legionnaires disease, Campylobacter jejuni diarrhea, Lyme disease, and Yersinia enterocolitica. New infectious diseases such as Ebola hemorrhagic fever, Lassa fever, enzootic hepatitis, variant Creutzfeldt-Jakob disease, and human ehrlichiosis, which have been reported abroad but not found in China, have become a "Sword of Damocles," causing widespread concern. At present, China is facing the double threats of old and new infectious diseases, and the battle to control them has entered a new stage.

II. Diagnostic principles for infectious diseases

Correct diagnosis, timely isolation, and effective treatment are the basis for preventing the spread of infectious diseases. Especially with severe infectious diseases such as plague and cholera, and major infectious diseases such as AIDS and SARS, the first case diagnosis is of great significance.

The diagnosis of infectious diseases should be a comprehensive analysis of epidemiology, clinical manifestations, and laboratory test data:

1. Clinical data: Including a detailed history and comprehensive physical examination for a thorough analysis. A preliminary diagnosis can be made according to the length of the incubation period, the nature of the onset, the characteristics of fever and rashes, poisoning symptoms, and specific symptoms and signs.

For example, fever with an obvious chill is common in severe bacterial infection (pneumococcal pneumonia, septicemic acute pyelonephritis, acute cholecystitis), malaria, and reactions to blood transfusions or infusions, but is rare in tuberculosis, typhoid fever, rickettsia diseases, and viral infections. However, fever is often accompanied by nonspecific symptoms such as dizziness, headache, fatigue, and loss of appetite, which have no differential significance for diagnosis, but locating local symptoms is an important reference. For example, fever accompanied by nervous system symptoms, including severe headache, vomiting, disturbance of consciousness, convulsions, and meningeal irritation, indicates a lesion is in the central nervous system, and encephalitis and cerebral meningitis should be considered. It is noteworthy that in elderly patients with severe infections, there are often changes in consciousness, and the body temperature is not necessarily high. Therefore, when inquiring about medical history and performing physical examinations, we should distinguish the key points, focus on the main line, analyze and think at the same time, and always make a differential diagnosis in the process of understanding medical history.

As another example, respiratory infectious diseases characterized by acute fever and a rash are also called acute eruptive infectious diseases. Chickenpox, rubella, scarlet fever, and measles are common, and those susceptible are mainly infants and children. As the appearance of the rash has a certain regularity with the time of fever, it is important for differential diagnosis in clinical practice. Chickenpox and rubella cause a rash on days 1–2 of the fever, scarlet fever on day two, smallpox on day three, and measles on day four. In rubella, there will be enlargement of the lymph nodes behind the ears, occiput, and neck. Chickenpox rash has centripetal distribution, i.e., it is mostly concentrated in the truncus. Measles rash starts from behind the ears and the hairline of the neck, gradually spreads downward, and finally reaches the limbs, palms, and soles of the feet, emerging completely in 3–5 days. Scarlet fever is an acute eruptive contagious disease caused by Group A β-type hemolytic streptococcus, and its important clinical features also include pale lips and a strawberry-like tongue.

2. Epidemiological data: Including the incidence area, time period, previous infectious diseases, contact history, vaccination history, and whether the disease occurs collectively or in families. The data also includes age, place of residence, occupation, living habits, history of living or traveling in epidemic areas, history of surgery, history of blood transfusion and blood products, trauma history, and contact history of animals such as cattle and sheep. All of this data is important for diagnosis, and sometimes even a small discovery can provide important clues. For example, when migrant workers returning from Africa and South Asia have fever and chills, imported infectious diseases such as malaria should be considered first.

3. Laboratory examinations and other auxiliary examinations: Laboratory examinations have special significance for the diagnosis of infectious diseases. In particular, the detection of pathogens can directly determine diagnosis, while immunological examinations, molecular biological examinations, ultrasound, CT, MRI, PET-CT, and other imaging examinations can also provide an important diagnostic basis.

For many infectious diseases, general laboratory tests are also helpful for early diagnosis. The increase in the total number of leukocytes and neutrophilia can be seen in most bacterial infectious diseases, such as sepsis. The total number of leucocytes in gram-negative bacilli infection often increases inconspicuously or even decreases, such as in brucellosis, typhoid fever, and paratyphoid fever. In most viral infectious diseases, the number of leucocytes decreases, and the proportion of lymphocytes increases, such as in influenza and viral hepatitis. However, the number of leucocytes in patients with epidemic hemorrhagic fever and epidemic type B encephalitis often increases. The total number of leucocytes is low or normal in the case of protozoan infection. The presence of abnormal lymphocytes in the blood is common in epidemic hemorrhagic fever and infectious mononucleosis. In helminth infection, eosinophils usually increase, such as hookworm and infection by schistosome. Eosinophil is common in typhoid fever and epidemic cerebrospinal meningitis. Patients with epidemic hemorrhagic fever and hepatic typhus usually have protein, white blood cells, and red blood cells in their urine. The former have membranous substance in their urine, while the latter is accompanied by jaundice, and positive urine bilirubin. The manifestations of intestinal viral infections are mostly watery stools or a small amount of mucus in the stool. Patients with bacillary dysentery and intestinal amebiasis often have mucopurulent bloody stool and jam-like stool. Meanwhile, the stool changes in toxic bacillary dysentery are not too obvious, but the poisoning symptoms (such as convulsion) are serious. The manifestations of bacterial intestinal infection are watery stool and bloody watery stool, or stools mixed with pus and mucus. Biochemical tests for liver and kidney function are helpful for the diagnosis of infectious diseases such as viral hepatitis and epidemic hemorrhagic fever.

Many infectious diseases can be diagnosed by detecting pathogens under a microscope or with the naked eye. Neisseria meningitidis, plasmodium, microfilaria, entamoeba histolytica and cysts, schistosome ovum, spirochetes, and other pathogens can be detected under a microscope; schistosome miracidium can be detected with the naked eye after hatching. The isolation, culture, and identification of pathogens (bacteria, fungi, viruses, and mycobacteria) in blood, urine, feces, cerebrospinal fluid, bone marrow, nasopharyngeal secretion, exudate, and biopsy tissues, as well as new and more specific immunology established in recent years (such as typhoid fever, brucellosis, and certain viral diseases) and molecular biological examination (such as PCR), are helpful for the diagnosis of infectious disease pathogens.

Traumatic diagnostic measures such as liver, bone marrow, skin, pleuroperitoneal membrane, lymph node, muscle biopsy, and histopathological examination have important value in the differential diagnosis of infectious and non-infectious diseases. Non-invasive diagnostic measures such as ultrasound, CT, MRI, and PET-CT reduce the need for invasive procedures. Ultrasound can show cardiac neoplasms and abnormalities of the pancreas, liver, kidney, and bladder; a CT scan can show abdominal tumors, retroperitoneal, substernal, and mesenteric lymph node abnormalities, and can also check the spleen, liver, kidney, adrenal gland, pancreas, heart, mediastinum, and pelvic lesions; MRI is superior to CT in detecting mostly unexplained fever, including of the nervous system.

III. Clinical diagnosis of intractable infectious diseases
Intractable infectious diseases refer to those that are difficult to diagnose and treat.

1. The causes of intractable infectious diseases
(1) Lack of experience: This can involve being new to clinical practice, lacking knowledge, insufficient clinical experience; blind confidence, no reporting, no consulting, no asking for instructions; no learning, not keeping up with trends, not being familiar with foreign patients with common or frequently-occurring diseases, such as malaria, paragonimiasis, echinococcosis, acariasis, and dengue fever. Although they are easy to diagnose in endemic areas, in non-endemic areas they can be misdiagnosed.

(2) Deficiencies of clinical data: This includes a deficiency of symptoms, signs, and auxiliary examinations, inaccurate data, and improper choices; excessive dependence on the results of auxiliary examinations, careless clinical observation, and neglecting the importance of symptoms and signs, such as spasmodic cough in pertussis, oral mucosal plaque in measles, rose rash in typhoid fever, skin ecchymosis in epidemic cerebrospinal meningitis, bulbar conjunctiva exudation, bleeding spots and scratch-like bleeding stripes in epidemic hemorrhagic fever, and eschar and ulcers in acariasis, all of which are helpful in establishing the diagnosis of specific diseases; a subjective lack or omission of necessary auxiliary examination; examination errors, mistakes, iatrogenic (such as drug reaction) causes of diagnosis difficulties, such as drug-induced leukopenia, platelet count reduction caused by EDTA anticoagulation in automatic whole blood cell counter, artificial pseudo fever, and "false" hematuria.

(3) Complicated clinical manifestations of an infectious disease: There are multiple clinical manifestations of an infectious disease, which may sometimes be unusual. For example, although clinically common, infectious mononucleosis can be acute or chronic; it can present with hepatitis, leukocytosis, hemolysis, and thrombocytopenia, which are easily confused with hematological diseases, making clinical diagnosis more difficult. There can be a combination of multiple manifestations if a lesion involves multiple organs and systems, which is difficult to diagnose. For example, hemophagocytic syndrome related to EB viral infection may present as high fever, hepatosplenomegaly, lymph node enlargement, pancytopenia, dysfunction of the liver, and coagulation, and rapidly progresses to multiple organ failure, which is easily confused with infectious diseases such as sepsis, typhoid fever, and epidemic hemorrhagic fever, as well as hematological diseases such as malignant histiocytosis and aplastic anemia.

(4) New infectious diseases: New infectious diseases such as SARS, AIDS, highly pathogenic avian influenza, Streptococcus Suis infection, and eperythrozoonosis have been

discovered, and the first diagnosis was very difficult. The first case of an imported infectious disease in a non-endemic area is also susceptible to misdiagnosis.

2. The thinking around the clinical diagnosis of intractable infectious diseases

Clinical thinking cannot be separated from the support of subject knowledge. Mastering the necessary basic theoretical knowledge of epidemiology and related medicine is a prerequisite for cultivating clinical thinking ability. The following general principles should be observed in the thinking process of clinical diagnosis of intractable infectious diseases:

(1) Seeking truth from facts

Collect detailed information and respect facts; note positive test results, but do not ignore the significance of negative results; do not overlook any subtle abnormalities, especially clinical symptoms that have not been reasonably explained, which often contain loopholes for diagnosis. Do not choose a certain far-fetched diagnosis at will.

Gathering a patient's medical history requires skill. Doctors do not simply listen to patients and record what they say, nor do they just ask questions and note the answers in some sort of tabular order. In the process of collecting medical history, doctors should make full use of all their knowledge and mobilize all their cognitive abilities to glean potentially significant data from a patient's body shape, posture, complexion, tone of voice, and expression in a highly concentrated way for timely analysis and thinking. Differential diagnosis should always be made in the process of understanding medical history.

Physical examination should be serious and have a clear purpose. By collecting medical history, doctors gain a preliminary understanding of a disease and come up with an idea for diagnosis, but it is still difficult to determine whether the diagnosis is true or not. By looking for positive or negative signs, the diagnosis can come closer to the actual condition. Physical examination with a clear purpose should be comprehensive, and should focus on key points, namely the point of doubt discovered in the process of collecting medical history. These signs should be examined, whether positive or negative, and should be concluded with confidence, which is of great significance for diagnosis.

It is necessary to understand and explain examinations in a reasonable manner. Although many cases can be diagnosed by medical history and physical examination, doctors always want to have special examinations for further support, as long as there are conditions. In most cases, this kind of support is absolutely necessary, and can make diagnosis more reliable, objective, and easy to quantify. However, it requires clinicians to fully understand the working principles, significance, accuracy, and error of various special examination instruments. If doctors lack knowledge in this field, it may lead to wrongful diagnosis in some cases.

Cooperating with medical technicians can improve the analytical quality of examinations. At hospitals with better conditions, there are often many auxiliary examinations for one case. If the examination results are inconsistent or even contradictory, clinicians should make an analysis of the doubtful points based on clinical manifestations, and strive to make a more practical diagnosis. Even if the conclusions of all auxiliary examinations are consistent, clinicians should consider whether they are consistent with patients' actual clinical manifestations. If medical technicians have a better understanding of patients' clinical conditions, it can be helpful for them in finding abnormalities and making a more accurate diagnosis.

The rate for the detection of malaria parasites, and filariform larvae and ova in feces during routine laboratory tests is very low. If the examiner knows that the patient is suspected of having a specific disease, the physician will surely have a higher positive diagnosis rate if he/she carefully searches for it. If the examiner knows that the patient has a high probability of having a disease, the positive diagnosis rate will definitely increase after searching. Clinicians should also understand the diagnostic criteria of medical and technical departments when applying for various examinations, as this is conducive to accurate judgments. For example, in the process of SARS diagnosis, we cannot diagnose it only on the basis of pulmonary shadow combined with other symptoms. We should emphasize that imaging should identify the specific characteristics of SARS that show up in imaging, i.e., the initial appearance of patchy infiltration shadow, unclear boundaries, rapid progress, and variability. Chest radiographs show severe symptoms but physical signs are not so serious.

(2) The principle of monism

One disease should be used to explain multiple clinical manifestations as far as possible. Some infectious diseases, such as epidemic hemorrhagic fever, high fever, hypotension shock, acute renal failure, gastrointestinal and intracranial hemorrhage in different stages, and severe hepatitis, can present as severe jaundice, hepatic encephalopathy, ascites, gastrointestinal bleeding, hepatorenal syndrome, and even DIC. These manifestations are caused by one disease, but when there are several diseases co-existing, doctors should distinguish between primary and secondary. They should not try to explain everything by monism, but consider dualism and even pluralism instead.

(3) Incidence rate and disease spectrum

When several diagnostic possibilities co-exist, common and frequently-occurring diseases should be considered first, especially common infectious diseases in epidemic areas. Secondly, rare diseases should be considered. For example, in the diagnosis of febrile diseases, comprehensive analysis and judgment are needed. First, judging from the nature of the lesions, is it an inflammatory disease? Is it infectious inflammation or non-infectious inflammation? Infection is generally considered to be the leading cause of acute fever, followed by neoplasia and vascular-connective tissue disease, which account for 90% of etiological diagnoses of fever of unknown origin. Systemic infections, localized abscesses, urinary system infections, and biliary tract infections caused by bacteria are the most common infections. Tuberculosis comes in second place, among which ex-pulmonary tuberculosis is far more prevalent than pulmonary tuberculosis. Fever is the main manifestation of malignant tumors, followed by lymphoma, malignant histiocytoma, and various solid tumors. Understanding and mastering the incidence rate and regularity of a disease's spectrum will be helpful to provide and enhance the logical thinking of clinical diagnosis and improve diagnostic accuracy.

However, rare diseases cannot be ignored. For example, a young woman with long-term fever accompanied by a rash, painful swelling of the superficial cervical and axillary lymph node, splenomegaly, leukopenia, and rapid erythrocyte sedimentation rate, had been suspected of having lymphoma, tuberculosis, and malignant histiocytosis. A lymph node biopsy confirmed the diagnosis of tissue necrotizing lymphadenitis.

In addition, attention should be paid to frequently-occurring diseases in special populations. For example, AIDS patients are prone to pneumocystis pneumonia and tuberculosis; patients who use immunosuppressants for a long time are prone to secondary fungal infections such as cryptococcal meningitis; patients who use antibiotics for a long time are prone to pseudomembranous enteritis because antibiotics inhibit the normal intestinal flora, and drug-resistant and illegible clostridium take the opportunity to breed.

(4) Considering organic diseases first

Consider organic pathological changes first, and then consider functional diseases.

(5) Considering benign diseases first

Before diagnosing malignant diseases, benign diseases must be ruled out.

3. The thinking around the clinical diagnosis of emerging infectious diseases

More than 30 new infectious diseases have appeared in the past 30 years. Learning how to detect new infectious diseases as early as possible is an important topic within the medical interface. For known diseases, diagnosis can be made quickly with clinical thinking. However, for emerging infectious diseases, there are major limitations. Unlike other diseases, infectious diseases have four basic characteristics, namely pathogens, infectiousness, epidemiological characteristics, and post-infectious immunity. Through understanding these characteristics, especially the epidemiological ones, doctors have successfully identified a variety of emerging infectious diseases.

For example, during the 40-day period from 5 February to 15 March 1982, 26 cases of acute diarrhea characterized by spastic abdominal pain and bloody stools were identified in Oregon, USA. Most patients had no fever or low fever. Among them, 25 cases were concentrated in seven small towns in one county. An outbreak of acute diarrhea with exactly the same characteristics as described above occurred in Michigan from 28 May to 27 June of the same year. A total of 21 cases occurred within one month. In order to find the possible causes of these two outbreaks, Riley et al. conducted systematic clinical, epidemiological, and laboratory studies on these two outbreaks. This provided a lot of evidence for determining the pathogens of the two outbreaks, and finally determined that the pathogen was a rare E.coli serotype $O_{157}:H_7$.

Another example: On 5 June 1981, the American newspaper *Morbidity and Death Weekly* reported that five previously healthy young gay men in Los Angeles had contracted pneumocystis carinii pneumonia. This kind of pneumonia used to be more common in elderly cancer patients receiving chemotherapy, and the incidence rate was equal between men and women. These reports attracted the attention of the US Centers for Disease Control and Prevention (CDC) and they began monitoring the situation. A few months later, it was found that 26 gay men were suffering from rare Kaposi's sarcoma. None of the patients had a history of cancer or chemotherapy. The main manifestation was a decrease in the number of helper T-lymphocytes. In 1982, this emerging disease was named Acquired Immune Deficiency Syndrome, or AIDS.

Some emerging infectious diseases have no significant differences in epidemiology or clinical and laboratory testing, and the course of the disease is short. They are therefore difficult to distinguish even through multi-level and systematic observation, such as some unexplained diarrhea. Therefore, the discovery of a new cause of disease can help with diagnosis. Some infectious diseases are recognized only after the cause is found, such as cryptosporidiosis. Compared with developed Western countries, China has a large gap in the field of pathogen diagnosis of emerging infectious diseases, and there is no perfect technology, method, or system for detecting and identifying unknown pathogen genes. Due to the lack of sensitivity and specificity, the current isolation methods for pathogen diagnosis of infectious diseases are often useless when the known pathogens cannot be isolated. According to statistics, the vast majority of unexplained outbreaks in China (estimated at more than 60%) have no etiological evidence, nor any possible investigation of pathogenic microorganisms at all. The technical level to discover new pathogenic microorganisms has not been reached. Among the 200+ pathogenic microorganisms of major significance for public health, only Chlamydia trachomatis and group B rotavirus were isolated and identified by Chinese scientists first. In the SARS epidemic of 2003, China was facing a worldwide and time-sensitive challenge. All-round gaps in the diagnosis, treatment, detection, pathogen isolation, and epidemiological investigation of emerging infectious diseases in China were fully exposed.

IV. The thinking behind the clinical treatment of infectious diseases

Clinical thinking in the treatment of infectious diseases is very important. The first aspect is specific immunotherapy, including the etiological treatment and the treatment of pathogenesis. The second is the appropriate symptomatic treatment of some prominent symptoms.

1. Etiological treatment

Among the measures for the treatment of infectious diseases, it is most important to find the cause and conduct etiological treatment. Anti-infective drugs have many dosages, many users, many expenses, and many problems. The rational application of anti-infective drugs is a common problem around the world. Clinicians and pharmacists should consider a patient's age, immune status, disease status, and differences in therapeutic drugs in the clinical thinking of anti-infective drug treatment, and establish an individualized treatment plan. Before using anti-infective drugs, the following factors should be considered:

(1)   When was the patient infected, and where is the infection site?
(2)   What is the severity of the infection?

(3) What are the main possible pathogens?

(4) How can pathogenic blood samples and results be collected and obtained? How can etiology and susceptibility reporting results be explained and used?

(5) For suspected (or determined) pathogens, what kinds of drugs (bacteria spectrum) are available? What are the specific varieties?

(6) What is the impact of the treatment of anti-infective drugs for concomitant diseases?

(7) Is there a history of previous medication (such as anti-infection) or drug allergies?

(8) Comparing the available anti-infective drugs with their antimicrobial spectrum, pharmacology, toxicology, pharmacokinetics, and pharmacodynamics, which have advantages?

(9) Comparing the efficacy/risk, and benefit/cost, what kind of medicine is preferable to use?

(10) What impact do the characteristics of the pathogens causing the infection and the individual differences in the patient's organ function and body condition have on the drug regimen?

(11) After a drug is selected, what is the basis for determining the dosage, the interval of administration, the route of administration, single or combined use, and the planned course of treatment? What is the basis for the designation of the appropriate program?

(12) How can we observe and judge the efficacy of drugs during treatment? How can adverse drug reactions be observed, handled, and prevented?

(13) How can the dosage regimen be adjusted if the condition changes? After the course of treatment, how can the efficacy of the medication plan be analyzed and evaluated?

(14) In addition to drug treatment, what other treatments are needed?

In clinical practice, antibacterial drugs are often abused (such as for viral diseases) or misused. Treating fever itself with antibiotics is probably the most common mistake. In fact, fever is not necessarily caused by bacterial infection. If there is no obvious basis for bacterial invasion, and if the condition allows, the use of antibacterial drugs should be suspended until clinical and laboratory tests prove the existence of infection.

For severe infections, it is often necessary to combine several antibiotics for treatment before understanding the susceptibility of pathogenic bacteria, that is, the de-escalation treatment method of a heavy hammer punch. It is often necessary to use a combination of antibiotics in the treatment of mixed infections. For certain infections, such as tuberculosis, combination medication is more effective than single medication, because this kind of bacteria is more resistant to monotherapy. When patients with leukopenia have severe pseudomonas aeruginosa infections, combined medication is also extremely effective. Importantly, using an aminoglycoside plus a penicillin against pseudomonas aeruginosa may be more effective than using any of these drugs alone.

Common inappropriate uses of antibiotics include: For viral diseases without complications; use of ineffective antibiotics; insufficient medication or overdose; improper medication route; continued use of the original antibiotic after the bacteria develop resistance; continued use of medication after severe toxicity or allergic reactions; stopping effective treatment prematurely; improper selection of antibiotic combination medication; over-reliance on medication and neglect of surgical treatment (such as drainage of local infections and extraction of foreign bodies). The above issues should be taken seriously.

2. Symptomatic treatment

While treating the cause, necessary symptomatic treatment should also be carried out. For example, if a high fever does not go away during treatment, antipyretic drugs can be given, but it is best to try physical cooling. For most of the cases with a definitive diagnosis, this is helpful to achieve ideal therapeutic effects.

3. Diagnostic treatment

If the diagnosis is unclear, diagnostic treatment can be performed, but a suspected diagnosis must be made before treatment. Diagnostic treatment is of no diagnostic value for most patients with fever. For patients who have a long-term fever of unknown cause, diagnostic treatment can be performed, with the exception of tumors, but a cautious attitude must be taken, and drugs with strong specificity, exact efficacy, and minimal side effects should be selected. Most of the drugs used for diagnostic treatment are antibiotics, antiprotozoal drugs, and antirheumatic drugs, such as metronidazole for hepatic amebiasis, antimalarials for malaria, and anti-tuberculosis drugs for tuberculosis. All of these drugs have side effects (such as drug fever, rashes, liver function damage, and hematopoietic organ damage), which can prolong the disease if used improperly. It should be noted that this method has its limitations. In terms of diagnosis, the general negative significance of the results of specific treatments is greater than the significance of the diagnosis. If the regular chloroquine treatment is ineffective for suspected malaria patients, the probability of malaria is considered to be very low.

(Li Lanjuan)

Fever and fatigue for 12 days, cough and shortness of breath for seven days

I. Medical history

Patient: Female, 27 years old, from Taiyuan in Shanxi Province. She was admitted to hospital after experiencing fever and fatigue for 12 days, and cough and shortness of breath for seven days.

On the afternoon of 21 February, the patient began to develop fever and fatigue, with no body temperature measurement, no chills, no expectoration, no nasal obstruction, and no runny nose. On 23 February, her body temperature rose to 39°C, accompanied by chills, headache, joint pain, and myalgia. She was diagnosed with an upper respiratory tract infection at the local hospital, and was treated with azithromycin and ribavirin, but her condition was not relieved. On 26 February, dry cough, shortness of breath, and wheezing appeared, especially when she was sitting down. When she lay down, the symptoms were relieved. She tested negative for Legionella pneumophila, Chlamydia pneumoniae, and Mycoplasma pneumoniae antibodies. On 2 March, the patient was transferred to another hospital. A chest X-ray examination showed lower lung inflammation on both sides, and she was given an intravenous drip of ceftriaxone sodium (Rocephin) and Imipenem and Cilastatin Sodium (Tienam). The symptoms did not decrease. On 4 March, she was treated with levofloxacin (Lailixin) and minocycline, and her body temperature dropped to 38°C. On 5 March, she was transferred to our hospital.

The patient was in good health, and had no history of chronic diseases of the heart and lungs. She denied a history of exposure to radioactive substances and toxicants, a history of drug allergy, and a history of exposure to infected water. She went to Guangzhou on a business trip ten days before the onset of illness. At that time, there was an epidemic of severe acute respiratory syndrome (SARS) in Guangzhou. She denied a family history of infectious and genetic diseases.

> **Thinking prompts:** This case is a patient with a fever. The fever itself can be caused by various problems such as infections, tumors, autoimmune diseases, and blood diseases. The general method of diagnosing the cause of fever is firstly to fully understand the patient's medical history. The following medical history is helpful to confirm the diagnosis: ① Fever: First of all, it is necessary to clarify the time of

the occurrence of fever. According to the duration of the fever, determine whether the patient has an acute fever (under two weeks) or long-term fever (more than two weeks). This patient started with 12 days of acute fever. The characteristics of fever also have a certain significance for differential diagnosis, including the onset, degree, duration, type, and whether it is accompanied by chills. ② Other symptoms accompanying fever, such as expectoration and sore throat caused by respiratory diseases; nausea, vomiting, constipation, or diarrhea from conditions of the digestive system; palpitations, precordial pain, dyspnea, and edema from the circulatory system. Lesions of each system accompanied by fever can often show specific characteristics, which can assist in further analysis of the lesion sites. This patient had a cough and shortness of breath along with a fever, indicating that the lesion may be in the respiratory tract. Further investigations should be made about sputum production, precordial discomfort, and edema of both lower extremities. ③ The treatment received and the reaction to it. The patient received treatment outside the hospital, so when asking about her medical history, the focus should be on the drugs she has used and how she reacted to them. This will be helpful to gain relevant information when receiving patients, which can help doctors to make a differential diagnosis, and inform preliminary treatment plans. ④ Residence or tourist history in specific areas (epidemic zones and pastoral areas). Fever is common in infectious diseases, so it is very important to ask about epidemiological history, including where the patient has been, whom they have been in contact with, and whether anyone around them has similar symptoms. On inquiry, it was discovered that this patient had been to a SARS epidemic area before the onset of her illness, which may have important clinical significance. ⑤ Other medical histories: Such as a history of tuberculosis and diseases related to immunodeficiency and sexual history. This information is very helpful for confirming causes. If some elements of a patient's medical history can be traced back to a certain source, the cause of the disease can often be found quickly.

II. Physical examination on admission

T 38°C, P 96 times/min, R 20 times/min, BP 14/9 kPa (1 mmHg = 0.133 kPa). Low mood, no skin stained yellow, no rash, no palpable swelling of lymph nodes, intact oral mucosa, no leukoplakia, and no swelling of tonsils. There was no deformity of the thorax; the percussion sounds of both lungs were clear; the breath sounds in the middle and lower parts of both lungs were thick during auscultation; no dry and wet rales or pleural friction sounds were heard. Examination of the heart, abdomen, and nervous system showed no abnormalities.

Thinking prompts: After understanding a patient's medical history, a further targeted, serious, detailed, and thorough physical examination is of great significance to diagnosis. Attention should be paid to the following during physical examination:

① The patient has a cough and shortness of breath. Therefore, cardiopulmonary examination should be the focus of the physical examination. A heart murmur may suggest that the patient has a problem with their heart function. The appearance of moist rales suggests that there may be exudation in the alveoli. During physical examination, the respiratory sounds in both lower lungs were found to be thick. However, no pleural fricative sound and no dry or wet rales were heard, which suggests that the lesion may be in the interstitium of the lungs. The exudation in the alveoli was not obvious. ② Never overlook any part of the body, including some easily missed parts, such as the mouth, throat, thyroid gland, and the tips of the fingers and toes. The patient in question was treated with a variety of antibiotics outside of the hospital. Therefore, we should check whether there is a double infection, and especially whether there are white spots in the oral cavity. ③ Special attention should be paid to distinctive signs, such as rashes, bleeding spots, lymph nodes, hepatomegaly, splenomegaly, joint swelling deformities, dysfunction, and local masses. The typical rash in fever patients can be decisive for diagnosis.

III. Auxiliary examination on admission

Thinking prompts: Routine examinations such as blood tests, urine and stool tests, and liver and kidney function tests should be completed first. Other examinations, such as biochemistry, biology, and imaging, should be given at the discretion of the attending physician. Fever has a complex etiology, especially when ① medical history and physical signs cannot provide any clues as to the cause; and ② some clues have been identified, but a diagnosis cannot be made.

In these cases, a comprehensive auxiliary examination should be made, including repeated blood culture, multi-site image examination, a puncture biopsy of lymphadenectasis, a puncture test of the thoracic cavity and abdominal cavity, bone marrow aspiration, and the detection of various autoimmune disease indicators and tumor markers. It should be noted that some inspections need to be repeated multiple times, and doctors should not give up if the first couple of inspection results are negative.

Routine blood test: WBC 5.3×10^9/L, N 75%, normal eosinophil, Hb 111 g/L, PLT 276×10^9/L, heterotypic lymphocyte 0.

Normal urine and stool. Normal liver and kidney functions.

ESR: 93 mm/h.

Antibody IgM of the Coxsackie virus, EB virus (EBV), and cytomegalovirus (CMV) were all negative, and the cold agglutination test was negative.

Arterial blood gas analysis: PO_2 84.2 mmHg, PCO_2 39.9 mmHg, SaO_2 98%.

Chest X-ray: Large, vague, and patchy shadows were seen in the central fields of both lungs, with clear edges. There was no significant increase in the hilar shadow. No abnormality was seen in the mediastinal cardiac shadow. Both diaphragmatic surfaces were smooth, and both costophrenic angles were sharp.

IV. Diagnosis

1. Preliminary diagnosis

The clinical manifestations of the preliminary diagnosis are acute fever, cough, shortness of breath, and other lung issues. The middle and lower parts of both lungs made thick respiratory sounds through auscultation, and no dry-wet rales and pleural friction sounds were heard. The chest radiograph at another hospital showed lower lung inflammation on both sides. Therefore, the initial diagnosis is acute lung inflammation, and the cause is yet to be investigated.

2. Diagnostic thinking

> **Thinking prompts:** Fever, cough, expectoration, hemoptysis, chest pain, and dyspnea are the main symptoms of acute lung inflammation, but acute lung inflammation does not necessarily have all of these symptoms. It is mostly caused by infection. Sometimes, it can also be caused by non-infectious factors, such as tumors and allergic reactions. Acute lung inflammation caused by connective tissue disease or chemical/physical factors is rare.

(1) Connective tissue disease: Connective tissue disease can cause acute lung inflammation, for which antibiotic treatment is ineffective. However, connective tissue disease can cause lung lesions as well as other clinical manifestations of the extrapulmonary organs. The patient in this case only showed lung lesions, and there was no damage to other organs, so connective tissue disease can be temporarily ruled out. For other pulmonary inflammation caused by chemical and physical factors, a history of contact with substances causing lung lesions was often found. In this case, such a history can be ruled out, so the possibility can be eliminated.

(2) Allergic reactions: Pulmonary inflammation caused by an allergic reaction includes eosinophil infiltration and pulmonary vasculitis. This type of illness mostly affects multiple systems. It has a short benign course, and increases eosinophils in the blood. This is not to be considered as the diagnosis for the patient in question.

(3) Tumors: Tumors can also cause fever, shortness of breath, and an irritating dry cough. Compression of the surrounding tissues can have corresponding manifestations. However, the patient in this case was young, and had no other corresponding manifestations except fever and shortness of breath. No space-occupying lesions were found in imaging examinations either at our hospital or the other one, so this possibility can be ruled out.

Therefore, on the basis of excluding non-infectious factors in the above analysis, infectious factors should mainly be considered, but further analysis of pathogeny is still required.

(1) Bacteria: Pulmonary inflammation caused by bacteria is the most common. Pathogenic bacteria include diplococcus pneumoniae, staphylococci, streptococcus, bacillus pneumoniae, and mycobacterium tuberculosis. Bacterial pneumonia often starts with an aversion to cold or chills, high fever, sputum production, severe systemic symptoms, significantly increased WBC, and neutrophils in blood. Although the patient in this case had a fever, a routine blood test showed a slight increase in neutrophils and ESR, but there were no chills and no sputum. During the course of the illness, many different kinds of antibiotics were used, including carbapenems. If it was a bacterial infection, it should have been cured easily, but the patient's condition did not improve significantly. The possibility of bacterial infection can be ruled out. However, for further elimination, especially for the exclusion of specific infections, C-reactive protein (CRP), tuberculosis antibodies, tuberculin test (PPD), and dynamic observation chest radiographs can be tested. In this case, there was no significant increase in C-reactive protein, and multiple tuberculosis antibody and PPD tests were negative, so the possibility of bacterial infection can be ruled out. However, in the treatment of the illness, attention should be paid to possible bacterial superinfection.

(2) Fungi: Fungal infections often occur in patients with low immunity. The use of antibiotics and hormones is an important cause of fungal infection, and the diagnosis of deep fungal infection is often difficult. The patient in this case used a variety of antibiotics during the course of her illness, so fungal infections should be considered. A pulmonary fungal infection with oral infection usually manifests as oral mucosal leukoplakia, pharyngeal discomfort, and sticky white sputum. Fungal pneumonia often appears with fever, and sometimes with cough, with mainly white or rust-colored sticky sputum, or yellow, bloody, and chocolate-colored; chest X-ray can be patchy, with cotton-like shadows and changes caused by interstitial pneumonia. The patient in question has no oral leukoplakia, no sputum, and no previous manifestations of low immunity, so the possibility of fungal infection can be ruled out. However, in the course of treatment, the patient should be closely observed in case of double infection.

(3) Spirochete: Pulmonary hemorrhagic leptospirosis, with fever, pulmonary symptoms, no jaundice, and no significant liver and kidney damage occurs mostly in summer and autumn, and is sensitive to penicillin and cephalosporin antibiotics. There was no history of contact with infected water in this case, and the use of antibiotics outside of the hospital was ineffective, so the possibility of spirochete.

(4) Mycoplasma and chlamydia: The clinical manifestations of pulmonary infection caused by chlamydia and mycoplasma have few characteristics, and the condition can be mild or severe; chest symptoms are few; X-ray manifestations are relatively severe and varied; extrapulmonary symptoms are relatively common; the peripheral blood WBC is low; the serum-specific IgM antibody is positive after the onset of the illness; and the cold agglutination test result can be positive in some patients. In terms of clinical symptoms, mycoplasma, and chlamydia cannot be completely ruled out in this case. However, they are sensitive to azithromycin and quinolone antibiotics. The patient's condition did not improve after using

these antibiotics, and the chlamydia pneumoniae antibody, mycoplasma antibody, and cold agglutination test result were negative, so the possibility of mycoplasma and chlamydia can be ruled out.

(5) Viruses: There are many viruses that can cause pneumonia, including the influenza virus, parainfluenza virus, cytomegalovirus, adenovirus, coronavirus, some enteroviruses such as the Coxsackie virus and ECHO virus, as well as the herpes simplex virus, measles, and rubella. Viruses that were discovered in recent years include hantavirus and SARS coronavirus. There are different manifestations of pulmonary inflammation caused by specific viruses, some of which are slow onset, some of which are acute onset. The progress of pneumonia is rapid, but the signs are often absent, and the X-ray manifestations are also diversified. WBC in peripheral blood can be reduced, normal, or increased. Diagnosis mainly depends on the characteristic manifestations of viral infection and the exclusion of pneumonia caused by bacteria and other pathogens. The patient in this case started with fever, accompanied by pulmonary symptoms, absence of pulmonary signs, low WBC in the peripheral blood, and ineffective treatment with various antibiotics. Therefore, viral infection cannot be ruled out.

After initially considering viral infection, the specific type becomes an important issue in the diagnosis. After admission, the patient tested negative for Coxsackie, EBV, and CMV-IgM, which did not support the diagnosis of common enterovirus and EBV and CMV. However, when determining the results, it should be noted that in patients with immune deficiency, viral infection could not be completely ruled out, even if the antibody was negative. Therefore, if appropriate, virus isolation or a viral antigen test should be carried out.

The patient in this case had been on a business trip to the SARS epidemic area before the onset. A patient's exposure history during an epidemic period is very important for diagnosis. After the onset of her illness, her husband, son, and parents were successively hospitalized, with the same clinical manifestations.

The diagnostic criteria for SARS cases issued by the Ministry of Health of the People's Republic of China are as follows:

1. Epidemiological history

1.1 Has a history of close contact with a patient, or belongs to one of the infected groups, or has clear evidence of infecting others

1.2 Has been to or lived in a city where SARS patients were reported, and secondary infection occurred within two weeks before the onset of the illness

2. Symptoms and signs

Onset is acute, with fever as the first symptom; body temperature is generally over 38°C, with occasional chills; fever may be accompanied by headaches, joint pain, muscle pain, fatigue, and diarrhea; cough without catarrhal symptoms in the upper respiratory tract; mostly dry cough, less sputum, occasionally bloody sputum; chest tightness; severe cases may have respiratory acceleration, shortness of breath, or obvious respiratory distress. Pulmonary signs are not obvious, but in some cases, moist rales may be heard, or signs of pulmonary consolidation may be found.

3. Laboratory examination

The white blood cell count in the peripheral blood has either decreased or not increased, and the lymphocyte count has often decreased.

4. Chest X-ray

There are varying degrees of flaky or patchy infiltrative shadows or reticular changes in the lung. Some patients progress rapidly and show large shadows in the lung; this often changes bilaterally, and the shadow absorbs and dissipates slowly. The lung shadow may not be consistent with the symptoms and signs. If the test result is negative, the patient should be re-examined after 1–2 days.

5. No obvious effect of antibacterial drug treatment

Suspected diagnostic criteria: 1 + 2 + 3 or 2 + 3 + 4

Clinical diagnostic criteria: 1.1 + 2 + 4 or more, or 1.2 + 2 + 3 + 4 or 1.2 + 2 + 4 + 5

Therefore, the patient in this case meets the diagnostic criteria for SARS.

Further diagnosis depends on etiological examination, including virus isolation, serological examination, and monitoring of the virus and viral antigen. Therefore, the detection of SARS (SARS-CoV) RNA and the quick detection of serum-specific antibodies will further confirm the diagnosis.

V. Treatment

After admission, oxygen inhalation, growth factor injection, gamma globulin, and thymopentin were given to improve the patient's immunity. IFNα anti-virus and levofloxacin were given to prevent infection and to supplement energy. On the third day after admission, the patient's body temperature returned to normal, and symptoms such as cough and shortness of breath had obviously lessened. Dynamic chest X-ray examination showed that the flaky blurred shadows on both lungs were gradually absorbed at intervals of two days. On 11 March, the chest X-ray showed that there were small, light shadows in the left middle lung field and the right middle lower lung field, and the inflammation had been obviously absorbed compared with how it was on admission. Routine blood and arterial blood gas analysis had returned to normal. The patient was declared clinically cured and discharged from hospital.

There is no specific therapy for SARS at present. Theoretically, antiviral therapy targets pathogens, but no effective specific anti-SARS-CoV drugs have been found. Therefore, comprehensive treatment is the main way to prevent secondary infection. This case did not become severe, and after comprehensive treatment, the patient's condition gradually improved.

VI. Lessons learned

In early November 2002, a serious, acute, and mainly pulmonary infectious disease appeared in Guangdong, China, and quickly spread to 24 provinces, autonomous regions, and municipalities directly under the central government, as well as 32 countries and regions in Asia, America, and Europe, causing outbreaks around the world. As with most infectious diseases, the spread was fast, the incidence was rapid, and the mortality rate was high. It attracted significant attention all over the world, and was known as atypical pneumonia in China. Following joint research on virus morphology, molecular biology, serology, and animal experiments of its pathogen by 13 network laboratories in nine countries around the world, the WHO announced in Geneva on 16 April 2003 that a new coronavirus called SARS coronavirus (SARS-CoV) was the pathogen of SARS – an acute and severe infectious disease dominated by pulmonary lesions.

SARS-CoV belongs to Nidovirales, Coronaviridae, and Coronavirus. Its genome is a single-strand positive-strand RNA composed of about 30,000 nucleotides. The composition of SARS-CoV is similar to a classic coronavirus. Epidemiological studies show that SARS patients are the main source of infection, and there is also a super-transmission phenomenon. Short-distance respiratory droplet transmission is the main mode of transmission, and people are generally susceptible to the SARS virus. At present, the pathogenesis is not completely clear, and the lesions can involve multiple organs – mainly the lungs and immune system. Clinical manifestations are usually non-specific – often fever accompanied by chills, headaches, and joint pain. Respiratory symptoms are usually a dry cough and chest tightness. In severe cases, patients have difficulty breathing, and some may have digestive tract symptoms.

This case was a patient with an emerging infectious disease. Therefore, during treatment in an external hospital, a timely and clear diagnosis could not be made. When treatment with various antibiotics was ineffective, it was finally diagnosed as SARS in combination with the patient's epidemiological history. After symptomatic treatment, the patient finally recovered. However, if there had not been any epidemiological data, the diagnosis would have been more difficult. Moreover, the patient was not diagnosed in good time, and did not realize the infectivity of SARS, which led to the collective onset of SARS within her family. For emerging infectious diseases, early diagnosis, early isolation, and early treatment are extremely important. Although China's Ministry of Health has issued diagnostic criteria for SARS, the focus should be on clinical diagnosis. It should be noted that the criteria for diagnosis or suspected diagnosis are not perfect. Firstly, it is difficult to determine a patient's contact history; secondly, even if some cases meet the clinical diagnostic criteria, the possibility of infection from other pathogens cannot be ruled out. In the early stage of the illness, positive serum antibodies are low, which means that this is not a suitable method of early diagnosis. The specific SARS-CoV antibody increased significantly only after ≥ 11 days. The detection of SARS-CoV RNA in the blood, airway secretions, urine, and feces by RT-PCR is of early-stage diagnostic significance, with good specificity but poor sensitivity. Therefore, the possibility of SARS cannot be ruled out by just a negative result. Virus isolation requires strict laboratory conditions, which are difficult to achieve in ordinary clinical laboratories. Moreover, it takes a long time and has a low positive rate.

At present, there is no specific treatment for SARS. Comprehensive treatment is the main method. This includes strict respiratory isolation and close monitoring of changes. Patients should stay in bed, avoid fatigue, avoid hard and severe coughing, and receive oxygen through a nasal catheter at an early stage. Patients with a high fever should be given physical cooling measures such as ice compresses and alcohol sponge baths. The heart, liver, and kidney function should be protected. Early SARS is not easy to distinguish from community-acquired pneumonia, so the application of antibiotics has different diagnostic significance for patients suspected of having SARS. Quinolones and macrolides antibiotics (such as azithromycin) can be used, because quinolones and azithromycin are effective for common respiratory tract bacterial infections as well as for mycoplasma, chlamydia, and legionella pneumoniae, which can cover common respiratory tract infections. At present, no effective anti-SARS-CoV drugs have been found. The main clinical applications are protease inhibitors such as ribavirin and oseltamivir phosphate capsules (Tamiflu). Glucocorticoid is highly beneficial for reducing lung injury and pulmonary interstitial fibrosis, and can prevent or reduce hypoxemia, ARDS, and multiple organ dysfunction syndrome. The use of glucocorticoid may further weaken a patient's immune function and lead to infection from drug-resistant bacteria and/or fungi. It is very important to master the indication, dosage, and course of glucocorticoid treatment. Severe SARS cases should be supported by artificial ventilation as early as possible to improve hypoxia and treat respiratory failure, which plays an extremely important role in relieving illness, improving the recovery rate, and reducing mortality.

SARS has been listed in the Law of the People's Republic of China on the Prevention and Control of Infectious Diseases, and its preventive measures are still to isolate the source of infection, cut off the route of transmission, and protect the susceptible population. At present, there is no effective vaccine.

(Wang Huifen & Su Haibin)

Low-grade fever in the afternoon for two months, cough and hemoptysis for five days

I. Medical history

Patient: Male, 48 years old, born in Fuyang in Anhui Province. He was admitted to hospital due to low-grade fever in the afternoon for two months, and cough and hemoptysis for five days. He stayed at the hospital from 16 September to 27 October 2002.

In mid-July 2002, the patient developed a fever without obvious inducement, peaking at 38.1°C, with a slight aversion to cold, no obvious chills, and no other accompanying symptoms. Generally, his body temperature started to rise in the afternoon, and reached its peak at 17:00–19:00. His body temperature fluctuated between 37.5°C–37.9°C, once reaching 38.1°C. The fever usually lasted for about 2 hours, and could not be relieved. He perspired significantly as it subsided. Five days before admission, he suddenly developed a severe cough with blood in his sputum. The amount of hemoptysis sputum was about 120 ml that night. Since then, there has been blood in the sputum. The amount of sputum was 200–300 ml every day and night, accompanied by pain in the right side of his chest. It was more obvious during deep breathing, without obvious chest tightness and shortness of breath. Since the onset of the illness, the patient has had no nasal congestion, runny nose, obvious chest tightness, palpitation, or shortness of breath; no nausea, vomiting, abdominal pain, or diarrhea; no frequent micturition, urgent urination, pain in urination, rash, joint swelling and pain, gingival hemorrhage, or epistaxis. Since the onset of the illness, his appetite and sleep have been poor, normal urination and defecation, and significantly decreased body weight by about 11 kg.

The patient was normally in good health, and denied any medical history such as tuberculosis, hypertension, and diabetes. He was a heavy smoker. He had smoked 600 cigarettes per year for more than 20 years, but did not drink. He was a long-term resident of Fuyang rural areas, engaged in agricultural labor.

> **Thinking prompts:** The patient's medical history is relatively complete, and suggests a diagnosis of tuberculosis or lung cancer. However, in fact, there are many illnesses with the symptoms of moderate fever, cough, and hemoptysis, most of which are pulmonary infectious diseases. This group of symptoms also shows in

bronchiectasis, bronchial cancer, or lung cancer. In other words, infectious or non-infectious pulmonary diseases can be manifested as fever and hemoptysis, which is often the first consideration in a differential diagnosis. Generally speaking, we hope to use unification, i.e., to explain a set of symptoms by a disease, but also including atypical symptoms, and even complications that accompany it. However, the clinical manifestations of the so-called extra-pulmonary disease in the lung will make differential diagnosis more complicated. This requires us to consider the disease as being as complicated as possible. We should ask for as thorough and comprehensive a medical history as possible, and dig out any clues in the course of the disease that may change the conclusions drawn by intuition and common sense.

Medical history follow-up: One year earlier, the patient suffered from acute bacillary dysentery, with abdominal discomfort, and diarrhea, 5–7 times a day, with a small amount of pus and blood, accompanied by tenesmus, but no chill and no fever, and no obvious abdominal pain. Local rural doctors gave oral treatment of norfloxacin (usage and dosage unknown). After three days, the symptoms were relieved and the patient decided to stop taking the medicine. Thereafter, his symptoms often recurred, but were milder. Diarrhea occurred two to three times a day, and the feces were yellowish and pasty, with a small amount of mucus and blood, and sometimes lower abdominal pain. The local doctor diagnosed it as chronic bacillary dysentery, but it was not treated because the patient did not cooperate. The patient was normally strong and capable of performing heavy manual labor, and his physical fitness significantly decreased after the onset of illness, so he could only engage in light manual work. The patient enjoys raw cucumber, tomato, and fruit, and likes to eat liquor-preserved crabs.

Thinking prompts: This very significant information was not recorded in the patient's current or past medical history, indicating that the resident completely ignored these crucial details. It is precisely the neglect of these details that led to the diagnosis of lung disease. Indeed, if there were no clinical manifestations other than these lung issues, it would not be wrong for us to first consider a diagnosis of pulmonary (bronchial) tuberculosis or a malignant lung tumor. It is precisely because we obtained the medical history of gastrointestinal diseases that we asked more questions, particularly whether the shift from acute bacillary dysentery to chronic bacillary dysentery is related to this lung manifestation of fever, cough, and hemoptysis. Are these two diseases occurring in two systems, or is the same disease manifested in more than two organs or systems? This brings us back to the aforementioned question of unification or dualization. Obviously, this case is very complicated, and it is still difficult to draw a conclusion without thorough physical and auxiliary examinations. However, it is this important missing medical history that leads us to consider a different, more complex diagnosis and makes it possible to avoid misdiagnosis.

II. Physical examination after admission

Body temperature 37.7°C, pulse 87 times/min, breathing 23 times/min, blood pressure 120/75 mmHg. Clammy complexion, as in chronic consumptive disease; clear consciousness but low spirit. Skin elasticity slightly poor; thin subcutaneous fat, but no edema. There was no yellow staining on the skin mucosa anywhere on the body, and no rashes such as petechia, ecchymosis, macula, or papule were observed. No subcutaneous nodules, and small superficial lymph nodes throughout the body. No yellow staining of the sclera, and no edema of the bulbar conjunctiva. No tenderness of the sternum, normal cardiac dullness, normal heart sounds, heart rate of 80 beats/min, good rhythm, grade 2–3 soft systolic murmur audible at the apex of the heart, and no pathological murmur heard in other valvular regions. Slight shortness of breath, normal bilateral vocal fremitus, and clear percussion sound. The right lower posterior chest showed dullness on percussion. Diminished respiratory sound, and fine moist rales could be heard occasionally, but no pleural friction. No varicose veins were observed in the abdomen, which was flat and soft. No obvious muscle tension was observed, and no mass was felt. Mild tenderness of the lower abdomen on both sides, no obvious rebound tenderness, no intestinal type and peristalsis wave, 0.5 cm below right rib of liver, soft, no tenderness. The spleen was not palpable below the costal margin. No obvious percussion pain in the liver and spleen area, negative Murphy sign, negative shifting dullness, and normal bowel sounds. There was no obvious percussion pain in either renal area, no deformity of the limbs, normal muscular strength and muscular tension, no swelling or movement restriction in joints, negative meningeal stimulation sign and pyramidal tract sign.

> **Thinking prompts:** The patient is a middle-aged male with a long-term low fever in the afternoon and obvious night sweats. Five days before admission, he experienced coughing, hemoptysis sputum/coughing up bloody phlegm, and chest pain. Weight loss has been obvious since the onset of his illness. He has a history of chronic bacillary dysentery, as well as suspected contaminated food. Diseases including tuberculosis, endobronchial tuberculosis, bronchodilatation (combined with infection), bronchial cancer, lung cancer, pulmonary amoebiasis, chronic bacillary dysentery, amoebic dysentery, and inflammatory bowel disease must be included in the diagnosis or differential diagnosis range. Therefore, the physical examination should highlight the chest and abdomen, and also note the manifestation of benign illnesses such as special infections, as well as possible signs of malignant diseases. For example, note the location and nature of positive signs during chest observation, palpation, percussion, and auscultation, including whether there is any deformity of the thorax. Pay special attention to whether there is mass on palpation of the liver and spleen during the abdominal examination. At the same time, adequate evaluation should be made of the patient's nutritional status, whether the superficial lymph nodes are swollen, whether his skin is yellow, whether he has a rash, and whether his joints are red and swollen, with deformed or restricted movement. These things cannot be ignored.

III. Auxiliary examination upon admission

Routine blood examination: WBC 7.9 × 10^9/L, N 0.81, L 0.18, E (eosinophil) 0.01, PLT 230 × 10^9/L, RBC 2.8 × 10^{12}/L, Hb 86 g/L.

Routine stool examination: WBC 4–5/HP, RBC full field, occult blood (++), no amoebic cysts and trophozoites were found.

Routine urine test, liver and kidney function, and electrolytes were normal. C-reactive protein was normal.

ESR 58 mm/h.

ECG was normal.

Chest radiograph: Bulky shadow on the right lower lung, high density, thickening of right pleura, small pleural effusion at costophrenic angle, slight elevation of the right diaphragm.

Abdominal B-ultrasonography: The liver was slightly enlarged. A 3.0 × 2.7 cm space-occupying area was found in the right posterior lobe. No abnormalities were found in the gallbladder, spleen, kidney, or pancreas. No abnormal masses or enlarged lymph nodes were found in the abdomen.

The PPD test was negative. Antacid staining of the sputum smear and a tumor cell search were negative three times each.

> **Thinking prompts:** With an improved medical history and physical examination, auxiliary examination must be comprehensive and targeted. The focus of the auxiliary examination in this case should be on imaging of the chest, lungs, and abdomen, as well as routine and special examinations of the sputum and stool. Routine examination includes routine blood and stool examination, ESR, C-reactive protein, a PPD skin test, a tuberculosis antibody test, a sputum smear examination, blood and stool culture, chest X-ray on plain film, and an abdominal B-ultrasound examination. Bronchoscopy, fiber colonoscopy, and chest and abdominal CT can be performed if necessary. Phlegm retention liquid to check exfoliated cells, sputum, and stool for amoeba trophozoites can also be considered.

IV. Analysis of Ward-round upon admission

1. Diagnostic thinking

(1) Tuberculosis: The patient is a middle-aged male with a long-term low fever in the afternoon and obvious night sweats. Five days before admission, he experienced coughing, hemoptysis sputum/coughing up bloody phlegm, and chest pain, and weight loss was obvious since the onset of his illness. A physical examination revealed chronic consumptive facial features, and percussive dullness of the lower right lung. Diminished respiratory sound, with occasional fine moist rales. An auxiliary examination found that the blood sedimentation had increased rapidly. A chest radiograph showed a shadowy mass in the right lower lung; the density was high, the right pleura was thickened, and the costophrenic angle had a small amount of pleural effusion, so the possibility of pulmonary tuberculosis had to be considered. Although the

PPD skin test was negative, tuberculosis infection was not excluded, and the test could be repeated after two weeks. Although the patient's sputum smears were negative for acid-fast staining three times, tuberculosis infection could not be ruled out. The positive rate of acid-fast staining was very low, and the overall rate was about 20%, so the patient had to be tested again. Alternatively, the PCR method could be used to detect the DNA of tuberculosis bacilli. Detection of serum tuberculosis antibodies is also helpful in the diagnosis of tuberculosis. However, pulmonary tuberculosis often encroaches on the lung apex or the inferior lung apex area. It is rare to see effects on the inferior lobe of the right lung only. Infiltrating lesions can often be seen on the X-rays of patients with pulmonary tuberculosis. Calcification points or even cavities can be seen in the nodular lesions. Therefore, the diagnostic basis of pulmonary tuberculosis in this case is not sufficient. For the same reason, there is no strong evidence of endobronchial tuberculosis. A chest CT scan or fiberoptic bronchoscopy can be considered to find the lesion and extract the tissue for pathological examination, or to extract secretions for tubercle bacillus examination, so as to make a definitive diagnosis. The patient's gastrointestinal symptoms can be explained by intestinal tuberculosis, and can be clarified by gastrointestinal barium double radiography or fiber colonoscopy, but tuberculosis cannot explain the patient's liver lesions. If a definitive diagnosis cannot be made, diagnostic treatment for tuberculosis can be considered.

(2) Lung cancer: The patient is a middle-aged man with a long-term low fever. Before admission, he had a cough, hemoptysis sputum/coughing up bloody phlegm, and chest pain. Since he fell ill, he had obviously lost weight. He had smoked 600 cigarettes per year for more than 20 years. During physical examination, he was found to have chronic consumptive facial features, percussive dullness of the lower right lung, diminished respiratory sound, and occasional fine moist rales. A chest radiograph indicated a blocky shadow in the lower right lung, with high density. Therefore, the possibility of lung cancer should be considered. Accelerated ESR, anemia, and apical murmurs can be explained by chronic lung cancer. However, there is no cytological and/or histological evidence at present, so it is important to continue further sputum aspiration for exfoliative cell examination, or a chest CT scan to clarify the nature of the lesion. If necessary, fiberoptic bronchoscopy may also be considered, with tissue taken for pathological examination or a cell brush smear. Examination of the bronchus rinse precipitation may be considered. As there is only one lung lesion, if it is a tumor, the primary mass is generally considered. What is the relationship between the intrahepatic mass and intrapulmonary mass, or is it liver metastasis of lung cancer? Is it lung metastasis of liver cancer? Are they all metastatic tumors, or two different tumors? Or are there other problems like abscesses from infectious diseases, or amoebiasis? These questions are best answered by pathological evidence.

(3) Bacterial pneumonia and lung abscess: Although the patient had a fever, cough, hemoptysis sputum/coughing up bloody phlegm, and chest pain, and the chest radiograph indicates a lumpy shadow in the right lower lung, with high density, thickening of right pleura, and a small amount of pleural effusion in the costophrenic angle, the possibility of

bacterial pneumonia and a lung abscess should be considered clinically. However, the patient experienced a slow onset of illness, mild toxic blood symptoms such as chills, no expectoration of pus, and low peripheral blood picture, so the possibility of bacterial pneumonia and lung abscess can be ruled out. His sputum can be sent for bacterial culture to provide a clear diagnosis. Special attention should be paid to bacterial infection secondary to other illnesses such as bronchodilatation, bronchial cyst, lung cancer, and tuberculosis.

(4) Liver cancer: The patient is a middle-aged male with a long-term low fever, and his body weight has decreased significantly since falling ill. Physical examination revealed chronic consumptive facial features, 0.5 cm under the right rib of the liver, and the chest X-ray showed a slight elevation of the right diaphragm; abdominal B-ultrasonography suggested a slight enlargement of liver, and a space-occupying area of 3.0 cm × 2.7 cm was seen in the right posterior lobe. The possibility of liver cancer should be considered. Further examinations such as testing AFP levels, abdominal CT, B-ultrasonography, or CT-guided liver puncture pathology may be performed for definitive diagnosis. See (2) for its relationship with intrapulmonary placeholders.

(5) Bacterial liver abscess: The patient had experienced a low fever for a long time, and his body weight had decreased significantly since falling ill. Physical examination revealed chronic consumptive facial features, 0.5 cm under the right rib of the liver, and the chest X-ray showed a slight elevation of the right diaphragm; abdominal B-ultrasonography suggested a slight enlargement of liver, and a space-occupying area of 3.0 cm × 2.7 cm was seen in the right posterior lobe. The possibility of bacteria should be considered. However, the patient in this case had a slow onset of illness; cold and other toxic blood symptoms were light, with no pain in the liver area; his peripheral blood picture was not high, so a bacterial liver abscess can be ruled out. It can be clearly diagnosed by blood culture, pathological examination of a lesion puncture and bacterial culture, and special attention should be paid to secondary infection on the basis of a liver cyst. If the space occupation of the liver and lung are bacterial, the possibility of migratory lesions should be considered. If this is the case, the systemic toxic blood symptoms should be more obvious. The possibility of a bacterial liver abscess is relatively small, but it is still necessary to perform a careful physical examination and necessary auxiliary examination to rule it out completely.

(6) Amoebiasis: The patient is a middle-aged male with long-term low fever in the afternoon, and night sweats, cough and hemoptysis sputum/coughing up bloody phlegm five days before admission; chest pain, significant weight loss since the onset of illness, history of chronic mucus, bloody stool, and a history of eating contaminated food. Physical examination found chronic consumptive facial features, lower right lung percussion voiced sound, diminished respiratory sound, occasional fine moist rales, mild tenderness in the lower left and lower right abdomen, no obvious rebound pain, 0.5 cm under the right rib of the liver, and no obvious tenderness and percussion pain in the liver area. Auxiliary examination: Routine stool examination: WBC 4–5 pcs/HP, RBC full field of view, occult blood (++), rapid blood sedimentation, chest radiographs suggest a lumpy shadow in the lower right lung, high density,

right pleura thickening, a small amount of pleural effusion in the costophrenic angle, mild elevation of the right diaphragm; abdominal B-ultrasonography suggests slight enlargement of the liver, and a 3.0 cm × 2.7 cm space-occupying area can be seen in the right posterior lobe. Amoebic dysentery, an amoebic liver abscess, or an amoebic lung abscess are highly likely, although no amoebic cysts or trophozoites were found in the patient's feces. The specimens should be kept for inspection. Note that the specimens must be fresh. The faster the inspection, the better. Note whether there are Charcot-Leyden crystals, which can help with the diagnosis. The concentration method can be used to improve the detection rate. In addition to feces, pleural effusion can also be sent for inspection. Lung and liver puncture (if there is pus) can also be sent for inspection. If a cyst and trophozoites can be found, the diagnosis is obvious, except for the possibility of other amoebic protozoa. Amoebiasis is caused by Entamoeba histolytica, and there are commensal nonpathogenic amoebae (Entamoeba dispar) in the human body. Their life history and morphology are similar, so they are easy to misdiagnose. The infection rate of the latter is more common than that of the former. Further tests are therefore required, such as serological tests for specific antibodies to the histolytic enzyme; specific DNA probes and PCR techniques can be used to determine the histolytic enzyme DNA in the stool for definitive diagnosis. The detection rate of specimen isolation and culture is generally not high in most subacute or chronic cases, so it can be omitted. If the above-mentioned examination cannot be performed, a colonoscopy may be considered; materials should be scraped from the ulcer surface for microscopic examination, offering more chance of finding trophozoites.

(7) Trematodiasis: The patient is a middle-aged male with long-term low fever and night sweats. Five days before admission, he developed a cough and hemoptysis sputum/coughing up bloody phlegm, and chest pain. He has a history of chronic mucus and bloody stools. He likes to eat liquor-preserved crabs. Physical examination found chronic consumptive facial features, lower right lung percussion voiced sound, diminished respiratory sound, fine moist rales, mild tenderness in the lower left and lower right abdomen, no obvious rebound pain, 0.5 cm below the right rib of the liver, and no obvious tenderness or percussion pain in liver area. Auxiliary examination: A chest radiograph showed a shadowy mass in the right lower lung with high density, right pleura thickening, a small amount of pleural effusion in the costophrenic angle, and slight elevation of the right diaphragm; abdominal B-ultrasonography showed a slight enlargement of the liver, and a space-occupying area of 3.0 cm × 2.7 cm in the right posterior lobe. The possibility of paragonimiasis should be considered. However, no other damage to the subcutaneous nodules, central nervous system, or genitourinary system were found in this case, and there was no increase in eosinophils in the peripheral blood picture. Therefore, the basis for supporting the diagnosis of trematodiasis is not sufficient. Further examination should be conducted to make a definitive diagnosis. Sputum and feces can be checked for paragonimus eggs. Intracutaneous test and immunoserology, or lung and/or liver histopathology, can also be performed to find eggs, juvenile worms, adult worms, or eosinophilic granuloma lesions for diagnosis.

(8) Pulmonary mycosis: The patient is a male with a long-term low fever in the afternoon and

obvious night sweats. Cough, hemoptysis sputum/coughing up bloody phlegm, and chest pain appeared, and weight loss was obvious before admission. Physical examination revealed chronic consumptive facial features, percussive dullness of the lower right lung, diminished respiratory sound, and occasionally slight fine moist rales. The auxiliary examination found that the blood sedimentation had increased rapidly. The chest radiograph showed a shadowy mass in the right lower lung; the density was high, the right pleura was thickened, and the costophrenic angle had a small amount of pleural effusion. The possibility of pulmonary mycosis should be considered. Common pathogens are Candida albicans, Aspergillus, new cryptococci, and mucor. However, the patient is healthy, with no serious diseases, and no long-term treatment with antibiotics, hormones, and immunosuppressants. Therefore, the possibility of mycosis is low. A sputum smear for fungal hyphae examination can be used to make a definitive diagnosis.

(9) Hydatid disease: Before admission, the patient had a cough, hemoptysis sputum/coughing up bloody phlegm, and chest pain. The auxiliary examination found that there could be an isolated space-occupying area in the liver and lungs. Moreover, the patient lived in rural Fuyang for a long time, engaged in agricultural labor, and also came into contact with animals such as dogs, pigs, cattle, and sheep. Therefore, the possibility of hydatid disease should be considered. However, it does not explain the patient's long-term low fever. No clear round cyst on the edge was seen on ultrasound examination, and there was no spot on the head joint. Hydatid disease does not usually affect the pleura. The patient has not traveled or worked in an epidemic area, and there has had been no epidemic in his local area. Therefore, Hydatid disease can be ruled out. This can be clarified by percutaneous testing, serum immunological examination, and circulating antigens.

(10) Chronic bacillary dysentery: One year earlier, the patient suffered from abdominal discomfort and diarrhea, 5–7 times a day, with a small amount of pus and blood, accompanied by tenesmus, but no chill and no fever, and no obvious abdominal pain. Local rural doctors gave an oral treatment of norfloxacin, and after three days, the symptoms were relieved and the patient decided to stop taking the medication. Since then, his symptoms often recurred, but were milder. Diarrhea occurred two to three times a day, and the feces were yellowish and pasty, with a small amount of mucus and blood, and sometimes lower abdominal pain. It was not treated. The patient has a suspected history of contaminated eating. Clinical manifestations should be highly suspicious of the possibility of chronic bacillary dysentery. However, the patient was found to have mild tenderness in the lower left and lower right abdomen. The routine examination was mainly red blood cells, and there were few white blood cells and no pus cells or macrophages. This did not support a diagnosis of chronic bacillary dysentery. A stool sample should be left for fecal culture. If necessary, a colonoscopy can be performed and mucus purulent secretions can be taken for culture to improve the diagnosis.

(11) Nonspecific ulcerative colitis: The patient has recurrent mucus bloody stools with pain in the lower abdomen, wasting, and anemia. The possibility of nonspecific ulcerative colitis should be considered. An X-ray barium enema and colonoscopy can be performed for a definitive diagnosis.

(12) Colorectal cancer: The patient is a middle-aged male with recurrent mucus and bloody stools, accompanied by pain in the lower abdomen, wasting, and anemia. Routine stool examination: WBC 4–5 pcs/HP, RBC full field of view, occult blood (++). The possibility of colorectal cancer should be considered. There is a single space-occupying area in the liver and lung, and the possibility of metastasis of colorectal cancer is small. Determination of carcinoembryonic antigens and related antigens of bowel cancer, manual anal examination, X-ray barium enema, and colonoscopy can help the diagnosis of colorectal cancer.

(13) Chronic schistosomiasis: The patient has recurrent bloody stools with mucus, accompanied by tenesmus. B-ultrasonography suggests that the liver is slightly enlarged, and the possibility of chronic schistosomiasis should be considered. However, the general symptoms of chronic schistosomiasis are relatively light. The liver is mainly enlarged in the left lobe, often accompanied by splenomegaly, with an obvious elevation of eosinophils. Moreover, the patient denies a history of exposure to infected water. Therefore, the possibility of chronic schistosomiasis is low. The incubation of fecal metacercariae, the deposition test of rectal mucosa biopsy eggs and ring eggs, or the detection of circulating antigens are helpful for differential diagnosis.

V. Treatment
1. Ward-round analysis two weeks after admission
According to the above analysis, after admission, the patient was given cefuroxime to prevent and control infection, followed by hemostasis such as hypophysin, aminomethylbenzoic (para-aminomethylbenzoic acid), and general symptomatic support treatment. There was no obvious relief of symptoms such as coughing up bloody phlegm. At the same time, relevant inspections were carried out. The sputum smears were negative for acid-fast staining, fungal hyphae, and exfoliated cells three times. DNA (PCR) of TBB was negative three times. Sputum bacteria culture was negative three times. Shigella dysenteriae was not found in 3 stool cultures. Amoebic cysts and trophozoites were not found in 3 stool tests, and paragonimiasis eggs were not found in 3 sputum and stool tests. The patient tested negative for tuberculosis antibodies, schistosome ring egg precipitation, and circulating antigen. AFP and carcinoembryonic antigens were normal. One week later, a chest X-ray, B-ultrasound, and CT examination showed liquefaction in the lesion, suggesting a pulmonary abscess and liver abscess. A right pleural puncture failed due to less effusion; the liver abscess was punctured under the guidance of B-ultrasound, and dark brown and viscous pus was extracted, which was mixed with bean dregs and necrotic tissue, and had the smell of rot. Amoebic trophozoites were found in the pus. Therefore, it is diagnosed as amoebiasis (intestinal amoebiasis, hepatic amoebic abscess, pulmonary amoebic abscess), with a further check for positive amoebic antibodies (ELISA method). So far, the diagnosis is clear. Cefuroxime treatment was stopped, switching to levofloxacin (0.2 g, intravenous drip, two times a day) and metronidazole treatment (1.0 g, intravenous drip, two times a day), and strengthening symptomatic support treatment. After four days of treatment, the patient's gastrointestinal symptoms, such as abdominal pain, diarrhea, mucus bloody stool,

and tenesmus, were relieved. A week later, the routine stool examination was normal, and the occult blood was negative. Blood routine: WBC 6.5×10^9/L, N 0.77.L 0.22, E 0.01, PLT 239×10^9/L, RBC 3.0×10^{12}/L, Hb 98 g/L, further supporting the diagnosis. Because the liver abscess is fluidized, puncture drainage guided by B-ultrasomotonography was performed, and metronidazole was used for flushing. Systemic treatment is the same as before.

Amoebiasis is caused by Entamoeba histolytica. Entamoeba histolytica has two forms: Cysts and trophozoites. The trophozoite is the causative factor. It invades the intestinal wall and causes dysentery symptoms. It can also cause parenteral amoebiasis with the migration of blood and lymph from the intestinal wall or directly spread to parenteral tissues (liver, lung, brain); the cyst is the source of its transmission. It is only formed in the human intestinal cavity, cannot be formed in the organs outside the intestinal cavity, and is discharged with the feces. Enteral and parenteral infections are classified according to the location of infection. Enteral infection can be characterized by acute and chronic amoebic dysentery, and parenteral infection is common with an amoebic liver abscess. The existing anti-amoebiasis drugs mainly act on trophozoites, and most of them act weakly on cysts. Although no cysts were found on pathogenic examination, both trophozoites and cysts should be considered during treatment. Since amoebiasis in this case invades the intestinal tract, liver, and lung at the same time and forms chronic amoebic dysentery, liver abscess, and lung abscess, the course of anti-infective treatment should be sufficient.

The most commonly used amoebicides currently in clinical use and their properties are as follows:

(1) Nitroimidazoles

1) Metronidazole: This has a strong elimination effect on enteral and parenteral amoeba trophozoites. It is currently the first choice for treating enteral and parenteral amoebic diseases. After oral administration, the product is absorbed in the small intestine. The plasma concentration reaches the peak at 1 hour, with a half-life period of 6–7 hours. The general treatment dose is 0.4–0.8 g/time, three times a day, 5–10 days for intestinal amoebiasis, and ten days for liver abscess. 50 mg/(kg·d) for children, three times a day, seven days. Intravenous administration was started at 15 mg/kg and then repeated at 7.5 mg/kg every 6 to 8 hours. Metronidazole has good oral absorption and colon drug concentration, meaning that it has a poor curative effect on patients with asymptomatic cyst discharge.

2) Tinidazole: This product is absorbed quickly. Its plasma concentration is 1 time higher than that of metronidazole. The half-life period is longer (10–12 hours). The side effects are few, and the curative effect is better. The dose is 2 g/d, 30–40 mg/(kg·d) with children. Other drugs of the same kind (including ornidazole and secnidazole) have a longer half-life period and good efficacy for all types of amoebiasis.

(2) Ipecine (emetine): Ipecine has a direct elimination effect on amoeba trophozoites, and has an extremely high curative effect on tissue trophozoites, but has no significant effect on intestinal amoebae. Due to the high toxicity of the drug, the treatment amount is close to the poisoning amount, and there is a cumulative effect, which can produce side effects such as

myocardial damage, blood pressure decline, and arrhythmia. It is used sparingly, and has been replaced by its derivative, dehydroemetine. The dose for adults is 1.25 mg/kg per day, no more than 90 mg/d, and it is injected into the deep subcutaneous tissue twice a day for 3–10 days.

(3) Diiodoquinoline: This drug can directly eliminate enteral amoeba trophozoites, but is ineffective for cysts and parenteral amoebic disease, and needs to be used with an in-tissue amebicide. The adult dose is 0.6 g/time, three times a day. The children's dose is 30–40 mg/(kg·d), over 15–20 days.

(4) Diloxanide: This product is the most effective at eliminating cysts at present, and can directly kill amoebic trophozoites. It is effective for patients with asymptomatic cyst discharge, and can also be used to treat chronic amoebic dysentery. It has a poor therapeutic effect on acute amoebic dysentery. Combined with metronidazole, it can prevent recurrence, and has no effect on parenteral amoebiasis. The adult dose is 0.5 g/time, three times a day, for ten days.

(5) Nitazoxanide: This drug is effective against intestinal tract protozoa. Diarrhea caused by Entamoeba histolytica and Giardia is treated with oral nitazoxanide 500 mg/time, two times a day for three days in a row. The results are observed in a randomized, double-blind trial. Diarrhea stops within seven days of treatment, with mild side effects.

(6) Chloroquine: This product is an antimalarial drug, which also has an eliminating effect on amoeba trophozoites. Oral absorption is rapid and complete. Drug concentration in the liver is much higher than that in plasma, and the distribution on the intestinal wall is small. It is ineffective against enteral amoebiasis, and is used to treat parenteral amoebiasis. It is only used for amoebic liver abscesses when metronidazole is ineffective. It should be combined with enteral anti-amoebiasis medicine in case of recurrence. In the treatment of invasive rectal colitis, the dosage is chloroquine (matrix) 600 mg, 300 mg, 150 mg, three times a day for 14 days, and the dosage for the treatment of a liver abscess is chloroquine (matrix) 600 mg, once a day for two days, then 300 mg once a day for 2–3 weeks.

(7) Antibiotics: Antibiotics mainly affect the growth and reproduction of amoebae by inhibiting the intestinal symbiotic bacteria, and are especially effective for amoebic dysentery with bacterial infection. Antimicrobials include tetracyclines, paromomycin, and fluoroquinolone.

Considering the specific condition and actual effects of treatment on the patient, anti-amoebic metronidazole was selected, supplemented with anti-bacterial levofloxacin, with diloxanide added at a later stage to eliminate the cysts and the source of infection.

2. Ward-round analysis after four weeks of treatment

The patient's low fever subsided, and cough, bloody phlegm, and chest pain were relieved after two weeks of treatment. Routine blood examination: WBC 5.7×10^9/L, N 0.72, L 0.27, E 0.01, PLT 215×10^9/L, RBC 3.2×10^{12}/L, Hb 103 g/L, ESR 36 mm/h; routine stool examination normal, occult blood negative, no amoebic cysts or trophozoites found in the feces; chest radiograph examination indicated that the pleural effusion had been absorbed, and the lung abscess had obviously reduced. B-mode ultrasound tomography indicated that the liver abscess had obviously been absorbed. The original anti-amoeba treatment was continued for four weeks, and diloxanide was added (0.5 g/time, three times a day for ten days) to destroy the cysts.

VI. Condition at discharge

The patient was treated with metronidazole and anti-infection levofloxacin as well as symptomatic support. After four days of treatment, the abdominal pain, diarrhea, mucus/bloody stool, and tenesmus and other gastrointestinal symptoms were relieved. One week later, the routine stool test was normal, and the occult blood was negative. Then, the patient was treated with B-ultrasonic-guided puncture and drainage of the liver abscess rinsed with metronidazole. After two weeks of anti-infection treatment, the low fever subsided, and cough, hemoptysis sputum, and chest pain were relieved. Routine blood examination: WBC 5.8×10^9/L, N 0.72, L 0.28, PLT 227×10^9/L, RBC 3.8×10^{12}/L, Hb 114 g/L, ESR 30 mm/h; routine stool examination normal, occult blood negative, no amoebic cysts and trophozoites found in feces; chest radiograph examination indicated the absorption of pleural effusion, the absorption of the lung abscess, the recovery of the right diaphragm, and the absorption of the liver abscess. The patient was discharged from hospital after stopping the drugs for three days without abnormalities.

VII. Follow-up

After discharge, the clinical manifestations such as fever, abdominal pain, diarrhea, cough, and expectoration were monitored, and routine blood and stool tests were checked every month for amoebic cysts and trophozoites and occult blood. Chest radiographs and abdominal B-ultrasounds were performed every three months. The patient was followed up for one year. During the follow-up period, no symptoms re-appeared. The routine blood and stool tests were normal. The occult blood was negative. Amoebic cysts and trophozoites were not found. After three months, the blood sedimentation was normal. The chest radiograph only showed slight thickening of the right pleura. The lung abscess completely healed. There were no abnormalities on the abdominal B-ultrasound.

VIII. Lessons learned

Amoebic dysentery, also known as intestinal amoebiasis, is a major infectious gastrointestinal disease caused by dysentery symptoms after the invasion of the colon wall by pathogenic Entamoeba histolytica. The lesions are mostly in the ileocecal colon, and tend to recur and become chronic. Protozoa can also become parenteral amoebiasis from the intestinal wall to the lymph nodes through blood flow or directly to organs such as the liver, lung, and brain. Amoebic liver abscesses are the most common, and there are many reports of amoebic lung abscesses. In recent years, due to poor dietary hygiene, amoebiasis has increased, and sufficient attention must be paid to it. The clinical manifestations of this case are very similar to other common diseases such as tuberculosis and tumors at first glance, but the patient's history of chronic diarrhea and mucus/bloody stool was initially neglected in the medical history, which led to an incorrect diagnosis. Therefore, the collecting of correct and comprehensive medical history and epidemiological data plus physical examination are very helpful for diagnosis, especially for patients with atypical clinical manifestations or secondary bacterial infections.

Secondly, if the patient has a lung and liver abscess, and a detailed auxiliary examination is not performed to make differential diagnosis (in this case, the diagnosis was made by finding amoeba trophozoites in pus), but empirical medication is prescribed (metronidazole is often used as a broad-spectrum antibiotic to eliminate anaerobic bacteria), it may lead to an incorrect diagnosis. The consequence may be that amoebic disease is treated by mistake and cured, but the amoebic cyst is not eliminated, and it may form an infectious source, thus causing the spread of the disease.

Thirdly, we should also note the identification of pathogenic amoebiasis (Entamoeba histolytica) and non-pathogenic amoebiasis (Entamoeba dispar) in the intestine to prevent misdiagnosis, because their life history and morphology are similar, and the infection rate of the latter in the population is much more common than the former. Significant progress has been made in the laboratory diagnosis of amoebiasis, including the detection of amoeba antigens (e.g., detection of Gal/GalNAc adhesion agglutinin antigens in a patient's serum and saliva by ELISA), and the determination of specific antibodies in serum by pure amoebic antigens or monoclonal antibodies. Specific DNA probes and PCR techniques can be used to determine the histolytic enzyme DNA in stool and abscess suction. This case was based on the patient's clinical manifestation. Trophozoites were found in the liver pus, and were confirmed by hematology tests and effective treatment.

(Zhang Ruiqi & Miao Xiaohui)

References

Chen, Haozhu. *Practical Internal Medicine.* 12th ed. Beijing: People's Health Publishing House, 2005.

Li, Zongming. *Differential Diagnosis of Clinical Symptoms.* 3rd ed. Shanghai: Shanghai Science and Technology Press, 1995.

Lin, Zhaoqian. *Diagnosis and Case Analysis of Febrile Diseases.* Beijing: People's Health Press, 1999.

Ma, Yilin. *Infectious Diseases.* 4th ed. Shanghai: Shanghai Science and Technology Press, 2005.

Xia, Mengyan, Gao Fei, and Li Xiaojing. "Progress in the Experimental Diagnosis of Amoebic Disease." *Foreign Medicine – Clinical Biochemistry and Examination Division* 23, no. 2 (2002): 91.

Recurrent fever for nine months, headache for six months

I. Medical history

Patient: Male, 43 years old, from Datong in Shanxi Province. He was hospitalized from 21 June 2006 until 6 November 2007 with recurrent fever for nine months, and headache for six months.

In September 2005, the patient had a fever of up to 38.2°C with no origin, and no other concomitant symptoms. His temperature decreased to normal after one month of intermittent intravenous antibiotic use. In December 2005, he had a fever again, accompanied by a headache. He went to a hospital and his spinal fluid pressure was found to be 330 mmH$_2$O (1 cmH$_2$O = 98.07 Pa). After considering the possibility of meningitis, he was dehydrated and treated with anti-infection drugs, but the symptoms were not relieved. Cryptococcus was found in his cerebrospinal fluid, and there was HIV Ab positive in his blood after review.

Follow-up history: The patient had a blood transfusion in 1998.

Thinking prompts: The patient is an adult male who went to see a doctor for fever and headache. With these symptoms, be alert to the presence of nervous system infection. In this case, look closely at the nervous system, especially meningeal irritation, and perform a lumbar puncture and CT examination of the skull. Cerebrospinal fluid should be checked for routine testing, biochemicals, bacterial culture, fungal culture, antacid staining, ink staining, latex agglutination testing, and cytology tests should be carried out.

The following conditions should be considered: ① Viral meningitis: Rapid onset, and high fever can be accompanied by myalgia and abdominal pain; the sugar and chloride in the cerebrospinal fluid do not decrease, and protein is below 1 g/L; after 2–3 weeks, these symptoms can be relieved. ② Purulent meningitis: Acute onset with high fever and chills; cerebrospinal fluid leukocytes are significantly increased, mainly neutrophils; sugar reduction is more obvious than in tuberculous meningitis; pathogenic bacteria can be found in cerebrospinal fluid smear and culture. ③ Fungal meningitis: Clinical manifestations and changes in the cerebrospinal fluid of cryptococcal meningitis are similar to tuberculous meningitis. Diagnosis depends on ink staining, culture, and antigen detection of cerebrospinal fluid. ④ Tuberculous meningitis: A recent history of close tuberculous contact; there may be tuberculous foci in other parts of the body; intracranial hypertension, signs of meningeal irritation, and other neurological symptoms and signs; cerebrospinal fluid examination results conform to the manifestation of non-purulent meningitis. ⑤ Brain abscess: Headache, vomiting, and optic papilla edema are the main manifestations, and CT is helpful for diagnosis.

Cerebrospinal fluid manifestations of common meningitis are shown in Table 3-1:

Table 3-1 Cerebrospinal fluid manifestations of common meningitis

Type of meningitis	Pressure	Leukocyte count (10^6/L)	Protein	Chloride	Sugar
Bacterial	Raised	Hundreds or more than 6,000, mainly neutrophils	Raised, 1–2 g/L	Decreased	Decreased
Tuberculous	Raised or slightly raised	25–500, Few up to 1000+, mainly lymphocytes	1–5 g/L or higher	Decreased	Decreased
Viral	Normal or slightly raised	10–100, mainly lymphocytes	Normal or slightly raised	Normal	Normal
Fungal	Moderately or significantly raised	10–500, mainly lymphocytes	0.2–5 g/L, average 1 g/L	Decreased by more than half	Decreased

Cryptococci were found in the patient's cerebrospinal fluid, and the diagnosis of cryptococci meningitis was considered. The susceptible population of cryptococcal meningitis includes those with serious basic illnesses or abnormal immune function such as diabetes, renal failure, cirrhosis, malignant lymphoma, leukemia, sarcoidosis, systemic lupus erythematosus, recipients of organ transplantation, and long-term, heavy users of immunosuppressants such as glucocorticoids. The incidence of cryptococcosis secondary to AIDS is 5%–10% in the United States and up to 30% in developing countries. After a diagnosis of cryptococcal meningitis, the existence of potential primary diseases should be considered.

At present, the patient's diagnosis is clear: AIDS complicated with cryptococcal meningitis.

II. Treatment after the first transfer

On 24 January 2006, the patient was transferred to a hospital and examined: CD4$^+$ T cells 10/mm^3, plasma viral load 11,000 Copies/ml. Amphotericin B antifungal treatment was given, after checking the negative result of the brain/spinal fluid cryptococcus. Later, this was changed to fluconazole. Antiviral therapy was given after 30 days of antifungal therapy: Lamivudine, Zidovudine, and Efavirenz (Stocrin).

> **Thinking prompts:** At present, the antifungal treatment guidelines for HIV infections complicated with cryptococcal meningitis are: Amphotericin B [0.7–1 mg/(kg·d)] combined with flucytosine [100 mg/(kg·d)] for two weeks, then fluconazole (400 mg/d) for ten weeks. Then, whether to maintain treatment is decided according to the patient's clinical condition.
>
> The common dose of amphotericin B is 0.5–0.7 mg/(kg·d). Specific usage: The doses in the first three days were 1 mg, 3 mg, and 5 mg respectively, and they were added to 500 ml of 5% glucose solution for an intravenous drip for 6–8 hours. If there were no serious adverse reactions, it could be increased by 5 mg every day from the fourth day until the daily dose reached 25–35 mg. After that, the dose was maintained for intravenous drip. The course of treatment was judged according to the curative effect, which generally took 2–3 months. A total dose of 2–3 g or more has a better curative effect. During the administration of amphotericin B, look out for adverse reactions such as drug reactions, chills, fever, loss of appetite, nausea, vomiting, and other pyrogen reactions; organ damage, mainly kidney function damage, but also myocardial and liver damage; electrolyte disorders. This medication can damage the renal tubules and cause hematuria, proteinuria, azotemia, and hypokalemia. Thrombophlebitis can also be caused by taking medication too quickly.
>
> Prevention and treatment of adverse reactions: Symptomatic treatment such as promethazine or antinfan (indometacin suppositories) was given before instillation. Liver and kidney function tests, electrolyte tests, and an electrocardiogram were performed during the course of medication.
>
> At present, antiviral treatment for AIDS is mostly combined with drugs known as highly-active antiretroviral therapy (HAART). Its composition can be mainly composed of two nucleoside reverse transcriptase inhibitors and combined with one NNRTIs or protease inhibitor.
>
> The indications and timing of the initiation of antiretroviral therapy in adults and adolescents are shown in Table 3-2.
>
> Antiretroviral therapy was initiated after 30 days of antifungal therapy. If anti-retroviruses are detected within 30 days of a diagnosis of cryptococcal meningitis, 30% of patients are susceptible to immune reconstitution inflammatory syndrome. In the first weeks or months of antiviral therapy, the patient may have an increased immune response to the pathogen of an opportunistic infection due to the increased

CD4$^+$ T cell count. This condition can be manifested as a new clinical disease. After antiviral therapy is initiated, the patient may have: ① a therapeutic paradoxical response: After the antiviral therapy is initiated, the treatment-related condition paradox becomes more serious; or ② an exposure response: After the immune function is recovered, the concealed infection appears with an obvious clinical manifestation.

Table 3-2 Indication and timing of antiretroviral therapy

Clinical staging	CD4$^+$ T cell count (n/mm^3)	Recommendation
Acute stage of infection	Regardless of the CD4$^+$ T cell count	Consider treatment
Stage of asymptomatic infection	A) > 350, regardless of the capacity of viral load B) between 200 and 350	A) Regular re-examination and temporary non-treatment B) Regular re-examination; start treatment if one of the following conditions occurs: CD4$^+$ T cell count drops more than 30% within one year Plasma viral load > 100,000 Copies/ml Patients require treatment urgently Ensure compliance
Stage of AIDS	Regardless of the CD4$^+$ T cell count	Perform therapy

Immune reconstitution inflammatory syndrome in cryptococcal meningitis is a clinical manifestation similar to the recurrence or aggravation of cryptococcal meningitis, such as reoccurrence of fever, headache, or neck pain in AIDS patients within eight weeks after the initiation of HAART, or no later than six months. At this time, cerebrospinal fluid pressure increases, and the number of cells increases, but a cryptococcus culture is negative. This is due to the gradual recovery and reconstruction of immune deficiency after HAART treatment, that is, the number of CD4$^+$ T cells gradually increases, the HIV viral load continues to decline, and the specific immune response begins to recover. The resulting inflammatory response is strengthened, resulting in inflammatory syndrome of immune reconstruction, which is easily confused with the recurrence or aggravation of cryptococcal meningitis. Therefore, HAART should be started after 4–8 weeks of antifungal therapy.

III. Treatment after the second transfer

On 1 April 2006, the patient was automatically discharged to a hospital. His cerebrospinal fluid (CSF) was examined for the new cryptococcus antigen (+). The CSF latex coagulation test result was 1:512. The blood CD4+ T cells were 17/mm³. The viral load was < 50 copies/ml. HAART treatment and fluconazole + flucytosine antifungal treatment were continued.

On 28 April, the drug was changed to amphotericin B liposome 200 mg/d × 40 days. Cryptococcus still appeared in the CSF after re-examination, and the dose was raised to 300 mg on 5 June. There was no change in the CSF. The patient was admitted to our hospital for further diagnosis and treatment.

IV. Treatment after re-transfer

Antiretroviral therapy was continued after admission: Amphotericin B liposomal combined with flurocytosine for antifungal therapy, mannitol for dehydration and reduction of craniofacial pressure, and compound sulfamethoxazole–2 tablets/day to prevent pulmonary PCP infection. A large number of cryptococcus neoformans (antigen 1:512) were found after repeated lumbar punctures and ink staining. From 25 August, 200 mg of fluconazole was injected intravenously once a day. 38 CD4+ T cells/mm³ were reviewed on 29 August. From 31 October, recombinant growth hormone (4 IU, once daily, subcutaneous injection) was administered for seven months. On 28 March 2007, 38 CD4+ T cells/mm³ were reviewed. Lumbar puncture CSF pressure > 330 mmH₂O; cerebrospinal fluid routine, and normal biochemistry; ink staining (−). Latex agglutination test 1:8. Discontinued recombinant growth hormone on 17 May. Interleukin-2 (2 mU) once daily, subcutaneous injection, five days per week for four weeks was added on 28 May. After six months of treatment, CD4+ T cells increased to 144 cells/mm³, cranial pressure was 230 mmH₂O, and the CSF latex agglutination test was 1:2. The clinical symptoms improved, and amphotericin B was discontinued. The total amount of amphotericin B was 15.8 g, and the total amount of amphotericin B liposome was 17.65 g. There were no toxic and side effects of amphotericin B during treatment.

Thinking prompts: After four months of antiretroviral treatment, the CD4+ T lymphocyte count did not increase significantly, and the cryptococcal infection did not improve significantly after antifungal treatment.

Difficulties occurred during the treatment. After antiretroviral treatment, the viral load of most AIDS patients is controlled to be undetectable, and there is immune reconstitution, showing an increase in CD4+ T cell count, and reducing opportunistic infections and malignant tumors. However, after antiretroviral therapy, the viral load of some AIDS patients has not been measured, but the CD4+ T cell count does not increase, which is called incomplete immune reconstitution.

Amphotericin B liposome is effective in the treatment of cryptococcal meningitis, and has fewer side effects than amphotericin B, but its high price greatly restricts its clinical application. At present, these drugs tend to be prescribed to patients who cannot tolerate amphotericin B, or cannot use amphotericin B due to renal insufficiency (blood creatinine greater than 221 μmol/L), or patients whose treatment with amphotericin B failed in the acute phase. The recommended dose is

4–6 mg/(kg·d), and the course of treatment is three weeks.

There was no significant increase in the CD4$^+$ T cell count after treatment with a growth hormone. After switching to Interleukin-2, the number of CD4$^+$ T cells increased. It has been reported that Interleukin-2 increases CD4$^+$ T cells by down regulating immune activation and T cell proliferation.

Because cryptococcal meningitis is difficult to control in this case, the dosage of amphotericin B is high. Adverse drug reactions should be closely monitored.

V. Follow-up

After discharge, the patient was generally in good condition without discomfort such as fever and headache. HAART and fluconazole were continued.

VI. Lessons learned

When diagnosing cryptococcal meningitis, be wary of susceptibility factors, especially HIV infections. In this case, antiretroviral treatment was initiated after 30 days of antifungal treatment when HIV infection was combined with cryptococcal meningitis. When incomplete immune reconstruction occurs, cryptococcal infection is not easy to control. Interleukin-2 treatment is recommended.

(Guo Fuping & Li Taisheng)

Recurrent fever for five weeks, numbness of limbs with progressive exacerbation of dyspnea for one month

I. Medical history

Patient: Female, 25 years old, from Harbin in Heilongjiang Province. She was hospitalized from 18 April to 12 May 2006 for recurrent fever for five weeks, numbness of the limbs, and progressive exacerbation of dyspnea for one month.

On 10 March 2006, the patient developed an unexplained fever of up to 37.8°C, with no other concomitant symptoms, and no improvement after self-administration of roxithromycin. On 17 March, she began to experience numbness of the limbs, and was hospitalized with a preliminary diagnosis of Guillain-Barré syndrome. The patient did not receive further diagnosis and treatment. On 26 March, the limb numbness worsened, and the patient could not walk on her own. She was given emergency treatment at our hospital.

Physical examination: Right-side neuro-facial paralysis, grade 5 muscle strength of both upper limbs. Tendon reflex of biceps brachii and triceps not elicited, grade 3 to 4 muscle strength of the proximal end of both lower limbs, grade 5 muscle strength of the distal end. Achilles tendon and knee tendon reflex not elicited. An emergency lumbar puncture was performed, pressure 158 mmH$_2$O. Routine cerebrospinal fluid test: Protein (+), total number of cells 28/mm^3, leukocytes 12/mm^3, mononuclear 4/mm^3, polynuclear 8/mm^3. Cerebrospinal fluid biochemistry: Protein 90.2 mg/dl, glucose 46 mg/ml, Cl$^-$ 122 mmol/L. Myoelectric illustration of peripheral neurogenic lesions. No abnormality was found on a CT scan of the patient's head. Guillain-Barré syndrome was considered, to be treated with normal human gamma-globulin and symptomatic support.

Thinking prompts: The patient is an adult female, experiencing numbness of the limbs and disordered mobility of both lower limbs. It is necessary to conduct a neurological examination, blood potassium tests, lumbar puncture, brain/spinal fluid, and a CT scan of the skull. The diagnosis on admission was contingent upon the following: ① The patient had a history of upper respiratory tract issues before the onset of her current illness, manifested as symmetrical lower limb dyskinesia, peripheral hypoesthesia, and protein cell separation in the cerebrospinal fluid, so Guillain-Barré syndrome was considered to be likely. ② Acute myelitis: The patient had no conduction tract sensory disturbance, persistent rectum/bladder dysfunction, or issues with the pathological pyramidal tract, so acute myelitis was temporarily ruled out. ③ Periodic paralysis: The patient experienced no flaccid paralysis of limbs, and blood potassium was normal, so periodic paralysis was temporarily ruled out. ④ Functional paralysis: The patient had neurological signs, so functional paralysis was not initially considered.

Acute Guillain-Barré syndrome (GBS) – an acute inflammatory demyelinating polyneuropathy – is an autoimmune disease. Its etiology remains unknown. Many scholars believe that infection factors before the onset of the disease may be an important cause of GBS. In recent years, the relationship between Campylobacter jejuni (CJ) infection and GBS has attracted increasing amounts of attention. In addition, GBS has been reported after infection by various pathogens, and the correlation with some cases is unclear. The basis for a diagnosis of GBS is as follows: ① Most cases have a nonspecific or viral infection history before the onset of the disease. ② About 75% of the cases reach a peak within one week; 25% of the cases reach a peak after 2–3 weeks. ③ Symptoms usually start with weakness of the lower limbs, gradually descending into paralysis, especially of the upper limbs. ④ Most patients have severe sensory abnormalities and disturbances, especially in the distal part of the limbs.⑤ About half of all cases are accompanied by cranial nerve palsy, mostly including the facial nerve. ⑥ Other autonomic nervous manifestations such as sweating, redness, swelling, palpitation. ⑦ The protein content of the CSF increases, but the number of CSF cells is normal.

Treatments for GBS include the following: ① Hormone therapy: Widely used, but controversial. International data indicates that a conventional dose of hormone cannot prevent the development of the disease nor shorten its course. ② Immunoglobulin therapy (IVIG): A high dose and short course of intravenous immunoglobulin has proven to be effective, and should be implemented as early as possible before respiratory muscle paralysis. ③ Plasma exchange therapy (PE): Beginning in the 1970s, the curative effect has been widely recognized, and PE can shorten the course of treatment and reduce the severity of the disease. The common side effect is hepatitis after plasma transfusion. ④ Immunosuppressants: Cyclophosphamide is used for severe GBS, with poor hormonal side effects; some people advocate for the use of cyclophosphamide to prevent the worsening of the disease, but it is cytotoxic, so it is generally not the first choice. Azathioprine is a mild immunosuppressant that mainly suppresses T lymphocytes, and has a relatively slow effect. It can be used to treat chronic GBS. It can also be used in the acute phase when other drugs are ineffective or contraindicated, but its cytotoxicity cannot be ignored. ⑤ Other treatments: In a clinical setting, 10% compound glycerin

500 ml every day can be used for intravenous treatment of GBS. There are also reports of hyperbaric oxygen therapy on the basis of conventional treatment. In addition, Traditional Chinese Medicine, including acupuncture and moxibustion, has achieved a certain curative effect in the treatment of GBS. In this case, the patient was treated with human gamma-globulin.

II. Development and treatment measures

On 29 March 2006, sudden dyspnea occurred, and SaO_2 decreased from 90% to 75%. Endotracheal intubation and ventilator-assisted breathing were given, and cefuroxime sodium (Cefuroxime) was added to fight infection and nutritional support. On 12 April, spontaneous breathing gradually recovered.

During the period of emergency treatment at our hospital, HIV-Ab was tested twice (+) and sent to the Beijing Center for Disease Control for two HIV antibody confirmation tests (−). There was a Follow-up of the patient's medical history. Prenatal examination in April 2005: HIV-Ab (−). Her husband had an extramarital affair and was suspected of HIV infection. From April 2005 to January 2006, they claimed not to have had sex. Since 18 February, she has had intermittent sexual contact with her husband.

> **Thinking prompts:** A small number of patients develop Guillain-Barré syndrome very quickly; muscle weakness reaches a peak within 12–48 hours, and life-threatening respiratory muscle weakness occurs at the same time. In case of respiratory failure, mechanical ventilation should be given in good time to help the patient pass through the dangerous period.
>
> The patient's husband had a history of extramarital sexual contact. Although the confirmatory test was negative, HIV infection could not be ruled out. According to the patient's medical history, the onset was in accordance with the acute stage of HIV infection.
>
> Acute infection usually occurs about 1–2 weeks after exposure to HIV. During the acute infection period, a large number of HIV copies and CD4[+] T cells decrease sharply. Around 50%–70% of infected patients had the clinical symptoms of HIV viremia and acute damage to the immune system. The main manifestations were systemic, skin, nervous system, and intestinal symptoms. Systemic symptoms include fever, sore throat, night sweats, arthralgia, lymphadenopathy, and hepatosplenomegaly. The main manifestations of skin damage are rashes, mostly non-itchy red macular papules, and occasionally diffuse urticaria or hydro herpes. Rashes occur mostly on the face and trunk, but can appear all over the body in severe cases. In cases of nervous system injury, about 9% of patients have acute HIV meningitis. The clinical manifestations are fever, headache, vomiting, and meningeal irritation. The number of monocytes and protein content in cerebrospinal fluid examination increases. Twenty to 40% of AIDS patients have peripheral neuritis.

The symptoms can appear in different stages of the disease. The most common symptoms are symmetrical hypoesthesia or numbness of the feet. Some patients feel slight pain. In addition, there is acute multiple neuritis or Guillain-Barré syndrome. The former is seen in the early stage of HIV, and the latter in the late stage. The first symptom is weakness in muscle activity, followed by a change in sensation. Physical examination showed myasthenia and decreased reflexes, increased protein in the cerebrospinal fluid, increased lymphocytes, and mononuclear cell infiltration and demyelination in a nerve tissue biopsy. Common gastrointestinal symptoms include nausea, vomiting, diarrhea, and oral and esophageal candidiasis.

Generally speaking, the acute symptoms of HIV last 2–4 weeks. However, the clinical symptoms in most infected patients are generally very mild and transient infection symptoms like a cold or mononucleosis. After symptomatic treatment or even without treatment, they can return to normal after two to three weeks. Therefore, many people are not clinically sure of the true acute infection stage.

The diagnosis of HIV infection should be confirmed by two positive ELISA screening test results and confirmed by Western blot.

III. Further examinations and results

Detection by branch DNA amplification: HIV viral load was 13,900 copies/ml. Lymphocyte subsets: The proportion and count of $CD4^+$ T cells decreased ($169/mm^3$), the proportion and count of $CD8^+$ T cells increased significantly and there was obvious abnormal activation (the proportion of $CD8^+$ $CD38^+$, $CD8^+$ HLA-DR$^+$ increased significantly), the proportion of $CD4^+$ and $CD8^+$ was inverted, and the expression of $CD4^+$ $CD28^+$, $CD8^+$ $CD28^+$ was normal.

Thinking prompts: In most HIV-infected people, the virus takes three months to turn serum antibodies positive. The ELISA method is sensitive and easy to operate, but there will be some false positives, so at present, it is only a preliminary screening. Western blot is the most specific and sensitive method of confirming HIV infection, but the operation is more complex than ELISA, and it is only used as a confirmatory test.

In the acute stage of infection, the level of the virus directly predicts the speed of HIV developing into AIDS. When the viral load in the plasma is less than 4,350 copies/ml, 8% of patients develop AIDS within five years. When the viral load in plasma is 4,350–36,270 copies/ml, 62% of the patients develop AIDS within five years. When suspected of acute HIV infection, check HIV RNA combined with HIV antibody diagnosis. Acute HIV infection often presents as HIV RNA positive and HIV antibody negative or suspicious. When HIV RNA is less than 10,000 copies/ml, it is a false positive. T lymphocyte subsets and HIV viral load should be improved.

The main immunopathological changes in HIV AIDS patients are a decrease in

CD4$^+$ T cells and their pure subsets, a decrease of CD28 expression, and the abnormal activation of cellular immunity. Studies have found that HIV infection can increase the expression ratio of CD38 and HLA-DR on CD8$^+$ T cells. CD8$^+$ CD38$^+$ and CD8$^+$ HLA-DR$^+$ are called activated subsets. Abnormal immune activation often indicates that there may be a microbial infection (such as HIV, CMV, or EBV), and the degree of activation is related to the severity of the infection.

The lymphocyte subsets of this patient were consistent with the immuno-pathological features of HIV/AIDS, and the HIV viral load was increased, so the possibility of HIV infection was considered. They were sent to CDC again for tests to confirm HIV.

IV. Treatment and follow-up after diagnosis

HIV confirmatory test (+) on 25 April 2006. Highly effective antiretroviral therapy was begun: Stocrin + Combivir. Numbness of the limbs and dyskinesia of both lower limbs gradually improved. The patient was discharged when her condition improved.

Follow-up: After six months of antiviral treatment, the number of CD4$^+$ T cells was 500/μl. HIV RNA could not be detected, antiviral therapy was stopped, and regular follow-up was recommended.

Thinking prompts: When HIV seroconversion occurs within six months, the patient can be given antiviral treatment. In the antiviral treatment of the acute stage of HIV infection, the HIV RNA level, CD4$^+$ T cell count, and drug toxicity should be detected. The goal of treatment is to reduce HIV RNA to undetectable levels. Stocrin is a mixture of lamivudine and zidovudine, and is a nucleoside antiretroviral drug; combivir is a non-nucleoside antiretroviral drug. The most common adverse reactions to zidovudine are myelosuppression and gastrointestinal discomfort. The adverse reactions to stocrin are: Central nervous system toxicity, such as dizziness, headache, insomnia, rashes, liver damage, and hyperlipidemia. The adverse reactions to lamivudine are fewer. Check the routine bloods, liver function, and blood lipid during treatment, and change the treatment plan if necessary.

V. Lessons learned

This is a rare case of acute HIV infection characterized by Guillain-Barré syndrome. As HIV infection can affect all systems of the body, we should be alert to the possibility of HIV infection in clinical work. Note a patient's epidemiological history. If he/she is clinically highly suspected of HIV infection, the review of HIV antibodies should be repeated.

(Guo Fuping & Li Taisheng)

Sore throat, fever, and fatigue for three days

I. Medical history

Patient: Male, 25 years old; admitted to hospital with a sore throat, fever, and fatigue lasting three days. The sore throat and fever occurred after the fatigue. His highest body temperature was 38.5°C with chills, no shivering, no cough or expectoration, and no obvious chest tightness or shortness of breath. He was given an intravenous drip of penicillin and dexamethasone for two days, but it did not work. He came to our hospital on 19 May 2007 and was admitted with acute tonsillitis.

> **Thinking prompts:** The patient has a short illness with an acute onset, and no serious symptoms except pharyngeal issues and fever. Therefore, the initial opinion is that he has an upper respiratory tract infection, pharyngitis, or tonsillitis. However, general upper respiratory tract infection has a self-limiting tendency. The common bacteria causing tonsillitis is streptococcus, which is sensitive to penicillin. Therefore, we should make sure that we distinguish it from other illnesses, especially pharyngeal fungi and pharyngeal diphtheria. We should ask whether there are basic conditions present such as diabetes, transplantation status, and immune function defects. We should also identify whether there is a history of long-term antibiotic use, and find out where the patients come from and whether their vaccination history is complete.

II. Physical examination and auxiliary examination

Physical examination: T 38.6°C, P 86 times/minute, looked seriously ill in the face, pained expression, speaking as if there was something in his mouth object in the mouth; slurred speech. There was no abnormality in the lung examination; heart rate 86 times/minute, with an even rhythm. No pathological noise was detected in the valve area of the heart. The liver and spleen could not be palpated below the costal margin. Local examination: Swelling of the left side of the neck, hard and tender; congestion of throat, left tonsil I° swelling, right side I° swelling.

After admission, the patient underwent a complete examination, including a routine blood test, C-reactive protein (CRP), erythrocyte sedimentation rate (ESR), biochemistry, EBV, CMV antibodies, and throat swab culture to determine the nature of the infection (bacterial, viral or fungal), as well as a chest X-ray and ECG.

The pharyngeal swab examination found that the tonsil surface was covered with white pseudo-membrane, which could not be peeled off easily, and bled after peeling.

Laboratory examination: Hb 150 g/L, WBC 12.8×10^9/L, L 15%. CRP 20 mg/L, ESR 30 mm/h, EBV, CMV antibody (−); blood biochemistry normal. Chest X-ray and ECG normal.

III. Diagnosis

Initial diagnosis: Pharyngeal diphtheria? Upper respiratory tract infection? Pharyngeal fungal infection?

Thinking prompts: When a patient has a short-term fever, the first consideration is infectious fever. White blood cells and neutrophils in the routine blood test are high, as is CRP, so the first consideration is bacterial or fungal infection. White blood cells are mostly normal in viral infections; only in epidemic hemorrhagic fever, infectious mononucleosis, and cytomegalovirus infection do they increase. The tonsil surface of the patient in question is covered in a white pseudo-membrane, which cannot be peeled off easily, and bleeds after peeling. This is a characteristic clinical feature of diphtheria. A further bacterial smear and culture can be performed. Therefore, the initial diagnosis is pharyngeal diphtheria. However, the diagnosis of infectious diseases depends on etiology; the diagnosis of bacterial infection depends on the results of bacterial culture; and viral infections can be detected by specific antigens or antibodies. Diagnosis before bacterial culture diagnosis is only clinical. Moreover, pharyngeal diphtheria is a rare disease at present. If bacterial culture or treatment is ineffective, other possibilities must not be ignored. It should be considered as different from the following diseases:

1. Upper respiratory tract infection caused by a viral infection. Tonsillar enlargement and catarrhal symptoms can appear in the respiratory tract, especially in patients with EB virus and CMV infection. The white blood cell count in the routine blood test can exceed the normal range. However, except for pharyngeal symptoms, there is no obvious lymph node enlargement in other parts of the patient's body, and the peripheral blood lymphocytes and monocytes are low, so the possibility of EB virus and CMV infection is not high. In other viral infections, CRP is generally low, and white blood cells do not rise, so it can be ruled out.

2. Fungal throat infections (such as thrush). Fungal infections are usually secondary in patients with a history of long-term antibiotic use, diabetes, transplant status, low immune function, or history of defects. After a detailed inquiry, the patient has none of the above-mentioned history, and the onset process is short, so the possibility of it being a fungal infection is not supported. Thrush is characterized by low fever and white flakes attached to the oral mucosa, which can spread to the pharynx and is peeled off easily. However, this patient's pharyngeal

swab culture membrane cannot be peeled off easily, so it is not a fungal infection.

   3. Ulcerative membranous pharyngitis. In this illness, there are necrotic ulcers and pseudo-membranes in the pharynx. It is often accompanied by gingivitis, bleeding easily, and a bad smell in the mouth. Fusobacterium and spirochete can be found in the throat swab smear. This patient had a white membrane only in the pharynx, so ulcerative membranous pharyngitis was ruled out.

IV. Diagnosis and treatment

The patient was instructed to take complete bed rest, with an intravenous penicillin drip, dexamethasone, vitamin C, and an energy solution, and an intramuscular injection of 80,000 units of diphtheria antitoxin on the day of hospitalization. The pseudo-membrane began to shrink, and partially shed after 33 hours, and the pharyngeal swab culture indicated diphtheria bacilli 48 hours after admission, disappearing completely after one week. The patient was discharged on the eighth day.

V. Ward-round analysis one week after admission

1. Diphtheria is an acute infectious disease caused by strains of bacteria called Corynebacterium diphtheriae that make a toxin. Its clinical features are the formation of a pseudo-membrane in places such as the pharynx, larynx, and nose, as well as fever, fatigue, nausea, vomiting, headaches, and other systemic poisoning symptoms. Serious cases can be complicated with myocarditis. The main points of diagnosis for diphtheria are as follows:

(1) Understanding the epidemiological data in detail: Including age, season, history of contact with diphtheria, whether the full vaccination course was carried out in the past, and whether there was diphtheria epidemic in the patient's area.

(2) Clinical manifestations generally have the following characteristics:

   1) The onset is slow, and fever and sore throat are not obvious; however, the symptoms of systemic poisoning are serious, and there is a typical diphtheria pseudo-membrane in the throat.

   2) Severe bloody secretions in the nasal cavity, along with cervical lymphadenopathy, and poisoning symptoms.

   3) A diagnosis can be made if the bacterial culture is positive, but diphtheria cannot be ruled out if the bacterial culture is negative.

2. Diphtheria should be differentiated from the following diseases:

(1) Streptococcal tonsillitis: Acute onset, high fever, sore throat, punctate, yellow exudate on the tonsil.

(2) Vincent's angina: Pharyngeal necrosis, ulcers, pseudo-membrane, gingival necrosis, and inflammation.

(3) Acute laryngitis: Severe symptoms, dyspnea; periodic symptoms, mild during the day and severe at night; no pseudo-membrane in pharynx.

(4) Allergic laryngeal edema: A sudden onset with a history of allergic reactions.

3. Diphtheria treatment:

(1) Anti-infective treatment: Penicillin is the first choice. Usage: 3.2 million units of intravenous drip or injection, 2–3 times a day, for 7–10 days. If the patient is allergic to penicillin, erythromycin can be used instead.

(2) Diphtheria antitoxin usage: One intramuscular injection or intravenous injection, with the correct dosage. Patients with simple diphtheria of the nose or tonsils need 20,000–30,000 units; those with simple diphtheria of the larynx need 30,000–40,000 units; those with diphtheria of the pharynx and larynx need 40,000–60,000 units; those with diphtheria of the larynx and trachea need 60,000–80,000 units; those with diphtheria of the nose, mouth, pharynx, larynx, and trachea need 80,000–120,000 units. After 12 hours, if the symptoms do not improve, another injection of the same or lower amount can be administered.

For prevention, 1,000–2,000 units can be injected at a time, or 1,000–2,000 units and 0.5 ml of diphtheria toxin can be injected subcutaneously in two places. Toxoid or 0.5 ml antitoxins can be injected after one month, and the whole immunization course can be given one week later using toxoid. It should be noted that an allergy test must be performed before administering the vaccination, which can cause nervous system reaction, epilepsy, and other adverse reactions in children.

VI. Condition at discharge

The patient's body temperature normal; no pharyngeal pain, cough, expectoration, chest tightness, or palpitations identified; during the physical examination, the pharynx was not congested, the tonsils were not enlarged, and cardiorespiratory auscultation was normal. The routine blood test and CRP were normal.

VII. Lessons learned

The most common characteristic of diphtheria is that the pseudo-membrane cannot be peeled off easily, and bleeds easily when removed. Diagnosis can be made through a positive bacterial culture, but a negative bacterial culture does not rule out diphtheria. Once it is diagnosed, diphtheria antitoxin should be used as quickly as possible.

(Yan Dong & Huang Jianrong)

Fever for more than ten days, with dysarthria and limited limb movement for five days

I. Medical history

Patient: Male, 55 years old, from Shanghai. He was hospitalized on 19 May 2008 with a fever of more than ten days, accompanied by dysarthria and limitation of limb movement for five days. On 7 May 2008, the patient had a fever of no obvious cause, reaching 40.9°C, accompanied by an aversion to cold, chills, dizziness, and abdominal pain. He was hospitalized locally to fight infection treatment, but his fever and chills persisted. On 15 May, he had dysarthria, limited limb movement, and double incontinence. No cough, expectoration, chest pain, or vomiting and diarrhea were experienced since the onset. He was transferred to our hospital for further treatment. On admission, he was relatively conscious, but he was occasionally confused, with a lack of appetite and incontinence.

The patient underwent mitral valve replacement for rheumatic valvular disease five years earlier and his postoperative recovery was satisfactory.

> **Thinking prompts:** The patient is a middle-aged male, with a short illness and acute fever, accompanied by significant neurological symptoms, hemiplegia, and aphasia. Because of his prosthetic valve replacement, his stroke and paralysis were initially considered to be cardiogenic, especially infective endocarditis. At this time, the diagnostic basis should investigate whether there is progressive anemia, congestive heart failure, arrhythmia, and embolism in the course of the disease (the common embolic sites include the brain, kidneys, spleen, and coronary artery, with corresponding cerebral embolism, lower back pain, abdominal pain, hematuria, pain in the left upper abdomen or left shoulder, left pleural effusion and splenomegaly, and myocardial ischemia or myocardial infarction).

II. Physical examination on admission

T 38°C, R 25 times/min, P 92 times/min, BP 135/80 mmHg. Acute facial appearance, depression, shortness of breath, immobile (had to be carried onto the ward), cooperated with the physical examination, no skin or mucous membrane stained yellow, no ecchymosis. Surface-level lymph nodes not enlarged. Equal pupil size, sensitive to light, tongue in the middle, soft neck, a small number of fine moist rales heard from the bottom of both lungs. Heart rate 92 beats/min, rhythm, mitral valve area can be heard with metal valve sound, abdominal distension, abdominal softness, upper abdominal tenderness. Shifting dullness (−), mild edema of lower limbs, muscle strength of right upper limb and both lower limbs 0–1, muscle strength of left upper limb 3, meningeal stimulation sign (−), right Babinski's sign (+), left Babinski's sign (−).

> **Thinking prompts:** During physical examination, check for manifestations of small vasculitis caused by microthrombus or the immune mechanism, such as bruises to the skin mucous membrane, sub-nail hemorrhage, Osler knots, and Janeway damage. Look for a heart murmur, and observe any changes to the murmur during follow-up. Because infective endocarditis often coexists with septicemia, we should also note the manifestations of septicemia such as rashes, hepatosplenomegaly, and migratory abscesses.

III. Auxiliary examination on admission

Blood routine: WBC 13.7×10^9 /L, N 89%, Hb 104 g/L, PLT 144×10^9/L. Blood culture once (+): Staphylococcus aureus (report from other hospitals, no drug sensitivity results).

ECG: Atrial fibrillation, incomplete right bundle branch block.

Chest X-ray: Increased markings of both lungs, possibility of right lower pneumonia, postoperative changes to the heart.

The opinions of our hospital's consultants on CT scans from other hospitals: ① A plain CT scan of the head showed bilateral subcortical infarction. Multiple infarctions occurred in the left frontotemporal occipital lobe and right parietal lobe. ② A lung CT scan showed pneumonia and bilateral pleural effusion (small amount). ③ Changes after mitral valve replacement. ④ The left atrium and left ventricle were enlarged, especially the left atrium. ⑤ An abdominal CT scan showed multiple splenic infarctions, no abnormal liver, and thickening of the gallbladder wall.

Echocardiography: After mitral valve replacement, the mechanical mitral valve was normal; moderate pulmonary hypertension with mild tricuspid regurgitation.

Abdominal B-ultrasound: Gallbladder enlargement, splenomegaly, multiple hypoechoic lesions in the spleen; the liver and kidneys were normal; intestinal cavity effusion, with a small number of ascites.

Routine urine examination: Red blood cell full field, white blood cell 3–5/HP, protein (+ + +). The abnormal rate of red blood cells in the urine was 72%. The clearance rate of endogenous creatinine was 92.4 L/24 h.

Liver function: Total bilirubin 25.1 μmol/L, albumin 33 g/L; the rest was normal.

Renal function was normal.

ESR: 73 mm/h.

Electrolyte: Hypernatremia, blood sodium 147 mmol /L.

Thinking prompts: A diagnosis of septicemia is based on blood culture or bone marrow culture. A positive blood culture result is also one of the main diagnostic criteria for infective endocarditis. It is one of the two main Duke diagnostic criteria, and evidently very important for diagnosis. It is the most direct basis for diagnosis, and it can also provide a Follow-up as to whether bacteremia continues. In acute cases, 2–3 blood samples should be taken within 1–2 hours before the application of antibiotics. In subacute cases, 3–4 blood samples should be taken 24 hours before the application of antibiotics. In cases where patients have previously used antibiotics, blood culture should be taken at least every day for three days in order to improve the positive rate. The best time to take blood is when shivering or when a sudden rise in body temperature occurs. Take 10–15 ml of blood each time, change the puncture site, and strictly disinfect the skin. Routine aerobic and anaerobic cultures need to be done. For patients who have had an artificial valve replacement, long-term indwelling venous catheters, urinary catheters, or the application of broad-spectrum antibiotics, hormones, immunosuppressants, and illegal drugs, fungal cultures also need to be done. In addition to routine blood and urine routine examinations, chest X-ray, electrocardiogram, abdominal B-ultrasound examination, and echocardiography are standards in the Duke criteria besides blood culture, which is the main examination method for endocardial involvement. Echocardiography can detect the location, size, number, and shape of lesions, and is also helpful to diagnose heart and valve diseases, detect the valve damage, understand the status of implanted mechanical or biological valves, observe various suppurative cardiac complications, and evaluate the severity of valve regurgitation and left ventricular function. It can be used as a reference to judge the prognosis and determine whether to operate.

IV. Diagnosis and treatment
1. Preliminary diagnosis and diagnostic ideas

(1) Staphylococcus aureus septicemia: The patient is a middle-aged male with acute onset. The total number of white blood cells and the proportion of neutrophils are significantly increased, and there is no acute infection limited to a certain system. The possibility of septicemia should be considered. The patient has a history of prosthetic valve replacement, and had a high chance of gram-positive bacterial infections. He had obvious toxemia symptoms, anemia, multiple cerebral vascular embolisms, and migrating abscesses (lung, spleen, and kidneys) during the course of his illness –strong evidence of infection. A blood culture showed that Staphylococcus aureus was the basis of diagnosis.

(2) Infective endocarditis: The patient had a fever of unknown origin after prosthetic valve replacement for more than one week, so the possibility of a diagnosis of infective endocarditis should be borne in mind. According to Duke's clinical criteria, the patient met five minor criteria: Predisposing factors (heart history, prosthetic valve replacement) + fever (body temperature $\geq 38°C$) + vascular signs (cerebral artery embolism) + immune system signs

(manifestations of glomerulonephritis including hematuria and proteinuria) + microbiological evidence (positive blood culture, but only once, not meeting the main criteria). Infective endocarditis can be diagnosed.

(3) Multiple cerebral embolisms: There are nervous system symptoms such as dysarthria, limb paralysis, and fecal incontinence. A CT scan of the head shows multiple infarctions, and the diagnosis is clear.

(4) Rheumatic heart disease, after mitral valve replacement.

2. Treatment

The patient had a high fever, aphasia, limited limb movement, double incontinence, and gross hematuria. Re-examination of the CT scan of his head showed a large area of infarction on the left side. The patient had abdominal distension, a pot belly, tenderness, no rebound tenderness, active bowel sounds, and suspicious positive shifting dullness. The possibility of peritonitis and toxic enteroparalysis should be considered. Levofloxacin and metronidazole were given to treat abdominal infection and correct the electrolyte disorder. Because the patient had hypernatremia, fusidic acid was not a suitable treatment, and it was not appropriate to use teicoplanin for proteinuria. The effect of fosfocina alone was not good, and rifadin could affect the metabolization of Warfarin. The patient was given linezolid + fosfocina for one week, and his body temperature dropped. However, because of the high price, the family asked to stop using it. Because the clearance rate of endogenous creatinine was 92.8 L/24 h, which was still in the normal range, 0.8 g Norvancomycin was given intravenously every 12 hours. One week later, the patient's serum creatinine increased to 145 mmol/L, and the dosage of Norvancomycin was reduced by half. The patient's condition improved. His consciousness gradually became clearer. Abdominal distension significantly reduced, as did defecation and flatulence. His body temperature gradually decreased. Later, the patient was automatically discharged due to funding problems, and was transferred to a local hospital for further treatment.

V. Lessons learned

The patient's history was typical of staphylococcal septicemia with infectious endocarditis. The diagnosis was quick and clear, but the treatment was not ideal. For patients with complications such as multiple migratory foci, which make it difficult to cure, and it is also necessary to consider the multiple drug resistance of bacteria. Staphylococcus aureus is one of the most common pathogens causing community and nosocomial infections. In recent years, infections caused by methicillin-resistant Staphylococcus aureus (MRSA) have increased globally. The epidemiology of Staphylococcus aureus (especially MRSA) has four main trends. First, in many countries, the infection caused by multiple resistant strains (especially MRSA) has received a lot of attention; second, the detection rate of MRSA is relatively low in some countries; third, MRSA appears in communities; finally, vancomycin-intermediate and vancomycin-resistant Staphylococcus aureus has appeared.

The multiple drug resistance of MRSA is very serious. It is not only resistant to methicillin, but also insensitive to antimicrobial drugs such as β-lactams, aminoglycosides, fluoroquinolones, tetracyclines, macrolides, and lincomycin. It is only sensitive to glycopeptide antibiotics. Therefore, both hospital-acquired MRSA (HA-MRSA) and community-acquired MRSA (CA-MRSA) are the first-line drugs of choice for the treatment of MRSA. However, vancomycin cannot effectively reduce the carrier rate of MRSA in patients, nor can it significantly reduce the mortality rate of MRSA infection. On the contrary, the failure rate of vancomycin in the treatment of MRSA infection is high all over the world. So far, there are only a few reports of vancomycin-mediated Staphylococcus aureus (visa) and vancomycin-resistant Staphylococcus aureus (VRSA) infection, which cannot explain the high failure rate of vancomycin in the treatment of MRSA infection. In 1996, Hiramatsu et al. noted for the first time that heterogeneous vancomycin-resistant Staphylococcus aureus (hVRSA) infection could lead to a failure of vancomycin treatment in the world, attracting attention of the global medical field. This finding provides a reasonable explanation for the failure of vancomycin treatment in MRSA infection.

Heterogeneous vancomycin intermediate Staphylococcus aureus (hVISA) is considered to be the precursor of VISA, which means that the offspring contains a small amount of vancomycin resistance mediators (MIC ≥ 4 μg/ml). However, their mother cells are sensitive to vancomycin (MIC ≤ 2 μg/ml). At present, VISA and VRSA are rare, while hVISA may be more common, especially in persistent MRSA bacteremia and endocarditis. The difference between VISA/hVISA and VRSA is that VISA and hVISA do not contain drug resistance genes such as VanA. They are related to the selection pressure of vancomycin, and the thickening of cell walls is an important mechanism in drug resistance. The potential clinical importance of hVISA is that it is associated with the failure of vancomycin treatment, and develops into VISA under selective vancomycin pressure. With the increase in MRSA infection, vancomycin will be widely used in clinical settings. Although there are no reports of VISA and VRSA in China, with the wide application of vancomycin, MRSA will inevitably develop into VISA or VRSA. Therefore, clinical microbiology laboratories should strictly monitor the drug resistance of MRSA, and advocate for the rational use of antibiotics to slow down the emergence of VISA or VRSA.

Multidrug resistant Staphylococcus aureus is a major challenge. Treatment is difficult and expensive, but it is gratifying that there are some effective new antibiotics. The new antibiotics that can significantly improve the prognosis of this kind of drug-resistant bacteria include linezolid, daptomycin, quinupristin-dalfopristin, and tigecycline.

Quinupristin-dalfopristin is a Streptocin antibiotic. It is a mixture of quinupristin and dafeptine at the ratio of 30:70 – two semi-synthetic derivatives of pristinamycin. Its mechanism of action is to inhibit the synthesis of bacterial protein and bind to a 50S subunit of a bacterial ribosome. Dalfopristin inhibits the early stage of protein synthesis, while quinupristin inhibits the late stage. Dalfopristin can also change the configuration of a ribosome and enhance the affinity between quinupristin and ribosomes, so they have a synergistic effect. The drug acts as a strong bactericide on MRSA, and has strong tissue permeability. At present, due to its only being an injectable drug, as well as its high cost and adverse reactions (myalgia, arthritis, and thrombophlebitis), its clinical application is limited.

Linezolid was the first oxazolidinone antibiotic, and was synthesized in 1987. Its mechanism is to inhibit the synthesis of bacterial protein, bind with a 50S subunit of a bacterial ribosome, and prevent the 50S subunit from binding with a 30S subunit mRNA to form a 70s complex. This drug acts in the early stage of protein synthesis. Although it is similar to the action sites of macrolides and tetracyclines, their action mechanisms are different. Chloramphenicol inhibits the formation of peptide-bonds, while linezolid inhibits the formation of the initial complex. Therefore, cross resistance is unlikely. Linezolid has only an antibacterial effect on Staphylococcus, so its curative effect is limited. The main advantage of linezolid is that it can be administered orally and intravenously. Like quinoluptin-dafopritine, the cost of linezolid is higher than conventional therapy. The cost of daily intravenous or oral linezolid is seven times that of intravenous vancomycin. It has been reported that continuous use of linezolid can lead to myelosuppression, but this can subside after withdrawal.

Daptomycin is a lipopeptide antibiotic with a cyclic polypeptide structure. It is a 13-membered amino acid cyclic lipopeptide with a decyl side chain, and has a new antibacterial mechanism. The mechanism of action is dependent on calcium ions entering the bacterial plasma membrane, including the multi-step process of membrane depolarization, and has no inhibitory effect on lipoteichoic acid. Because of this unique mechanism of action, there is no cross resistance between daptomycin and other antibiotics. For this reason, daptomycin has attracted more attention than other antibiotics. Many antibiotics only have effects on growing bacteria, daptomycin has effects on both growing and stable bacteria. This feature makes it possible to treat deep painless infections such as endocarditis and osteomyelitis. The importance of its clinical application includes its activity against Staphylococcus aureus that is resistant to linezolid, quinupristin-dalfopristin, and teicoplanin. Daptomycin has fast germicidal efficacy, and can kill more than 99.9% of MSSA (methicillin sensitive Staphylococcus aureus) and MRSA within 1 hour of treatment. It is difficult for MRSA to develop resistance to daptomycin in single passage and continuous passage tests. The disadvantages of daptomycin are high cost, no oral dosage form, poor permeability of lung tissue, and possible transverse muscle pain.

Tigecycline (9-tert-butyl glycyl amino minocycline) is a representative drug of glycyl tetracycline. Tigecycline is the first glycyl tetracycline and the first new tetracycline analogue to be marketed in the 30 years since minocycline was introduced. The main active sites of tigecycline and tetracycline antibiotics are bacterial ribosomes. Compared with tetracycline and minocycline, tigecycline has a stronger affinity, which reduces the possibility of rapid resistance to tigecycline. The unique advantage of tigecycline is that it can stably resist the resistance mechanism of common tetracyclines. It has been proved that tigecycline has activity against strains containing the TET gene (gene-encoding tetracycline resistance). Up to now, no tigecycline-resistant isolates have been obtained by prolonged exposure to a sub-moderate concentration of tigecycline under laboratory conditions. At present, tigecycline has no oral dosage form, and is only given intravenously. Tigecycline has significant activity against Staphylococcus aureus (MIC_{90} is 0.25–0.5 μg/ml) and Staphylococcus aureus which is intermediately resistant to glycopeptides.

Infections caused by Staphylococcus aureus (especially MRSA) will continue to be a major challenge for clinicians worldwide. At the same time, the emergence of drug-resistant forms is closely related to the use of new antibiotics. Therefore, we should not put too much emphasis on finding and developing new antimicrobial agents. Despite the presence of vancomycin- and teicoplanin-resistant Staphylococcus aureus, non-intestinal glycopeptide antibiotics can still be used as the main drugs for the treatment of systemic infections. For MRSA infections that do not respond to vancomycin treatment, the choice of therapeutic drugs depends on the site of infection, antimicrobial activity, pharmacokinetics and safety, potential drug resistance, and treatment cost. Linezolid is more effective than vancomycin in the treatment of pneumonia and infections of the skin and soft tissue. It can be administered orally or intravenously, making it more suitable for long-term outpatient treatment. Daptomycin has a bactericidal effect on the whole growth period of bacteria, especially for the treatment of deep infections (such as endocarditis and osteomyelitis caused by MRSA), but daptomycin is not recommended for use in the treatment of pneumonia. Tigecycline is suitable for the treatment of complex intra-abdominal infections and complex skin infections in adults. In short, in order to prevent the rapid emergence of drug-resistant strains of Staphylococcus aureus, antibiotics should be used wisely to control infection.

(Jin Jialin & Weng Xinhua)

Recurrent fever for more than one year, and swelling and pain in the right lower limb for more than one month

I. Medical history

Patient: Male, 62 years old, admitted on 10 January 2008 due to repeated fever for more than a year, and swelling and pain in the right lower limb for more than a month.

In the middle of January 2007, the patient had a fever with no obvious cause, and a temperature of between 38°C and 39°C. Before each attack, he had an aversion to cold, chills, and lower back pain. After taking analgin or indomethacin, his body temperature went back to normal. One month later (14 February 2007), an emergency CT scan at a tertiary hospital identified an abdominal aortic aneurysm. On the same day, an abdominal aortic aneurysm stripping and stent implantation were performed, and supportive treatment such as postoperative hemostasis and anticoagulation were given. Fever occurred again two weeks later, with a body temperature of 37°C–38°C, an aversion to cold, and chills, which lasted for 3–5 days each time. The fever recurred after ten days, and was relieved after taking NSAID. The patient was hospitalized again on 20 April, and was given anti-inflammatory and symptomatic support treatment (details unknown). He was discharged on 30 April after improvement. After discharge, he experienced intermittent fever, mainly low. In the two weeks prior to his admittance to our hospital, his fever was frequent, with an interval of 1–2 days, and a body temperature of 39°C–40°C. His aversion to cold and chills was obvious. Oral antipyretics and indomethacin were able to relieve it. Neutrophils increased in every blood test performed during an episode of high fever. He remained at our hospital for further diagnosis and treatment. In the course of his illness, he was in good spirits, and had a good appetite; no cough, expectoration, frequent micturition, urgent micturition, painful micturition, abdominal pain, diarrhea, red and swollen joints; his body weight dropped by nearly 15 kg.

He had suffered from type 2 diabetes for ten years, and his blood glucose was controlled at about 8 mmol/L. He had experienced primary hypertension for 20 years. He underwent high ligation and stripping of the varicose veins in his right lower extremity, and stent implantation for an abdominal aortic aneurysm.

Thinking prompts: Careful inquiry about the patient's medical history should be carried out, along with a comprehensive physical examination. Assessing whether there is a primary infection focus or an inducement of infection before fever is the key point of inquiry, as it is helpful to analyze the types of possible infectious pathogens and facilitate the selection of antibacterial drugs in the process of formulating treatment plans. This includes skin and wound infection or trauma history before fever (suggesting Gram-positive cocci infection), upper respiratory tract infection (suggesting Streptococcus infection), urinary system infection, intestinal tract or biliary tract infection (suggesting Gram-negative bacilli or enterococci infection), artificial prosthesis device (possibly Staphylococcus epidermidis infection) or immunodeficiency (considering a special bacterial infection such as a fungal infection or Listeria-producing bacteria-infection).

Note any changes in a patient's mental state, and whether there are symptoms of septicemia, or systemic infection, such as general discomfort, muscle aches, loss of appetite, nausea and vomiting, abdominal distention, diarrhea, headaches, dizziness, apathy, irritability, anemia, hepatosplenomegaly, jaundice, toxic myocarditis, or acute renal failure. Migratory lesions are also common symptoms of septicemia, and should be carefully examined during physical examination. Common illnesses include subcutaneous abscesses, lung abscesses, liver abscesses, suppurative arthritis, and osteomyelitis.

This patient had been unwell for a long time, with repeated fever for more than one year. There is no definite localized focus, so the possibility of systemic infection is greater.

II. Physical examination

Body temperature 39°C, respiration 20 times/min, pulse 90 times/min, blood pressure 130/80 mmHg. Clear mind, generally in good spirits. Acceptable nutritional status; entered the ward on foot; automatic position; cooperated with the physical examination. No swelling of the superficial lymph nodes, no yellow staining or bleeding points on the skin and mucous membrane, no yellow staining on the sclera, no congestion or bleeding of the eyelids and conjunctiva, no swelling of the pharynx, soft neck, heart rate of 90 beats/min, audible murmur, soft and flat abdomen; the liver and spleen could not be palpated; no tenderness and rebound pain anywhere in the abdomen, shifting dullness (−), no edema in either of the lower limbs, physiological reflex present. Pathological reflex did not lead out.

III. Auxiliary examination on admission

Routine blood examination: White blood cells $20.34 \times 10^9/L$, neutrophils 87%, hemoglobin 83 g/L.

Blood culture (8 January 2008, this hospital): Negative.

Abdominal B-ultrasound: Chronic cholecystitis with cholesterol crystals and splenomegaly.

B-ultrasound of the right lower limb: Multiple lymph node enlargement in the right groin, dilation of the right superficial vein, rough thickening of the wall, and possibly large edema.

Chest CT scan: Increased lung markings, mediastinal lymph node enlargement, bilateral pleural thickening, obvious slight enlargement of the left side of the heart, a small amount of pericardial effusion, calcification of the aortic arch and coronary artery.

Abdominal CT scan (27 December 2007, at our hospital): Cholecystitis, calcification of the abdominal aorta adjacent to the intersection of the visible wall, and thickening of the soft tissue density shadow; an enhanced scan is recommended.

Routine urine test, liver function: Hypoproteinemia, albumin 25 g/L, the rest normal.

Renal function was normal. Antinuclear antibody (ANA) and antineutrophil cytoplasmic antibodies (ANCA) were (−).

ESR: 42 mm/h, CRP: 100 ng/L (3.25–8.2 ng/L).

Tumor markers (CA125, CA19-9, CY21-1, AFP, CEA, CA50): (−).

Glycosylated hemoglobin: 5.9%.

> **Thinking prompts:** When a patient has a fever of unknown origin, before excluding infectious diseases, blood culture is the most important etiological examination. In order to obtain a higher positive rate, blood should be collected before the administration of antibiotics and during shivering and high fever, and blood should be collected repeatedly for examination. When blood culture is negative and blood infection is suspected, a special culture medium should be used to cultivate special pathogens such as L-shaped bacteria, Legionella, Mycobacterium, Bartonella, and fungi. Routine examination of the blood and urine, erythrocyte sedimentation rate, abdominal ultrasound, and chest X-ray can be classified as routine examinations. In case of septicemia, migratory lesions, or heart, liver and kidney damage, or shock often occur. Cardiac ultrasound can be listed as a routine item, and auxiliary CT and MRI examinations can be performed when necessary.

IV. Diagnosis and treatment after admission
1. Initial diagnosis

The patient's body temperature exceeded 38.3°C for more than three weeks. After more than two weeks of in-hospital examination, the cause was still unclear. The patient could be diagnosed with a fever of unknown origin.

> **Thinking prompts:** There are two main causes of fever of unknown origin: Infectious diseases and non-infectious diseases. Among the non-infectious diseases, vascular

diseases of the connective tissue and neoplastic diseases are the most common. Infection, neoplastic diseases, and vascular diseases of the connective tissue make up the etiology of more than 80% of patients.

2. Possible diagnoses

On analyzing the patient's medical history, the following possible causes were identified:

(1) Septicemia: The patient experienced recurrent fever for more than one year, with a long illness, but without regular anti-infection treatment, and without symptoms and signs limited to a single system. He had a history of diabetes mellitus. The patient had low immunity, and had undergone high ligation and stripping of varicose veins in the right lower extremity, which may have been the source of infection. Combined with the patient's repeated peripheral blood leukocyte examination, the results showed that the total number of leukocytes and the proportion of neutrophils had increased. Therefore, the possibility of septicemia should be considered, and blood culture should be performed. At the same time, we should pay close attention to the progress of the disease and whether there are migratory lesions.

(2) Endocarditis: The patient had no heart murmur, typical skin lesions such as ecchymosis of the skin and mucous membrane, Osler's knot, and Janeway's lesion. He had a history of abdominal aortic aneurysm, so the possibility of bacterial aneurysm could not be ruled out. He should accept echocardiography and blood culture examination.

(3) Focal infection: An abdominal CT scan showed cholecystitis and increased hemogram, but the patient did not have abdominal pain, jaundice, or other manifestations. The physical examination did not identify corresponding abdominal tenderness, rebound pain, or other abdominal signs; liver function was normal. The diagnosis of simple cholecystitis does not explain the whole picture of the disease, so there is no evidence for the time being.

(4) Absorbed heat from a hematoma after the rupture of an abdominal aortic aneurysm, i.e., aseptic fever. The patient has a history of abdominal aortic aneurysm, and his body temperature gradually dropped to normal without antibiotics after his stent implantation. However, this cannot explain the repeated fever and high hemogram after the stent implantation. The possibility of this diagnosis is small, but his fever before implantation may be related to it.

(5) Infection related to stent implantation: With the patient's history and postoperative hemogram, the possibility of this is high. Further fungal and bacterial cultures are needed to make a definitive diagnosis, but they cannot explain the fever before stent implantation.

(6) Fever caused by a foreign body after stent implantation: This diagnosis is possible, but would not explain the infection.

(7) Vascular disease of the connective tissue: Non-specific vasculitis caused by auto-immune diseases is a common source of fever in the elderly, such as senile temporal arteritis and rheumatic polymyalgia. This patient has no corresponding clinical manifestations, such as temporal headache, intermittent mandibular dyskinesia, and visual impairment, or muscle pain and stiffness of the neck, shoulder girdle, and pelvic girdle. Immune indicators such as ANA

and ANCA were negative during auxiliary examination, so this diagnosis is not supported.

(8) Lymphoma: Intermittent fever of unknown origin, no superficial lymph node enlargement, but obvious recent weight loss. Peripheral blood smears were performed to find abnormal lymphocytes; superficial lymph nodes and abdominal and retroperitoneal lymph nodes were examined with B-ultrasound to make a definitive diagnosis, and a puncture biopsy was performed when necessary.

3. Examination results and treatment

On the third day after admission (12 January), the bacteria laboratory called to inform us of a growth of Gram-positive cocci and Gram-negative bacteria. Combined with stent implantation, cefepime (2.0 g intravenous drip, once every 12 hours) and pazufloxacin (0.5 g intravenous drip, once every 12 hours) were given. The patient's body temperature dropped. On 16 January, the patient had a high fever again, and obvious pain in the right lower limb. On examination, a 4 cm × 3 cm area of tender red skin with a high temperature was found on the medial side of the right calf, as well as a 3 cm × 2 cm area of tender red skin on the medial side of the right knee, and a 4 cm-diameter tender lump in the right groin. At the same time, five positive blood culture results all showed Streptococcus constellatus (penicillin sensitivity, erythromycin sensitivity, and clindamycin sensitivity).

Therefore, the diagnosis of Streptococcus constellatus septicemia was clear. On 16 January, teicoplanin (0.4 g IV, once a day), fosfocina (8.0 g IV, once every 12 hours), and rifampicin (0.45 g oral, once a day) were administered. A B-ultrasound of the right soft tissue mass showed inflammation and inguinal abscesses of the right waist, groin, scrotum, middle and lower segments of the lower limbs, and dorsum of the soft tissue of the feet.

On 22 January, the general surgery department was consulted for the incision and drainage of the right inguinal abscess. The patient's body temperature gradually decreased, and the multiple migrating abscesses in the right lower limb gradually subsided. Routine blood examination: WBC 6.3×10^9/L, neutrophils 66%, hemoglobin 98 g/L. C-reactive protein 29.4 ng/L.

V. Diagnosis at discharge

Streptococcus constellatus septicemia, type 2 diabetes, essential hypertension, and multiple abscesses usually occur after skin incision and drainage, and after abdominal aortic stent implantation.

VI. Lessons learned

In the early stage of his illness, the patient lacked the typical symptoms of septicemia, such as ecchymosis, hepatosplenomegaly, migratory abscesses, and septic shock, and there was no obvious invasion pathway. After irregular application of antibiotics, the patient showed intermittent low fever, which did not attract attention. This delayed the diagnosis and treatment. Therefore, the possibility of septicemia should be considered when the clinical manifestations include unexplained acute high fever, chills, and a significant increase in the total number of white cells and neutrophils without the symptoms and signs limited to a single system. Repeated blood culture is an important examination tool for diagnosis, especially before the administration of antibiotics and during shivering and high fever. Migratory purulent focus is more common in Gram-positive coccal septicemia. In addition to antibiotic control, the purulent focus must be cut and drained, and the course of treatment should be extended appropriately. In addition, the patient has a history of type 2 diabetes and hypertension, so there is a basis of low immunity, which is also one of the factors of predisposal to infection. It is necessary to manage blood sugar effectively, so that the infection can be easily controlled.

Streptococcus constellatus is an intermediate Streptococcus group, of which 38% are Streptococcus constellatus β Hemolysis. This group of bacteria mainly exists in the human oral cavity. It can be isolated from gingival crevices, dental plaque, and root canals, and also exists in the larynx and nasopharynx. It colonizes in the gastrointestinal tract. It can cause gingival abscesses, which lead to septicemia and endocarditis. It can also cause brain abscesses, osteomyelitis, suppurative arthritis, subcutaneous abscesses, and cellulitis. This group of Streptococcus is highly sensitive to penicillin, but a few resistant strains and some moderately sensitive strains have appeared in recent years. Therefore, penicillin should still be used to treat it, but cautiously under the guidance of drug sensitivity. With severe infections, penicillin should be combined with aminoglycosides, cephalosporin, clindamycin, and vancomycin, depending on the situation. In addition to antibacterial treatment, abscesses must be drained.

(Jin Jialin & Weng Xinhua)

Right upper abdomen discomfort for two months and skin-stained yellow for one week

I. Medical history

Patient: Male, Han, 43 years old, a cadre, married, working in the Altai region of Xinjiang. He was admitted to our hospital complaining of discomfort in his right upper abdomen for two months, and yellow-stained skin for one week.

The patient first felt discomfort in his right upper abdomen two months earlier but it did not affect his life so he was not concerned. One week before admission to our hospital, the color of his urine deepened; his stool was normal; his sclera was stained yellow, accompanied by nausea and vomiting, and discomfort in the upper abdomen. No diarrhea. Mild frequent micturition, no headache, no dizziness. An abdominal ultrasound examination at a local hospital found intrahepatic space occupation and multiple cysts. He came to our hospital for a definitive diagnosis. Since the onset of his illness, the patient had been in good spirits. His appetite, urine, and stool were normal.

The patient was in good health, and denied any history of infectious diseases such as hepatitis, tuberculosis, and typhoid. His vaccination history was unknown, and he denied any allergy to drugs or food. In 1986, he underwent surgery for traumatic liver rupture. During the operation, he received a transfusion of 800 ml blood.

> **Thinking prompts:** When a patient had right upper abdomen discomfort and jaundice, we should focus on the main symptoms and accompanying symptoms of the digestive system, such as stool characteristics and color, urine color, nausea, and fever.

II. Physical examination

Body temperature 36.2°C, pulse 84 times/min, breath 21 times/min, blood pressure 120/80 mmHg, body weight 81 kg, normal development. He was in an active position, with a relaxed expression, ruddy complexion, clear consciousness, and good spirits. His neck was symmetrical, and he had no sense of resistance. His jugular vein was not inflamed, and his thorax was symmetrical. A percussion examination of both lungs revealed a clear sound. His abdomen was flat and symmetrical. An L-shaped incision was made in his upper abdomen,

25 cm in length. No abdominal muscle tension, no tenderness, no mass. Liver not touched. Murphy sign (−). Spleen not touched.

> **Thinking prompts:** The patient's illness lasted two months, but the progress was slow. The general situation was good, with only mild jaundice. A B-ultrasound found intrahepatic space occupation and multiple cysts. Preliminary analysis showed that a tumor was more likely, and further imaging examination was required.
>
> In general, the following problems should be considered:
>
> (1) Liver cyst: The edge of the mass in the liver parenchyma is clear, and the density is uniform; there is no peripheral enhancement after contrast enhancement. Most cases are not accompanied by high fever and chills.
>
> (2) Liver abscess: High fever and chills are common, and the onset is urgent and severe. There is often a history of liver injury. This patient's CT scan result showed that the capsule in the liver was thick; the peripheral inflammatory reaction was severe, and the density of the mass was uneven.
>
> (3) Secondary liver cancer: Multiple round nodules in the liver with low-density shadow and surrounded by an edema zone. The primary lesion is extrahepatic, and is generally not difficult to distinguish.
>
> (4) Primary liver cancer: A solitary liver nodule with multiple round nodules and a low-density shadow surrounded by obvious edema bands. The patient may have ascites and a history of upper gastrointestinal bleeding. For this patient, laboratory tests show that α-fetoprotein has increased, which can generally be clarified in combination with CT imaging. Initial diagnosis after admission: The nature of the intrahepatic space occupation remains to be determined.

III. Auxiliary examination

Routine blood: White blood cells 15.40×10^9/L, neutrophils 83.20%, red blood cells 4.20×10^{12}/L.

Blood biochemistry (14 June): Potassium 3.05 mmol/L, sodium 138.40 mmol/L, glutamic pyruvic transaminase 86 U/L, glutamic oxalacetic transaminase 67 U/L, albumin 34 g/L, total protein 76 g/L, globulin 42 g/L, total bilirubin 83 μmol/L, conjugated bilirubin 52 μmol/L, Gamma-glutamyl transpeptidase 393 U/L.

CT (Figure 8-1):

(1) Multiple hydatid cysts in the liver with partial calcification, slight dilatation of the intrahepatic bile duct, gas accumulation in the left lobe of the liver, considering the possibility of hydatid rupture or infection, and enlarged spleen.

(2) CT angiography (CTA) showed that the portal vein was not developed, and the hepatic segment of the inferior vena cava was compressed and narrowed.

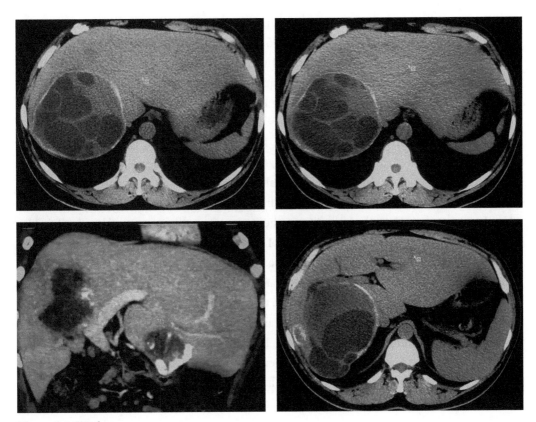

Figure 8-1 CT photos

Ultrasonography showed that there were multiple cystic lesions in the right lobe of the liver, solid lesions in the left lobe, and slight dilatation in the lower left outer segment.

IV. Ward-round analysis

The patient's diagnosis on admission was hepatic hydatid, with a definitive diagnosis of infection and biliary obstruction. His condition was fair. He experienced a fever in the afternoon, but his vital signs were stable and surgery was an option. The main complications of surgery included biliary fistula, perihepatic effusion, hydatid recurrence, residual cavity infection, and long-term tube-wearing affecting daily life. The following day, the patient was to undergo laparotomy and liver hydatid resection.

On 18 June, the patient decided not to have surgery. His test results from 17 June were as follows:

Blood biochemistry: Potassium 5.30 mmol/L, sodium 141.710 mmol/L, chlorine 103.7 mmol/L, calcium 2.29 mmo/L, alanine aminotransferase 64 U/L, glutamic oxalacetic transaminase 27 U/L, albumin 24 g/L, total protein 63.40 g/L, globulin 39.40 g/L, total bilirubin 80.80 μmol/L, conjugated bilirubin 44.60 μmol/L, unconjugated bilirubin 36.20 μmol/L, γ-glutamyl transpeptidase 276.00 U/L, bile acid 24.86 μmol/L, osmotic pressure 296.41 mosm/L.

Routine blood test: WBC 21.50×10^9/L, neutrophils 90.60%, erythrocytes 4.31×10^{12}/L, neutrophil count 19.48×10^9/L, hemoglobin 135.00 g/L, platelets 429.00×10^9/L.

Laboratory tests showed that the patient was suffering from biliary obstruction complicated with infection and severe liver impairment. In combination with clinical and laboratory tests, hepatic hydatid rupture or infection was considered. Surgery was to be performed as soon as possible.

V. Treatment

On 20 June, the patient underwent removal of a hydatid liver cyst, common bile duct exploration, T-tube drainage, and intestinal adhesion release under general anesthesia.

The surgery found intestinal adhesions to the liver, serious adhesions, an enlarged gallbladder, dark liver, cholestasis, free adhesion, exposure of the right lobe of the liver, separation of the right coronary ligament, a prominent hydatid in the seventh segment of the right lobe of the liver, and a smaller hydatid below it. Surgeons separated and resected the gallbladder in combination with antegrade and retrograde. Internal capsule removal was used to suck out effusion and cysts. Hypertonic liquid was inserted for 30 minutes, and the residual cavity was cleaned up. A hydatid was also found in the third segment of the liver. Effusion and cysts were sucked out by puncture. Surgeons opened the lower part of the common bile duct, and sucked out a small amount of yellow cystic fluid along with the cystic wall. They then cut the common bile duct and placed a T tube for drainage. The T tube was unblocked, and the operation was completed successfully.

> Thinking prompts: The patient had multiple hydatids in the liver, a history of surgery, severe abdominal adhesions, a greater separation surface, a large residual cavity in the liver, a hydatid breaking into the biliary tract, and biliary obstruction. Postoperative biliary obstruction symptoms improved, and the patient's jaundice was significantly lower than before operation. Since it was infectious surgery, the patient was given third-generation cephalosporins to fight infection.

VI. Postoperative examination

Examination on 25 June: Glutamic pyruvic transaminase 64 U/L, glutamic oxalacetic trans-aminase 37 U/L, albumin 20 g/L, total protein 58.00 g/L, globulin 38.00 g/L, total bilirubin 56.60 μmol/L, conjugated bilirubin 31.00 μmol/L, unconjugated bilirubin 25.60 μmol/L, γ-glutamyl transpeptidase 176.00 U/L.

Pathological results: (hepatic hydatid) Echinococcus granulosus.

> Thinking prompts: From the liver function test results, jaundice was significantly reduced, and the clinical treatment was satisfactory. Supportive treatment should be offered in the postoperative recovery stage.

VII. Lessons learned

This case is characterized by a slow onset. The first symptom was discomfort in the right upper abdomen with yellow-stained skin. The patient's general condition was good. An abdominal B-ultrasound examination showed intrahepatic space-occupying lesions. Further examination showed that leukocytes and neutrophils were significantly increased in the hemogram. A CT scan of the liver showed multiple cysts with calcification, gas accumulation in the lesions, and intrahepatic bile duct dilatation. Biochemical examination showed that transaminase increased slightly, while conjugated bilirubin and γ-Glutamyl transpeptidase increased significantly. Based on the above clinical manifestations and imaging features, combined with the patient living and working in an area where echinococcosis is common, excluding other space-occupying liver diseases, he can be diagnosed with hepatic echinococcosis. The main clinical manifestation of the disease is compression symptoms caused by hydatid cysts. The compression or rupture of the biliary tract caused by hydatid cysts often leads to biliary obstructions and infections, which is the most common complication. The diagnosis in this case is not difficult in terms of symptoms, signs, epidemic history, and imaging, but most cases of hepatic cystic echinococcosis have no obvious symptoms in the early stage, and clinical treatment is often given due to complications, which increases the difficulty of diagnosis and treatment.

The treatment of hepatic echinococcosis is mainly surgery, supplemented by drug therapy. For hepatic echinococcosis complicated with biliary tract infection, timely surgery and antibiotic treatment should be carried out.

(Shao Yingmei & Zhang Yuexin)

Repeated abnormal liver function for more than two months, and yellow-stained skin and sclera for six days

I. Medical history

Patient: Female, 39 years old, from Taizhou in Zhejiang Province. She was hospitalized between 8 November 2007 and 20 January 2008 for repeated liver dysfunction for more than two months, and yellow-stained skin and sclera for six days.

The patient was hospitalized for cancer of the left breast two months earlier at a local hospital. During hospitalization, she was found to be positive for surface markers of viral hepatitis B with mild abnormalities of liver function. The patient was diagnosed with cancer of the left breast and chronic viral hepatitis B (mild) at a local hospital, and underwent a mastectomy of her left breast after liver protection treatment. The patient's condition was stable after surgery. She received chemotherapy once a month ago at a local hospital. Her liver function before and after chemotherapy was unknown. Eleven days before admission, the patient developed fatigue and decreased appetite. She went to the local hospital again and her liver function was found to be abnormal. She was given liver-protecting and jaundice-relieving treatments such as diammonium glycyrrhizinate, reduced glutathione, and ademetionine. Six days earlier, her condition worsened, and she developed yellow staining of the skin and sclera. Sometimes, she developed nausea and vomiting after eating, with obvious fatigue and skin ecchymosis at the venipuncture site. There was no significant oliguria, no hematemesis or melena, no fever, and no change in consciousness.

The patient had previously been healthy. She had no history of acute hepatitis, nor food and drug allergies, blood transfusions, a contaminated diet, or genetic disease in her family. Her mother had a history of positive hepatitis B surface markers.

II. Physical examination on admission

T 36.8°C, P 76 times/min, R 21 times/min, BP 94/52 mHg, clear mind, low spirits, severe yellow staining of the skin and sclera, no liver palms and spider nevus, superficial lymph nodes without palpable swelling, trachea in the middle, clear respiratory sounds in both lungs, no dry and wet rales, strong heart sounds, heart rate 76 times/min, no murmur, slightly distended abdomen, positive mobile turbid sound, mild tenderness around umbilicus, no rebound pain. Her liver and spleen could not be palpated below the costal margin. There was percussion pain in the liver area. There was no edema in either of her lower limbs, and a neurological examination was negative.

III. Auxiliary examination on admission

Routine blood test: WBC 6.8×10^9/L, N 75.2%, Hb 96 g/L, PLT 123×10^9/L.

Liver function: ALT 263 U/L, AST 329 U/L, TB (total bilirubin) 219.6 μmol/L, CB (combined bilirubin) 114.3 μmol/L, TP (total protein) 56.2 g/L, A (albumin) 27.1 g/L. PT (prothrombin time) was 29.6 seconds.

Renal function: Cr 33 μmol/L, Bun 3.67 μmol/L.

Electrolytes: K^+ 3.74 μmol/L, Na^+ 130 μmol/L, Cl^- 103 μmol/L.

Gastroscope: Chronic superficial gastritis.

B-ultrasound: Right hepatic cyst, edema of the gallbladder wall with cholestasis, ascites.

IV. Preliminary diagnosis

1. Viral hepatitis B, chronic, severe (middle stage).
2. After operation of left breast cancer.
3. Drug induced hepatitis?

V. Ward-round analysis on admission

The patient presented with manifestations of severe hepatitis such as fatigue, lack of appetite, nausea, vomiting, and deepening jaundice. Combined with laboratory indicators such as serum bilirubin 10 times higher than normal and prothrombin time prolongation, the patient can be diagnosed with chronic and severe viral hepatitis B.

In order to judge the curative effect and estimate the prognosis, subacute severe hepatitis, and chronic severe hepatitis can be early, middle, and late stages according to their clinical manifestations:

(1) Early stage: Meeting the basic conditions of severe hepatitis, such as severe fatigue and gastrointestinal symptoms, rapidly deepening jaundice, serum bilirubin 10 times higher than normal, 30% < prothrombin activity ≤ 40%, or confirmed by pathology, no obvious encephalopathy or ascites

(2) Middle stage: Grade II hepatic encephalopathy or obvious ascites, bleeding (bleeding point or ecchymosis), 20% < prothrombin activity ≤ 30%

(3) Late stage: Refractory complications such as hepatorenal syndrome, massive hemorrhage of the digestive tract, severe bleeding (ecchymosis at injection site), severe infection, electrolyte disorder that is difficult to correct or hepatic encephalopathy above grade II, brain edema, prothrombin activity ≤ 20%

According to the clinical manifestations of this patient, she can be diagnosed with severe hepatitis (middle stage).

Thinking prompts: Chronic hepatitis B and chronic HBsAg carriers should be specifically analyzed when they have hepatitis. Severe hepatitis caused by drugs or other hepatitis viruses such as A and E should be ruled out. This patient had a history of chemotherapy, so liver injury caused by chemotherapy should be ruled out. However, the patient's liver function was repeatedly abnormal before chemotherapy, and was aggravated after it. Therefore, it should be considered that on the basis of chronic hepatitis B, viral activity leads to aggravated hepatitis. Consider the hepatitis virus series and exclude the possibility of superinfection of other hepatitis viruses such as A and E; HBV-DNA was checked, and virus replication was observed; urine glucuronic acid was detected to exclude the possibility of drug-induced hepatitis; an abdominal puncture was performed to check the ascites (routine and culture) to determine whether there was abdominal infection.

VI. Ward-round analysis seven days after admission

Three series of hepatitis B examinations: HBsAg positive, HBeAg positive, HBcAb positive; other hepatitis indicators were negative. HBV-DNA: 1.47×10^5 copies/ml.

Liver function: ALT 350 U/L, AST 402 U/L, TB 336 μmol/L, CB 183 μmol/L, A 27.4 g/L. Prothrombin time 30.2 seconds.

Urine glucuronic acid: Within the normal range.

Routine ascites test: WBC 80/μl, N 30%. Ascites culture was negative.

The patient's vital signs were still stable, but fatigue, nausea, and vomiting were obvious. Physical examination: The sclera had severe yellow staining, the abdomen was slightly swollen, positive mobile turbid sound, no obvious tenderness or rebound pain, and nervous system examination was negative.

In view of the above examination results, the current diagnosis excluded severe hepatitis caused by drugs or other hepatitis viruses such as A and E; chronic severe hepatitis caused by the hepatitis B virus should be considered. There was no evidence of abdominal infection. In terms of treatment, the conventional medical treatment or antiviral lamivudine was added. Because the patient's jaundice deepened and prothrombin time prolonged, artificial liver support treatment was used.

1. Timing of the antiviral treatment: According to APASL guidelines in 2008, HBeAg positive patients with ALT > two times the baseline value and serum HBV DNA level > 2.0×10^4 IU/ml (10^5 copies /ml); or HBeAg negative patients with ALT > two times the baseline value and serum HBV DNA level > 2.0×10^3 IU/ml (10^4 copies /ml) should be considered for treatment. If the patient has suffered or is close to decompensation of liver function, he/she should be treated as quickly as possible; otherwise, he/she should be followed up every 3–6 months.

Patients receiving immunosuppression or chemotherapy should be screened for HBsAg. If HBsAg is positive, a direct antiviral drug should be selected for preventive chemotherapy. The course of treatment should begin with immunosuppression or chemotherapy, and should stop at least 12 weeks after receiving immunosuppression or chemotherapy.

The latter is a very important suggestion, which is often ignored by doctors. HBsAg positive and abnormal liver function were found in this patient before chemotherapy, so according to the guidelines, antiviral treatment should be started before chemotherapy.

2. Selection of antiviral drugs: At present, there are two kinds of antiviral drugs on the market: Interferon and nucleoside analogues.

APASL guidelines suggest that patients can be treated with common interferon 5–10 mU, three times a week; peginterferon α-2a 90–180 μg per week; entecavir 0.5 mg/d; adefovir dipivoxil 10 mg/d; telbivudine 600 mg/d or lamivudine 100 mg/d. Thymosin-α 1.6 mg, twice a week can also be used. If liver function decompensation has occurred or will occur, lamivudine is recommended. In this case, entecavir and telbivudine can also be used.

According to the patient's wishes, lamivudine was used for antiviral treatment.

3. Artificial liver support system in severe hepatitis: In the half-century since Sorrentino put forward the concept of the "artificial liver" in 1956, it has made great progress. Research is based on the powerful regeneration ability of liver cells. An in vitro mechanical or physical and chemical device can temporarily assist or replace the severely diseased liver, remove harmful substances, and compensate for the metabolic function of the liver. This means that liver cells can be regenerated until the autologous liver recovers, or until a liver becomes available for transplantation. Due to the complex function of the liver, most artificial livers can only replace some functions, so it is also known as an artificial liver support system (ALSS).

At present, the artificial liver can be three types, namely, a non-biological artificial liver, a biological artificial liver, and a mixed artificial liver. A non-biological artificial liver performs plasma exchange, blood/plasma perfusion, hemodialysis, hemofiltration, molecular adsorbent recirculating system (MARS) and other methods for individual or combined application. When accompanied by hepatic encephalopathy, plasma exchange plus blood perfusion should be selected; when accompanied by renal failure, plasma exchange plus hemodialysis or hemofiltration should be chosen; when accompanied by hyperbilirubinemia, plasma bilirubin adsorption should be selected; when accompanied by water and electrolyte disturbance, plasma exchange plus hemofiltration or hemodialysis should be selected. Sometimes, more than three methods should be used in combination at the same time. Biological artificial livers and mixed artificial livers have achieved certain curative effects in animal experiments, and have been preliminarily applied in clinical practice, but their outcomes need further evaluation.

4. Indications and contraindications of artificial liver support systems

(1) Indications

1) Severe viral hepatitis: Including acute severe hepatitis, subacute severe hepatitis, and chronic severe hepatitis. In principle, the early and middle stages are better; prothrombin activity is 20%–40%, and the platelets are $> 5 \times 10^9$. Patients with late severe hepatitis and prothrombin activity $< 20\%$ can also be treated, but complications are common, so caution is advised.

2) Liver failure caused by drugs, poisons, surgery, trauma, or allergy.

3) Perioperative treatment of liver transplants for advanced liver disease.

4) Hyperbilirubinemia caused by intrahepatic cholestasis and postoperative hyperbilirubinemia, for which medical treatment failed.

(2) Contraindications

1) There is serious active bleeding, DIC.

2) Those who are highly allergic to drugs used in the treatment process, such as plasma, heparin, and protamine.

3) Patients with circulatory failure.

4) Patients with unstable cardiac and cerebral infarction.

5) Patients with severe systemic infection.

VII. Ward-round analysis one month after admission

One month after admission, the patient received liver protection medication such as compound glycyrrhizin, ademetionine, and Kuhuang, as well as enzyme lowering and jaundice treatment. She received lamivudine antiviral treatment, and artificial liver support twice. After treatment, the patient's symptoms improved, nausea and vomiting were relieved, and jaundice subsided to TB 125 μmol/L, CB 89 μmol/L, prothrombin time 27.0 seconds.

One week earlier, the patient had abdominal distention and pain after eating, and aggravated nausea. An abdominal X-ray showed incomplete intestinal obstruction, which was relieved after fasting, but then low fever and abdominal circumference increased. Many abdominal puncture examinations were carried out, and the routine WBC of ascites was about 320/μl, N 35%. Escherichia coli [extended spectrum β lactamase (ESBL) (+)] was cultured in ascites, and anti-infection treatment was given with sulperazon. Treatment was given to improve intestinal microecology such as bifidobacterium, lactobacillus acidophilus, and enterococcus triple viable bacteria (bifid triple viable).

Routine blood examination: WBC 10.4×10^9/L, N 80.5%.

B-ultrasound: Chronic liver disease, splenomegaly; multiple cysts were found in the right liver; edema of the gallbladder wall; moderate amount of ascites. During the two re-examinations, HBV-DNA was negative.

Liver function: ALT 31 U/L, AST 86 U/L, TB 216 μmol/L, CB 112 μmol/L.

After the above treatment, the patient's condition improved for a time, indicating that the above treatment was effective. However, in the course of treatment, symptoms such as abdominal pain appeared, which was confirmed as incomplete intestinal obstruction by abdominal X-ray, followed by fever and ascites, which was confirmed as primary bacterial peritonitis by an abdominal puncture examination.

Cases of severe hepatitis are often complicated with various infections due to low autoimmune function. Common infections include bacteremia, pneumonia, and peritonitis. The patient's infection symptoms are often atypical, such as irregular fever and a slight increase in peripheral blood leukocytes. Spontaneous bacterial peritonitis is common. Only half of patients have abdominal tenderness and rebound pain. The positive rate of ascites culture is low.

Spontaneous bacterial peritonitis (SBP) refers to an acute diffuse bacterial infection of the peritoneum without perforation of the abdominal organs, and other infectious causes such as inflammation (abscess, acute pancreatitis, or cholecystitis). It is a common but serious complication in patients with liver disease. Its occurrence and development are related to factors such as intestinal flora disorder, weakening of the intestinal mucosal barrier function, intestinal bacterial translocation, and low immune function. The predisposing factors included gastrointestinal bleeding, low concentration of ascites protein, and weakened intestinal peristalsis. The main mechanism of SBP may be that the intestinal bacteria enter the sub-serosal lymphatic vessels through the intestinal wall and then enter the abdominal cavity. SBP was mainly infected by a single strain. Gram negative aerobic bacteria are the most common, accounting for 70%–80%, and more than half of them are Escherichia coli. They can also be caused by Streptococcus and anaerobic bacteria. The pathogenic bacteria of SBP mainly come from the intestinal tract, but infections of the lungs, soft tissue, and urinary tract can also be secondary to SBP.

The typical clinical manifestations of SBP are chills, fever, abdominal pain and (or) abdominal distension, abdominal muscle tension with tenderness, rebound pain, and decreased bowel sounds. However, the clinical manifestations of patients with severe hepatitis complicated with SBP are atypical and varied, so the diagnosis of SBP is mainly based on the counts of polymorphonuclear granulocytes (PMN) in ascites and ascites bacterial culture. Although it is advocated that the culture of ascites bacteria should be carried out in a blood culture bottle to improve sensitivity, there are still about 60% of SBP cases with negative culture results. This makes the ascites PMN count an important index for the diagnosis of SBP, and the best diagnostic cut-off value is PMN $\geq 0.25 \times 10^9$/L.

Once a diagnosis of SBP is established, empirical antibiotic treatment should be started immediately. The initial antibiotic treatment should cover Streptococcus of Enterobacteriaceae and non-Enterococcus. Cephalosporin is the most studied injectable antibiotic for the treatment of SBP. Experiments show that compared with other antibiotics, cephalosporins are more effective in treating SBP. They have less nephrotoxicity and are less prone to double infection, so cephalosporins can be used as the first choice for injection. Oral quinolones are also effective for SBP patients without serious complications (no septic shock, intestinal obstruction, or serum creatinine > 6 mg/dl). They are similar to cephalosporins in cure rate, survival rate, and double infection. As far as this patient is concerned, the ascites is cultured as Escherichia coli (ESBL+), so it should be treated with carbapenems or compound antibiotics, such as ampicillin + sulbactam.

VIII. Condition at discharge

After anti-infection treatment, ascites gradually subsided and body temperature returned to normal. The patient continued antiviral and liver protection treatment, and got better. Her liver function was examined before discharge: ALT 34 U/L, AST 56 U/L, TB 83 μmol/L, CB 42 μmol/L, prothrombin time 16 seconds. HBV-DNA negative; B-ultrasound: A small amount of ascites.

IX. Follow-up suggestions

APASL guidelines suggest that ALT, HBeAg, and/or HBV DNA should be monitored at least every three months during treatment. For patients taking adefovir dipivoxil, renal function should be tested. Patients who use interferon must be alert to the side effects of interferon.

For oral antiviral therapy, if HBeAg seroconversion occurs in HBeAg-positive patients, and if two HBV DNA tests at least six months apart are negative, the drug can be stopped. In HBeAg-negative patients, the course of treatment of oral antiviral drugs is not clear, but if HBV DNA is negative after three consecutive tests every six months, the drug can be stopped.

X. Lessons learned

Patients with severe hepatitis are complicated cases, and are prone to multiple complications. Therefore, it is necessary to fully grasp the diagnosis and treatment measures of hepatitis, such as the indication of antiviral treatment, and the prevention and treatment of complications. In this case, early and timely artificial liver support therapy plays a key role in improving symptoms and increasing chances of survival.

(Wu Wei & Li Lanjuan)

Recurrent fever, chills, hyperhidrosis, and joint pain for three months

I. Medical history

Patient: Male, 20 years old, a Kazakh herdsman in a county in Xinjiang. He was admitted due to three months of repeated fever, chills, sweating, and general joint pain.

One month earlier the patient visited a local hospital, and no abnormality was found in his chest X-ray. He was suspected of septicemia, viral infection, and rheumatic fever. After being treated with antibacterial drugs (levofloxacin, cephalosporin, and ribavirin) and anti-rheumatic drugs for two weeks, he was discharged from the hospital with a normal temperature, and stopped taking drugs. In the past ten days, the above symptoms recurred and worsened, and he came to the superior hospital for treatment. He was admitted to the hospital with FUO (fever of unknown origin.)

> **Thinking prompts:** The characteristics of this case: ① Young male herdsman; ② Repeated fever, chills, hyperhidrosis, and joint pain for three months; ③ After antibacterial treatment in a local hospital, his temperature subsided, but the symptoms recurred after stopping medication. It is suggested that this is a systemic infection, for which antibacterial treatment is effective. The possibility of bacterial infection should be considered. For patients with long-term recurrent fever, hyperhidrosis, and joint pain, medical history and epidemiology should be looked into further. Physical examination should focus on the superficial lymph nodes, hepatosplenomegaly, rashes, and joint swelling.

The patient was a herdsman, whose family owned over 100 sheep and more than 10 cattle. He had delivered lambs four months ago. Some sheep had dystocia and suffered miscarriage, and he did not wear gloves while handling them. He was in the habit of drinking unboiled mountain spring water. Occasionally, when the skin on his limbs became damaged, he would treat it himself without disinfection.

II. Physical examination

Body temperature 38.6°C, pulse 96 times/min, respiration 24 times/min, blood pressure 110/70 mmHg, good growth and development. Facial features of acute illness, damp skin on head and trunk, no rash. Several slightly enlarged lymph nodes, about 1 cm in length, can be felt in the bilateral neck and armpit, with a soft texture, mobility, and no tenderness. No abnormality in the heart and lungs, 2 cm below the liver rib, and below and beside the spleen rib; no tenderness. No swelling, pain, or limited movement in the joints. Right testicle slightly enlarged and tender. The physiological reflex is present, and the pathological sign is negative.

III. Ward-round analysis on admission

The clinical features of this case were as follows: ① Young male herdsman; ② Repeated fever, arthralgia, and hyperhidrosis for more than three months; ③ Antibacterial treatment was effective, but the disease recurred after discontinuing the drug; ④ High body temperature accompanied by sweating, enlarged lymph nodes, and hepatosplenomegaly; ⑤ Swelling and pain in the right testicle; ⑥ No rashes or joint swelling; ⑦ A recent history of contact with cattle and sheep, with treatment of miscarriage and dystocia in sheep; no protective measures, and a history of drinking unboiled water.

The following diseases should be considered in the comprehensive analysis of the patient:

1. Diseases caused by contact with animals like cattle and sheep, such as brucellosis. Clinical manifestations of brucellosis include repeated fever; the course of the disease is long; typical wave-type fever; most patients have an irregular fever, with sweating as one of its more prominent features; hepatosplenomegaly and enlargement of the lymph nodes; joint pain mainly affecting the large joints; sacroiliac joints pain common. Men have swelling and pain in one or both testicles, and women have oophoritis or salpingitis with lower abdominal pain. The white blood cell and neutrophil numbers of patients with Brucella infection are normal or reduced; the Brucella agglutination test is positive, and Brucella can be detected through bacterial culture of the blood and bone marrow.

2. Infections related to skin injury or contaminated drinking water, such as septicemia, are characterized by sudden chills, fever that is high, remittent, irregular, or continuing, accompanied by general discomfort, headaches, joint pain, hepatosplenomegaly, and rashes in some patients, depending on whether the infected bacteria produce a rash toxin. Some patients have superficial enlargement of the lymph nodes, offering clues about infection according to the location. Leukocytes or neutrophils are obviously elevated, and a positive culture of blood or bone marrow bacteria can be used in diagnosis. If a bacterial infection occurs after drinking contaminated water, there are usually digestive tract symptoms such as abdominal pain, diarrhea, mucous stool, or bloody purulent stool.

3. Differentiation from infectious diseases of the lymph nodes and hepatosplenomegaly, such as infectious mononucleosis: The clinical manifestations of infectious mononucleosis are

fever that is irregular, remittent, or continuing, as well as angina and enlargement of the lymph nodes, especially in the neck; hepatosplenomegaly, and a rash in some patients. The number of white blood cells is normal or elevated, abnormal lymphocytes are often seen, and more than 10% of abnormal lymphocytes are helpful for diagnosis. A positive heterophil agglutination test and positive EB virus antibody have diagnostic significance. Infectious mononucleosis is caused by the Epstein-Barr virus. Antibacterial treatment is ineffective.

4. Differentiation from orchitis: The testicles are usually red and swollen, with obvious tenderness and fever. If the bacterial infection spreads, it can cause septicemia, often without hepatosplenomegaly.

5. Differentiation from rheumatic fever: Rheumatic fever has symptoms such as repeated fever, hyperhidrosis, wandering arthritis of the large joints, annular erythema or subcutaneous nodules, and carditis. The number of leukocytes and neutrophils increases. ASO (anti-streptolysin "o"): > 500 U, which is helpful for diagnosis. Bacterial culture negative.

6. Differentiation from leukemia and lymphoma: Acute leukemia is often characterized by fever, hemorrhage, progressive anemia, and enlarged lymph nodes, liver, and spleen. Some patients have retrosternal tenderness and significantly increased white blood cells. Leukemia cells can be diagnosed by a blood smear and bone marrow smear. Lymphoma is characterized by fever, night sweats, fatigue, and emaciation. Progressive painless enlargement of the lymph nodes is the most common manifestation, which can be confirmed by lymph node puncture or pathological examination.

IV. Auxiliary examination after admission

WBC 4.8×10^9/L, N 45%, L 50%, Hb 120 g/L, PLT 260×10^9/L.

ESR 35 mm/h.

Liver and kidneys biochemically normal, no abnormal findings in chest radiographs.

Abdominal ultrasound: Hepatosplenomegaly, no abnormal findings.

Bone marrow smear normal.

Brucella was cultured in blood and bone marrow. The result of the agglutination test for Brucella serum was 1:320 (positive).

> **Thinking prompts:** Emphasis should be placed on routine biochemical examination of the blood, liver, and kidneys, blood bacteria culture, bone marrow smear and bacteria culture, and chest X-ray examination. Because most patients have used antibacterial drugs before admission, in order to improve the positive rate of bacterial culture, only symptomatic and supportive treatment is given instead of antibacterial drugs when the condition allows.

V. Diagnosis

Brucellosis.

Diagnostic basis: The patient is a male herdsman with a history of close contact with cattle and sheep, and a history of delivering lambs; repeated fever, general joint pain, hyperhidrosis, testicular enlargement for three months, enlargement of the bilateral cervical lymph nodes, hepatosplenomegaly, and testicular enlargement, normal WBC. The results of the agglutination test of Brucella serum were positive. Brucella was cultured in blood and bone marrow.

VI. Treatment

Antibacterial treatment plan: Antibacterial treatment of brucellosis requires a combination of antibacterial drugs that can enter cells. Rifampicin 600 mg/d and doxycycline 0.2 g/d, taken orally twice for six weeks, are currently recommended by the WHO.

> **Thinking prompts:** Why does brucellosis recur after the patient improves? First, Brucella is an intracellular parasitic bacterium, and it is difficult for general drugs to enter the cells to work on it. The course of treatment of antibacterial drugs is too short. Only two weeks are not enough; the course should be at least six weeks. Second, the antibacterial effect of the selected antibiotics on Brucella is not ideal. Brucella is a gram negative bacillus, and is sensitive to antibiotics such as aminoglycosides, tetracyclines, and rifampicin.

Results: After being treated with rifampicin and doxycycline for one week, the patient's body temperature dropped to normal, and his symptoms disappeared after two weeks. After being discharged from hospital, the patient continued to take the medication for six weeks, and he was completely cured without recurrence at the six-month follow-up.

VII. Lessons learned

The course of this case is long, characterized by repeated fever, joint pain, and hyperhidrosis accompanied by enlargement of the lymph nodes, hepatosplenomegaly, and right testicular swelling and pain. Antibacterial treatment was initially effective, but there were relapses after the medication was stopped. From the clinical manifestations, the patient can be preliminarily diagnosed with a bacterial infection or septicemia, despite a routine blood test coming back normal. The patient is a male herdsman with a history of contact with cattle and sheep, and a history of delivering lambs. Therefore, the first consideration was the long-term fever, but the white blood cells were not high, as in animal-related zoonotic diseases. Positive bacterial culture in the blood or bone marrow is the key to making a definitive diagnosis. Therefore, especially for patients who have used a variety of antibacterial drugs, if the condition permits, do not use antibacterial drugs temporarily. Closely observe the fever and any clinical changes, and conduct bacterial culture of blood or bone marrow many times, as this can improve the positive rate. In this case, the patient had received antibacterial treatment, which was effective, but he relapsed after stopping the medication. Therefore, antibacterial drugs were not used this time, but blood and bone marrow cultures were performed, and a diagnosis was made quickly.

In addition, it is very important to select sensitive and effective antibacterial drugs for combination therapy, as well as a sufficient course of treatment for radical cure or elimination of intracellular parasitic bacteria such as Brucella, to prevent the recurrence of the illness.

(Zhang Yuexin)

Intermittent fever for ten years, splenomegaly for five years, joint pain for one year, and aggravation with swelling of the lower limbs for one month

I. Medical history

Patient: Male, 66 years old, Han, a farm worker in Xinjiang. His main complaints were intermittent fever for ten years, splenomegaly for five years, joint pain for one year, and an aggravation with swelling of the lower limbs for one month. He was admitted to hospital with FUO (fever of unknown origin).

Ten years earlier, the patient suddenly developed chills and a high fever lasting for one week, without obvious inducement. He was diagnosed with typhoid fever at a local hospital, and received anti-infection treatment (the specific medication is unknown), after which his body temperature returned to normal. After that, he had many episodes of chills, as well as a high fever without obvious inducement that retreated after sweating. This occurred several times a year, and was accompanied by fatigue. Each time, after being treated with antibacterial drugs and antipyretics (name and dose unknown) at local clinics, his fever dissipated and his symptoms were relieved, but a clear diagnosis was never made. The patient was not concerned because he could still work.

Five years earlier, he felt distention in the upper left abdomen, and a palpable mass without abdominal pain, accompanied by a low fever (37°C–38°C). At the local community hospital, he was found to have an enlarged spleen, but the diagnosis was still unclear. The patient then took Chinese medicine (name unknown) for six months, but the treatment failed.

A year earlier, the patient felt obvious abdominal distension, obvious enlargement of the left upper abdominal mass, and aggravation of symptoms such as low fever, fatigue, and joint pain. He was hospitalized again at a local secondary-level hospital. After repeated examinations, a Brucella serum agglutination test was positive, and a biopsy of inguinal lymph node aspiration showed lymphocyte proliferation and no abnormal lymphocytes. The patient was diagnosed with brucellosis, and was treated with rifampicin (0.3 g/d, twice a day) and tetracycline (1.5 g/d, three times a day) orally for nearly six months. He felt that his symptoms were not obviously relieved, but gradually aggravated, particularly fever, fatigue, joint pain, and emaciation (weight loss of about 7 kg). Edema of both lower limbs was obvious one month before admission, which affected his daily life, as he was unable to do farm work. Therefore, he came to our hospital for medical treatment.

Epidemiological history: Raising sheep at home and having a history of delivering lambs.

II. Physical examination on admission

T 37.7°C, P 80 times/min, R 22 times/min, BP 110/80 mmHg, body weight 65 kg. Bilateral cervical lymph nodes enlarged like walnuts, medium quality, good mobility, light tenderness. No yellow stains, rashes, or bleeding spots on skin and sclera. No abnormalities found in the lungs. Heart rate 80 beats/min, regular rhythm, and systolic level-2 blowing murmurs heard at the apex of the heart. Flat, soft abdomen. Liver could not palpated below the costal margin; spleen about 10 cm below the rib, and of medium quality. Abdominal percussion drum sound, negative shifting dullness, normal bowel sound. No redness, swelling, or restricted movement in the joints of limbs, and moderate pitting edema in both lower limbs. Physiological reflex present and pathological reflex negative.

III. Diagnosis

1. Analysis of condition on admission

The clinical features are as follows: ① 66-year-old male farm worker with a history of close contact with sheep and delivering lambs; ② Intermittent fever for ten years with hyperhidrosis, and progressive splenomegaly for five years; ③ Low fever, emaciation, enlarged lymph nodes in the neck, splenomegaly, and moderate pitting edema of both lower limbs; ④ Fever symptoms were relieved after antibacterial treatment, but recurred after drug withdrawal. Anti-Brucella treatment was ineffective in the past six months, and symptoms worsened for one month; ⑤ The many Brucella agglutination tests performed at the previous hospital were all positive; ⑥ No rashes, joint swelling or pain, ascites, or positive signs in the heart and lungs.

2. Possible diagnosis

Infection-related diseases such as brucellosis, tuberculosis, visceral leishmaniasis, malaria, and septicemia; diseases related to the immune system include rheumatic fever and adult Still disease; diseases related to hematological tumors including lymphoma and malignant histiocytosis.

3. Differential diagnosis analysis

(1) Long-term fever with hyperhidrosis and emaciation should be differentiated from tuberculosis, rheumatic fever, and autoimmune diseases.

1) Differentiation from tuberculosis: Pulmonary tuberculosis often shares symptoms with tuberculosis poisoning such as cough, expectoration, low fever in the afternoon, night sweats, and emaciation. Tuberculosis lesions can be found on chest radiographs, making it easy to differentiate. In addition to the above symptoms of tuberculosis poisoning, the lymph nodes

often swell and rupture, forming sinuses. Needle aspiration biopsy can identify pathological changes such as tuberculosis granuloma or caseous necrosis, and positive acid-fast staining or culture of tubercule bacillus can confirm the diagnosis. In addition to the symptoms of tuberculosis poisoning, there are often osteoarthritic symptoms in the tubercle of the bone joints. X-ray examination shows the characteristic lesions of the bone joint, while surgical pathological examination shows the specific pathological changes of tuberculosis granuloma, and can confirm the diagnosis. This case is similar to tuberculosis due to symptoms such as long-term fever, hyperhidrosis, emaciation, and enlargement of the lymph nodes. However, the characteristics of fever and hyperhidrosis in this patient were different from the low fever in the afternoon and night sweats of tuberculosis. Although the lymph nodes were enlarged, there was no rupture or sinus formation, no pulmonary symptoms and signs or osteoarthrosis. In addition, progressive enlargement of the spleen and moderate pitting edema of both lower limbs are not common signs of tuberculosis. Tuberculosis antibodies, a PPD test, and lymph node biopsy can be used for diagnosis. In this case, a lymph node biopsy conducted at the external hospital failed to find the characteristic pathological changes to the tubercles, so tuberculosis can be ruled out.

2) Differentiation from rheumatic fever: Rheumatic fever is a recurrent acute or chronic systemic connective tissue inflammation, which may be related to group A streptococcal infection. Typical rheumatic fever often features fever, migratory polyarthritis, subcutaneous nodules, annular erythema, and cardial (endocardial, myocardial, and pericardial) inflammation. The anti-O titer was higher than 500 U/L, white blood cells and neutrophils increased, bacterial culture was negative, erythrocyte sedimentation rate was rapid, and C-reactive protein increased. This case had none of the above symptoms and signs, especially no migratory polyarthritis, subcutaneous nodules, annular erythema, or cardial inflammation. The possibility of this disease can be ruled out.

3) Differentiation from adult Still disease: Adult Still disease is characterized by unexplained long-term fever, multiform rashes and variability, joint pain, enlarged lymph nodes, sore throat, increased white blood cells and neutrophils, rapid erythrocyte sedimentation rate, and negative blood culture, for which antibacterial treatment is ineffective. Adrenal glucocorticoid can obviously relieve symptoms. The patient of this case has no rash, no sore throat; antibacterial treatment was effective. The possibility of this disease can be ruled out.

(2) Long-term fever with progressive splenomegaly should be distinguished from illnesses such as sepsis, visceral leishmaniasis, malaria, malignant histiocytosis, and lymphoma.

1) Differentiation from visceral leishmaniasis: Visceral leishmaniasis is a chronic endemic parasitic disease caused by infection by Leishmania donovani, and is clinically characterized by long-term irregular fever, emaciation, and enlargement of the spleen, liver, and lymph nodes, especially progressive splenomegaly, accompanied by pancytopenia and increased serum globulin. In some cases, liver damage and even the manifestations and signs of liver cirrhosis can be found. The diagnosis can be confirmed through the bone marrow (positive rate of 85%), swollen lymph nodes, or spleen puncture (positive rate of more than 90%), Giemsa stain, or Wright's stain to find protozoa. Antibacterial treatment is not effective,

and antimony agent treatment is required. The patient in this case presented with long-term fever, and progressive enlargement of the lymph nodes and spleen, but antibacterial treatment was effective at the early stage of the disease, and no parasite was found in bone marrow and lymph node examination, so the possibility of visceral leishmaniasis could be ruled out.

2) Differentiation from malignant histiocytosis: Malignant histiocytosis refers to a malignant tumor of the hematological system, and is rare. The main manifestations include long-term irregular fever, progressive anemia, hepatosplenomegaly, and lymphadenopathy. A definitive diagnosis can be made with the discovery of malignant histiocytes in bone marrow examination. Antibacterial therapy is generally ineffective. This case was effectively treated with antibiotics at the early stage of the disease. The bone marrow smear showed no malignant histiocytes, and the course of the disease was ten years. It was unlikely to be malignant histiocytosis, which could be ruled out.

3) Differentiation from lymphoma: Lymphoma is characterized by progressive and painless lymphadenopathy, which may be accompanied by long-term or repeated fever, night sweats, emaciation, and hepatosplenomegaly. A lymph node imprint and a pathological section or lymph node puncture smear can be performed, and the diagnosis can be confirmed if lymphoma cells are found. The lymph node biopsy in this case was a lymph node proliferative lesion that was not treated with anti-tumor therapy, and the 10-year-long course of the disease did not resemble the outcome of lymphoma. This possibility can be ruled out.

4) Differentiation from septicemia: Septicemia is a serious infection with acute onset in clinic, including chills, high fever, rash, joint swelling and pain, and enlargement of the liver, spleen, and lymph nodes. Acute organ dysfunction may occur in severe cases, or even infective shock, disseminated intravascular coagulation (DIC), and multiple organ failure. The patient in this case suffered from chills, high fever, general discomfort, and joint swelling and pain in the early stage of the disease, and antibacterial treatment was effective, making it similar to septicemia. However, its course is as long as ten years, which is different from septicemia. It should be considered that it may be caused by chronic infection instead of general bacterial infection.

5) Differentiation from malaria: Malaria is a parasitic disease transmitted by mosquito bites. It is characterized in clinic by intermittent chills, high fever, sweating, splenomegaly, and anemia, and no enlargement of the lymph nodes. Plasmodium can be diagnosed with a blood smear. The patient in this case had none of the above-mentioned manifestations, and because Xinjiang is not a malaria-endemic area, and the patient had not been to a malaria-endemic area before illness, the possibility of malaria can be ruled out.

6) Differentiation from cirrhotic portal hypertension: The patient in this case had splenomegaly, edema of the lower limbs, and three series of hemocyte/blood cells and low albumin, which are different from liver cirrhosis. In China, liver cirrhosis is mainly caused by viral hepatitis, schistosomiasis, autoimmune liver disease, and heavy drinking. It usually manifests as chronic liver disease and related clinical symptoms and signs, but no long-term

repeated fever, hyperhidrosis, or lymphadenopathy. The patient had no history of hepatitis, lived in Xinjiang, had no history of contact with infected water, no history of schistosomiasis, and no history of heavy drinking, so the possibility of cirrhotic portal hypertension can be ruled out.

> **Thinking prompts:** In this case, due to fever, enlargement of the lymph nodes, and splenomegaly, the relevant examinations for bacterial infection should be emphasized.

IV. Auxiliary examination after admission

Routine blood test: WBC 6.3×10^9/L, N 30.5%, L 64.1%; Hb 111 g/L, PLT 66.4×10^9/L.

Tuberculosis antibodies negative. Blood culture negative three times.

ESR 30 mm/h.

Biochemical examination: Albumin 24 g/L, globulin 35 g/L, ALT and AST normal. CRP 17.2 mg/L, rheumatoid factor RF (+), anti-neutrophil antibodies (cANCA and pANCA) negative.

Abdominal B-ultrasound: Diffuse hepatic lesions, splenomegaly.

Bone marrow examination: High lymphocyte ratio, accounting for 58.5%. Some karyotypes were irregular, and megakaryocytes and platelets were few.

X-ray: Bilateral knee and elbow joint degeneration, no obvious abnormality in the pelvis.

According to clinical manifestations, epidemiological history, and laboratory examination results, the initial diagnosis of brucellosis (chronic stage) was correct. Blood and bone marrow cultures were performed immediately after admission, and one week later, the results of the bone marrow cultures reported Brucella positive, which could be diagnosed as brucellosis (chronic stage).

V. Treatment after admission

Before the results of the blood and bone marrow cultures were reported, physical cooling and symptomatic treatment were given, and the clinical manifestations of the patient were closely observed. Antimicrobial treatment was given after the examination results confirmed brucellosis. The antibacterial drug treatment plan is rifampin 600 mg/d orally divided twice, and moxifloxacin 400 mg/d orally. After one week, the patient's body temperature dropped to normal, and the symptoms were obviously relieved. After two weeks, the symptoms disappeared and he was discharged from hospital. He continued to take the medicine until the sixth week, and no recurrence occurred after six months of follow-up.

VI. Lessons learned

This case is chronic brucellosis, but in the early stage of the disease, due to atypical symptoms or insufficient understanding, it was not treated as such in time, which led to the development of the chronic form of the disease. In this case, the blood culture was negative and the bone marrow culture was positive many times, which suggested that bone marrow culture should be performed when the blood culture is negative, and the positive rate of the latter was obviously higher than that of the former. In this case, rifampicin and tetracycline failed to work, which may be due to the severe resistance of bacteria to tetracycline. According to overseas research reports, brucellosis is more resistant to tetracycline, which is rarely used now. Second-generation tetracycline drugs such as doxycycline or quinolones can be used instead. In vivo and in vitro tests have confirmed that quinolones have a better curative effect on brucellosis. Therefore, tetracycline was not effective in this case, and it is possible that it is also resistant to doxycycline. A combination of rifampicin and quinolones was used instead, and the effect was satisfactory. A history of close contact with sheep and cattle, especially delivering lambs, has important epidemiological significance for the diagnosis of brucellosis.

(Zhang Yuexin)

Fever for four days and disturbance of consciousness for one day

I. Medical history

Patient: Female, 28 years old, farmer from a Hangzhou suburb. She was admitted to hospital in April 2003, having suffered a fever for four days and disturbance of consciousness for one day.

The patient developed a fever after fatigue four days previously, and her body temperature fluctuated around 39°C, without nasal congestion, runny nose, sore throat, and cough. After being hospitalized locally for three days, the fever did not ease and there was irritability, so she was transferred to our hospital.

The patient was healthy and had no medical history. She was married, and had one child and a happy family life. Everyone was in good health. There had been reports of encephalitis caused by Coxsackie virus in the suburban counties of Hangzhou that month.

> **Thinking prompts:** The patient had an acute onset, and the main symptoms were fever and disturbance of consciousness, suggesting an infection of the central nervous system. Therefore, the patient's medical history should be investigated for common and frequently-occurring diseases that can cause central line infection, especially bacterial central line infection with acute onset. For example, asking patients whether they have been in contact with anyone suffering from meningoencephalitis, and whether they have had otitis media in the past. This will identify the possibility of bacteria invading the central nervous system. The two other common pathogens causing slow-onset central line infections are Cryptococcus neoformans and Mycobacterium tuberculosis. The former often exists in dust and pigeon feces, while the latter is related to a history of or contact with tuberculosis. In addition, we should inquire about positive symptoms and their evolution in patients with central line infections in order to make a preliminary assessment of their condition and prognosis.

II. Physical examination

T 39.6°C, P 122 times/min, R 20 times/min, BP 109/76 mmHg. Irritability, inability to answer questions, soft neck, no yellow stain on the skin and sclera, no bleeding points, no swelling of the superficial lymph nodes, no dry or moist rales in either lung, H 122 times/min, regularity, no murmur, soft abdomen. The liver and spleen could not be palpated below the costal margin; no percussion pain in liver area, shifting dullness (−), grade 5 muscle strength of limbs, normal muscle tension, left Babinski's sign (+), Kernig's sign (−), and Brudzinski's sign (−).

> **Thinking prompts:** Physical examination is mainly concerned with whether there are positioning signs, whether muscle strength and tension are normal, and pupil size and shape. If necessary, fundus examination can be performed to observe whether there is edema on the optic nerve papilla. Subcutaneous bleeding points often suggest bacterial septicemia.

III. Auxiliary inspection

Routine blood test: WBC 9.2×10^9/L, N 75%, L 20%.

Liver function: ALT 175 U/L, AST 81 U/L, TB 18 μmol/L, CB 7 μmol/L, other liver function indexes were normal.

CRP, ESR, CT, B-ultrasonography, chest radiographs were normal.

All indexes of cerebrospinal fluid examination were normal.

> **Thinking prompts:** Examination of the cerebrospinal fluid plays an important role in the identification of central line infection. Routine tests and biochemical indicators of the cerebrospinal fluid can roughly determine the kind of pathogen infection (virus, bacteria, mycobacterium tuberculosis, or fungi). Cerebrospinal fluid culture is very important for the acquisition of bacteria, fungi, and mycobacterium tuberculosis. Virus-specific serological examination can determine the kind of virus infection. Imaging changes of brain parenchyma and meninges can be observed by plain and enhanced MRI.

IV. Ward-round analysis at admission

1. Preliminary diagnosis

The patient had a fever for four days, disturbance of consciousness for one day, left Babinski's sign (+), normal cerebrospinal fluid indicators, and abnormal liver function indicators. Acute viral infection was suspected, complicated with viral encephalitis and liver damage.

> **Thinking prompts:** The patient had a short, acute-onset illness, so acute infection was considered. In addition to fever and disturbance of consciousness, she also had liver function damage, which indicates multiple organ damage. Infections that can cause multiple organ damage are often systemic or local bacterial infections with toxemia. Combined with infection indicators, CRP and cerebrospinal fluid were normal. No focus of infection was found in the patient's medical history,

and the possibility of bacterial infection was low. Therefore, viral infection was considered first. But which virus infection? A diagnosis that is accurate to specific pathogens is the most complete and ideal, but it is sometimes difficult to achieve in clinical practice.

2. Diagnostic thinking

The common pathogens causing encephalitis are epidemic cerebrospinal meningitis bacteria and epidemic encephalitis B (Japanese encephalitis B) virus, both of which occur in teenagers and children. However, due to routine vaccination in early childhood in China, the incidence of some infectious diseases in children decreases, but tends to increase in adults. Epidemic cerebrospinal meningitis spreads through the respiratory tract, and most often occurs in winter and spring. Meningeal injury is the main clinical manifestation (such as increased intracranial pressure and positive meningeal irritation signs), and the cerebrospinal fluid often changes accordingly. However, Japanese encephalitis B needs mosquitoes as the transmission medium. In regions with distinct seasons, the occurrence of Japanese encephalitis B has strict seasonality. In summer, damage to the brain parenchyma is the main clinical manifestation (consciousness, convulsions, changes in muscle strength and respiratory rhythm, and positive pathological reflex), and a small part of the cerebrospinal fluid can be completely normal.

According to the time of onset, clinical manifestation, and auxiliary examination in this case, infection from these two pathogens is impossible. To identify specific pathogens, it is necessary to re-recognize the four characteristics of infectious diseases (pathogen, infectivity, epidemiological characteristics, and post-infection immunity), which are all closely related to clinical practice. Finding pathogens is the gold standard for diagnosis. Epidemiological characteristics often indicate the source of prevalent infectious diseases, which is directly related to the diagnosis of some of them. When inquiring about a patient's medical history, we should bear in mind that for a pathogen with durable immunity after infection, no secondary attack is normally caused, and a second diagnosis of the same pathogen must be made cautiously. There were many cases of encephalitis caused by Coxsackie virus in the patient's living environment, suggesting that she may have been infected, causing brain and liver damage that can be determined by serological examination. Due to the lack of specific treatment for viral diseases, and because the course of the illness has exceeded four days, it is necessary to give symptomatic and supportive treatment instead of antiviral treatment. Note the stability of vital signs and prevent the occurrence of brain edema.

V. Ward-round analysis on day 3 of admission

After receiving symptomatic support treatment, the patient's body temperature gradually lowered, and the peak moved backward. Since the previous day, her highest body temperature was 38.4°C, her consciousness was clearer, and her answers were to the point. Babinski's sign on the left side (−). The previous day, she tested positive for Coxsackie virus IgM antibodies, so the diagnosis of encephalitis caused by Coxsackie virus was obvious.

Thinking prompts: Coxsackie virus, echovirus, and poliovirus constitute the classic enteroviruses. Poliomyelitis has been eliminated in China. Enteroviruses are mainly transmitted through digestive tract and close contact in daily life. Coxsackie virus and echovirus have many serotypes, which can cause different clinical manifestations leading to respiratory system damage, central nervous system damage, myocarditis, hepatitis, epidemic myalgia, epidemic hemorrhagic conjunctivitis, and hand, foot and mouth disease. They can also cause multiple organ injuries, and the severity of illness varies. Enteroviruses discovered after 1969 (enterovirus 68, enterovirus 69, enterovirus 70, enterovirus 71) are known as new enteroviruses. The new enterovirus 71, which was rife in Anhui Province in spring 2008, was characterized by a rash on the hands, feet, and mouth. Some sufferers died of complications such as encephalitis. It is worth mentioning that virus infection often has one characteristic, either pantropic affinity or relative affinity. Pantropic determines that the virus can invade multiple tissues at the same time; relative affinity determines that viral invasion often affects a certain tissue, while clinical manifestations are determined by whether the invading virus is dominant in pantropic or relative affinity, and the resulting pathophysiological changes. For example, the hepatitis B virus causes liver injury, but it can also have extrahepatic manifestations such as bone marrow suppression. Hemorrhagic fever with renal syndrome virus is characterized by kidney damage, but also by lung, liver, and brain damage.

VI. Ward-round analysis on day six after admission

The patient's body temperature gradually dropped to about 37.5°C in the four days after her admission to hospital, but suddenly surged to 39.7°C in the early morning of day 5. She did not complain of any other discomfort, was conscious, answered questions to the point, and did not elicit pathological reflexes. Routine blood examination indicated that WBC was 12.6 × 10⁹/L, N 79%, L 16%. Due to sudden fever, a B-ultrasound of liver, gallbladder and spleen was re-examined. The results showed that there was a 1.6 cm-long effusion under the left diaphragm. No abnormality was found in liver, gallbladder, or spleen. The fever was still high after a day of observation.

Thinking prompts: The patient's condition was improving, and her body temperature and consciousness were close to normal, so why did her body temperature rise again? Was the initial diagnosis too arbitrary? If this is the case, the patient's fever is saddle-type, which is most commonly caused by the dengue virus. However, the patient comes from a suburban county of Hangzhou, and has not visited Guangzhou and other places in recent months. Moreover, mosquitoes had not finished hibernation in Hangzhou when she fell ill, so she cannot be diagnosed with dengue fever. Was the initial diagnosis (Coxsackie encephalitis) correct, but complicated with bacterial infection on this basis? If so, what kind of bacterial infection is it? What about the infection site?

Could it be a more insidious bacterial infection such as a perianal infection? Is fever related to subphrenic effusion? Blood culture should be done before antibiotics are given. Antibiotics with a narrow antibacterial spectrum and better tissue distribution can be selected before the culture results are reported. Clindamycin can be given as diagnostic treatment, and anti-Gram-negative bacteria treatment should be ramped up when necessary. Look closely at the double diaphragm B-ultrasound. Is it post-infection fever? This is caused by an allergy after an infection, so antibiotic treatment is ineffective. Cortical hormone treatment should be given when, but infectious fever such as bacteria must be ruled out.

VII. Ward-round analysis on day 12 of admission

After 0.6 g of clindamycin through an intravenous drip twice a day, the patient's body temperature dropped significantly on the first day of treatment. During the treatment, it was suspected that the antibacterial treatment and body temperature drop were coincidental. Clindamycin was discontinued after two days of treatment, but the patient's body temperature increased the day after discontinuation. Two days after discontinuation, her body temperature jumped to 39.2°C again. Clindamycin was immediately re-applied, and her body temperature dropped significantly. On day 12, it was 37.7°C. The patient did not complain of discomfort, and no positive signs were found in an examination of her nervous system. Blood culture was performed after clindamycin treatment, and no bacterial growth was reported. That same day, a B-ultrasound examination showed that splenic tissues had mostly disappeared. Only a small amount of tissue remained in the splenic hilum, which was replaced by a liquid mass.

Thinking prompts: The patient's body temperature dropped significantly after treatment with clindamycin, especially after transient discontinuation. It rose again, then dropped quickly after re-application of clindamycin, which confirms an infection of Gram-positive bacteria complicated with a spleen abscess on the basis of encephalitis caused by Coxsackie virus. The source of the bacteria is considered to be the throat. Few reports exist of splenic abscesses. Since 1990, only around 100 cases have been reported. In this case, the liver, gallbladder, and spleen were normal on B-ultrasound at admission. The left subphrenic effusion occurred after one week, then the splenic tissues almost completely disappeared, which indicated the necessity of re-examining routine examinations when the cause of fever was unclear. The general surgery department was consulted immediately to remove the splenic abscess, otherwise it would likely have ruptured spontaneously, causing intra-abdominal infection and adhesion. So, how did the patient acquire a splenic abscess? Retrospective analysis shows that her immunity decreased after Coxsackie encephalitis and hepatitis, which caused Gram-positive bacteria such as Streptococcus to invade the blood from the throat. This resulted in bacteremia, i.e., bacteria remaining in the spleen, causing an abscess.

VIII. Discharge from hospital

No spleen abscesses were found during surgery, but a large liquid mass was found in the spleen area. The splenic hilar vessels were ligated, and the mass was taken out. When the mass was cut out, yellow-green liquid was found, which was sent for bacteria culture, but no bacterial growth was discovered. Two weeks after surgery, the patient recovered and was discharged.

IX. Lessons learned

1. The diagnosis of an infectious disease is often related to its four characteristics. The general principles of each textbook on infectious diseases will detail the spectrum, pathogenesis, common clinical manifestations, stage manifestations, and characteristics of each disease, and will lay out the basic concepts. When studying the various theories about infectious diseases, we should always think about the general theory, and draw inferences from others.
2. Consider or exclude bacterial infection, and perform an etiological examination before treatment. Otherwise, antibiotics will affect the culture results.
3. Choose antibiotics for diagnostic treatment with a narrow antibacterial spectrum, so as not to interfere with retrospective analysis, cause confusion, or hinder the accumulation of clinical experience.

(He Jianqin & Li Lanjuan)

Fever, fatigue, loss of appetite, with yellow urine for seven days

I. Medical history

Patient: Female, 4 years old, from the town of Shengfang in Hebei Province. She was hospitalized with fever, fatigue, loss of appetite, and dark yellow urine for seven days. She was at our hospital between 16 January and 15 February 2008.

Seven days previously, the pediatric patient had developed a fever without obvious origin, with a peak body temperature of 38.8°C, no chills and no intolerance of cold, no pharyngalgia, cough, expectoration, abdominal pain, diarrhea, frequent micturition, urgency, and pain. She was suffering fatigue and loss of appetite, and her food intake had decreased by a third compared with before, accompanied by nausea and several occurrences of vomiting. The vomit was gastric contents, and was non-projectile. Her urine was darker yellow than normal. The patient had visited a local clinic six days earlier, and was diagnosed with an upper respiratory tract infection. After an intramuscular injection of Alidine was given, her body temperature dropped slightly, but it did not return to normal, and fluctuated around 38°C. She took a course of oral amoxicillin for two days, and later changed to an anti-inflammatory treatment with ceftazidime for three days (the specific use of the drug is unknown). However, her body temperature was not controlled, and her urine color darkened further. Therefore, she was transferred to a hospital for treatment, where she was checked for abnormal liver function, and diagnosed with suspected hepatitis. She was transferred to our hospital and admitted through the outpatient service.

The patient was in a good physical condition and had no history of hepatitis or family history of liver disease or hereditary illnesses. She denied any contact with similar patients, and had no history of drug or food allergies. She had not received her immunizations at the right time.

> **Thinking prompts:** Asking for a patient's medical history is a diagnostic method that is used to understand the occurrence and progress of diseases in detail. A preliminary clinical judgment can be made after analysis, synthesis, and comprehensive thinking. It should include the onset of the disease, the main symptoms, etiology and inducement, the development and evolution of the disease, accompanying symptoms, diagnosis and treatment, and the general situation in the course of the disease.

First of all, in view of the chief complaint, we should inquire further about whether the onset was slow or acute, as well as the etiology or inducement, all of which have a bearing on diagnosis. The patient in case had a rapid onset, and a history of only seven days. There was no obvious cause or inducement before the onset of the disease, so the preliminary judgment is that the disease may either be acute, or an acute attack of a chronic disease. Secondly, the patient's first symptoms appeared almost at the same time. However, fever should be the entry point for asking about medical history. Note the length of fever and whether the onset was slow or acute, and whether there is an aversion to cold, chills, or sweating. For example, chills are often the first symptom of septicemia. Inquire about the pattern of body temperature changes, so that the fever type can be analyzed. Note that due to the wide application of antipyretics and antibiotics in clinics, the fever type of some illnesses can become atypical. The accompanying symptoms of fever are very important for judging the location of a lesion and analyzing the nature of a disease. For example, the patient in this case had no cough, expectoration, abdominal pain, diarrhea, frequent micturition, urgent micturition, and pain. The preliminary judgment was that there is no basis for diagnosing an infection of the respiratory tract, digestive tract, and urinary system at the onset of the disease, but the skin, lymph nodes, pharynx, heart, lungs, liver, spleen, and nervous system should also be examined. Fever is often the first manifestation of acute infectious diseases, so we should inquire about the patient's contact history and diet in detail, paying attention to the season and geographical location of the onset. Fatigue is often one of the accompanying symptoms of fever, and is characterized by endotoxemia or viremia in infectious diseases. Loss of appetite and nausea are digestive tract symptoms that often occur in the course of various diseases. If the patient has vomited, inquire about the time of occurrence, as well as inducing factors, the patient's relationship with food, drugs, and mental factors, and the characteristics of the vomiting. Intracranial high-pressure vomiting (projectile), often without a nausea aura, and signs of meningeal irritation can be picked up during physical examination. Jaundice can be three clinical types: Hemolytic, hepatocyte, and obstructive. In addition to noting the characteristics of jaundice, we can ask about the above three aspects. Jaundice accompanied by fever is more common in septicemia, acute icteric hepatitis, biliary ascaris, and hemolytic jaundice. The nature and color of urine and feces have certain implications for diagnosis. For example, with hemolytic jaundice, the urine is mostly the color of soy sauce. With hepatocellular jaundice, it is a strong tea color. The stool can be gray-white with obstructive jaundice, so attention should be paid to this during your inquiries. Look out for anemia, bleeding from the skin mucus, liver palm, spider nevus, and varicose veins in the abdominal wall. Also check the superficial lymph nodes, and look for liver and spleen enlargement, as well as masses in the gallbladder and abdomen through palpation. Hepatomegaly (strong but pliable in texture and tenderness) is common in acute hepatitis. Percussion can be used to identify ascites, which are common in hepatobiliary diseases.

In addition to understanding the occurrence and development of diseases, diagnosis, and treatment in the course of an illness are also very important. If the etiology of fever has not been determined, the application of antipyretics and antibiotics often interferes with the diagnosis, and makes subsequent treatment more difficult, especially for infectious diseases. The antibiotics used in the past are particularly important for clarifying the pathogen and guiding the application of antibiotics in the future.

II. Physical examination on admission

T 37.2°C, P 92 times/min, R 22 times/min, BP 90/60 mmHg, conscious, cried from time to time, uncooperative with physical examination, slight yellow staining of the skin sclera, no rash, pigmentation, bleeding spots, and spider moles all over the body, no superficial lymph nodes all over the body; pharyngeal congestion, bilateral II-degree enlargement of the tonsil without purulent secretions, soft neck, no resistance, no abnormality in cardiopulmonary auscultation, flat abdomen, no abdominal wall varicose veins, soft abdomen, no tenderness or rebound pain in the whole abdomen; liver and spleen palpable below the costal margin with discomfort, negative abdominal shifting dullness, and no finger concave edema in either of the lower limbs. No liver palm. Presence of physiological reflexes such as abdominal wall reflex and biceps brachii reflex, but pathological reflexes such as Kernig's sign and Brudzinski's sign were not elicited.

> **Thinking prompts:** To gain a better understanding of the patient's medical history and physical condition, perform a routine blood test, a c-reactive protein, ESR, and PPD test, blood culture, and Widal test to prompt viral or non-viral infection. Check the urine and stool to rule out an infection of the urinary system or intestinal tract. Check the liver function and myocardial enzymes for damage to liver cells and myocardial cells. Check virus typing (enzyme-linked immunosorbent) and the five types of hepatitis B (electrochemiluminescence immunoassay) to understand the common hepatotrophic and non-hepatophilic virus infections that cause abnormal liver function. Compared with enzyme-linked immunosorbent assay (ELISA), electrochemiluminescence immunoassay has the advantages of specificity of immunological reaction, sensitivity, precision, and accuracy of luminescence. It is one of the most sensitive indices for determining whether there is a hepatitis B virus infection.
>
> Because this patient had pharyngeal congestion and bilateral tonsil enlargement, a throat swab secretion culture should be performed to rule out bacterial and fungal infection of the respiratory tract. If septicemia occurs, there may be a local infection. Chest X-ray and abdominal color Doppler ultrasound

should be checked. Routine ECG should be performed to check for myocardial injury.

III. Auxiliary examination on admission

Routine blood test: WBC 27.46 × 10⁹/L, N 25%, L 62.6%, Hb 110 g/L, RBC 4.22 × 10¹²/L, PLT 167 × 10⁹/L, abnormal lymphocytes 11%.

Liver function: ALT 360.7 U/L, AST 205.9 U/L, GGT 244.2 U/L, ALP 538.7 U/L, A 34.4 g/L, TB 28.6 μmol/L.

Myocardial enzymes: LDH 818.1 U/L, CK 132.9 μmol/L, CK-MB 56 U/L, α-HBDH 724.4 U/L.

Virus typing (ELISA): HAV-IgM, HBsAg, anti-HCV, HDV-Ab, CMV-IgM and EBV-IgM all negative.

HBV immunological markers (electro chemiluminescence immunoassay): HBsAb positive, others negative.

No pathogenic bacteria were found in the throat swab secretion culture, and the blood culture and PPD test were negative many times over. The Widal test, ESR, C-reactive protein, routine urine, routine stool, chest X-ray, abdominal color Doppler ultrasound, and electrocardiogram were all normal.

IV. Ward-round analysis on admission

1. Preliminary diagnosis

The patient had an acute onset with an illness course of one week. The clinical manifestations were mainly fever and abnormal liver function. From the analysis of current laboratory tests, the specific causes were not clear. First of all, the duration of the fever and the fluctuations in body temperature did not constitute a diagnosis of fever to be investigated. However, due to the unclear cause of abnormal liver function, the patient was initially diagnosed with abnormal liver function. Fever can be infectious and non-infectious, and the causes of abnormal liver function can also be distinguished in this way.

Thinking prompts: There are many causes of fever, but generally speaking, there are two categories: Infectious and non-infectious diseases. Infections caused by various pathogens, (whether acute, subacute or chronic, local or systemic) can cause fever, such as viruses, bacteria, fungi, mycoplasma, chlamydia, spirochetes, and parasites. Non-infectious fever is more common in aseptic tissue damage, absorption of necrotic substances, antigen-antibody reaction, and endocrine and metabolic disorders. However, the duration of the fever in this case was under two weeks. It seems unreasonable to take the cause of fever as the starting point for diagnosis. Therefore, it is possible to identify infectious and non-infectious diseases one by one from the common causes of liver function damage combined with the causes of fever. The former is mainly viral hepatitis caused by hepatotropic virus, and EB virus, cytomegalovirus, mycobacterium tuberculosis, fungi, and parasites that mainly affect the liver. The latter includes alcohol, drugs, toxic liver diseases, and congenital metabolic liver diseases such as Wilson disease, α1-antitrypsin deficiency, and hemochromatosis.

2. Diagnostic thinking

(1) Non-infectious diseases

1) Alcohol, drugs, and toxic liver diseases: Firstly, it is easy to rule out alcohol-induced liver diseases. Although drugs and toxic liver injuries have received a lot of scholarly attention all over the world, they are often ignored or misdiagnosed in practical work. This is because the clinical manifestations of drug-induced liver disease are diverse, and can be manifested as acute or chronic liver cell injury, cholestasis, and vascular disease. The time from the onset of symptoms to receiving medication can be as short as four days or as long as eight weeks, and some people even present after seven days of withdrawal. However, liver cell injury can last as long as two months after drug withdrawal. On the other hand, clinicians have an insufficient understanding of drug-induced liver diseases. When patients are found to have abnormal liver enzymes, if the serum virus markers are negative, they are often diagnosed with non-A-E hepatitis or viral hepatitis with unknown causes, ignoring their history of drug taking. The patient in this case had taken medication at the beginning of her illness, but had no clear history of toxic contact. Her recent course of medication had been given after digestive tract symptoms appeared, but the non-hepatotropic virus infection had not yet been excluded, so drugs and toxic liver diseases were not considered for the time being.

2) Wilson's disease, α1-antitrypsin deficiency, and hemochromatosis in metabolic diseases: ① Patients with Wilson's disease have various manifestations of liver disease, which can be chronic hepatitis of unknown origin or fulminant liver diseases (very rare), the latter usually complicated with hemolytic anemia. The results of liver biopsy are inconsistent with laboratory changes, and some patients may have issues with their nervous system, bones, kidneys, and even heart as the first symptom. Therefore, for all patients with unexplained liver diseases under 30 years old, Wilson's disease should be considered as a possibility. Usually, a diagnosis of Wilson's disease is based on a decrease of the corneal Kayser-Fleischer (KF) ring and serum ceruloplasmin, and an increase of copper in the urine. However, the former can only be seen under a slit lamp. If patients have only liver disease but no symptoms of the nervous system, young patients (50%) can have no K-F ring, and the serum ceruloplasmin level of 5% does not decrease (> 20 mg/ml). In addition, due to incorrect urine sampling, unclean containers, or careless operation, the copper excretion in the urine can be less than 50–100 μg in a 24-hour period. However, some patients who do not have Wilson's disease may also have a decrease of the corneal Kayser-Fleischer (KF), decreased serum ceruloplasmin, and increased copper in the urine, but these conditions generally do not occur at the same time. In highly suspicious cases, multiple indices should be detected together, and a liver biopsy should be performed to measure the copper content of the liver tissue to aid diagnosis. Although the cause of abnormal liver function in this case was not clear, the patient

still had a fever and enlarged lymph nodes. Hematology showed that the number of abnormal lymphocytes had increased. These symptoms cannot be explained by Wilson's disease, and therefore, it is not currently being considered. ② α1-antitrypsin deficiency is common in older pediatric patients with chronic active hepatitis or liver cirrhosis, who may have a family history as well as a cough, shortness of breath, and repeated pulmonary infection. When the disease progresses, there may be abnormal transaminase, a significant increase in ALP, and a decrease in albumin. Protein electrophoresis can prompt α1 globulin to decrease. If necessary, the α1-AT content can be determined and Pi phenotype analysis can be used to confirm the diagnosis. Although the patient in this case had abnormal liver function in the clinic, this did not indicate an albumin decrease. The patient had no accompanying respiratory symptoms, so a diagnosis basis of α1-antitrypsin deficiency was not made. ③ Hemochromatosis is a group of rare congenital metabolic defects that are caused by excessive iron deposits in the liver, pancreas, heart, spleen, and skin, which lead to the destruction of parenchymal cells in varying degrees, as well as extensive fibrous tissue hyperplasia and organ dysfunction. Hemochromatosis usually involves the liver, and is manifested as hepatomegaly or abnormal liver function, while skin pigmentation is often the first symptom, and liver biopsy can aid diagnosis. In this case, in addition to abnormal liver function, a fever, enlarged lymph nodes, and abnormal hemogram can be seen in secondary hemochromatosis infection, but it is not the first manifestation, so the possibility of hemochromatosis can be ruled out.

(2) Infectious diseases

1) Viral hepatitis caused by a hepatotropic viral infection: The characteristics of hepatitis A are as follows: The incidence of hepatitis A is high in children who are not vaccinated on time. It is mostly spread in daily activities, because HAV enters the body through the mouth. It goes into the blood stream through the intestine causing viremia, and it will reach the liver in about a week. HAV replicates in the liver and also enters the blood circulation, causing low-concentration viremia. Therefore, fever and aversion to cold may appear at the beginning of the illness, lasting for about a week. After that, liver cell damage begins to appear. HAV may cause liver cell damage through immune mediation rather than directly. At this time, digestive tract symptoms and other pre-jaundice symptoms may appear such as loss of appetite, nausea, and vomiting, and serum ALT increases significantly. Etiological examination can show that anti-HAV-IgM is positive. Anti-HAV-IgG is negative in the acute stage, and turns positive in the recovery stage. In this case, there were digestive tract symptoms and fever at the onset of the illness. In the first week, transaminase showed a slight increase, but the virus typing examination showed that anti-HAV-IgM was negative. Viral hepatitis A infection would not cause more than 10% abnormal lymphocytes, so a diagnosis of acute hepatitis A could not be considered.

2) CMV infection: CMV is an infectious disease caused by the human cytomegalovirus. CMV infection is widespread in China, and mostly occurs in infants and young children. Because the digestive system is most frequently affected by CMV, CMV hepatitis is common. However, CMV infection cannot be diagnosed by clinical manifestations. Diagnosis should be assisted by

virus isolation or serum antibody level. Acquired infections mostly occur in pediatric patients with immunodeficiency, who may show hepatitis and mononucleosis. However, in this case the serum anti-CMV-IgM was negative, indicating that there is no active infection. Because of immune deficiency, or because young pediatric patients have a low ability to produce antibodies, false positives may appear. Molecular hybridization or PCR can be used to detect CMV mRNA or DNA-specific CMV fragments from blood samples to rule out the possibility of CMV infection.

3) Mycobacterium tuberculosis and fungal and parasitic infections: ① A primary infection of mycobacterium tuberculosis, which is common in children, usually starts in the lungs, and may manifest as a cough, expectoration, and low fever. A chest radiograph can indicate a dumbbell shadow, which is called a primary syndrome. A PPD test will be positive. However, the patient in this case did not have the above symptoms and imaging manifestations, and many PPD tests were negative after admission, so the possibility of mycobacterium tuberculosis infection was not considered; ② Fungal infections are generally seen in patients who have been treated with antibiotics for a long time or have low immunity, and the focus of the infection is mostly in the oral cavity and respiratory tract. There may be oral leukoplakia and dry and moist rales in both lungs, and there is no increase in white blood cells in general. In this case, fungal infection should not be considered; ③ Parasitic infections are either protozoa or helminth infections. In addition to the epidemiological history of mosquito bites, animal scratches, or contact with infected water, a hemogram can show a change in the mononuclear phagocyte system with a significant increase in eosinophils. This is not consistent with the patient's condition in this case, and was not considered.

4) Infectious mononucleosis (IM) is more likely to be considered: EBV infection mostly occurs in children and adolescents, and spreads through close oral contact. Patients in some cases have an unknown contact history, and may have clinical manifestations such as fever, sore throat, and hepatosplenomegaly. 70% of patients may have obviously enlarged lymph nodes, occurring about a week into the course of disease. Around one-third of cases have macules, papules, skin bleeding spots, or erythematous eruptions from scarlet fever. Myocarditis can also occur. The most prominent feature of infectious mononucleosis is that the mononuclear phagocyte system is involved, lymphocytes in the peripheral blood are obviously increased, and abnormal lymphocytes appear. EBV antibodies can appear in the serum. A heterophile agglutination test can be partially positive, and EBV DNA can be used when necessary. Because it is a self-limiting disease, the prognosis is good, and symptomatic treatment is used instead of special treatment. Antibiotic treatment is ineffective for EBV. When liver injury occurs, it can be treated as viral hepatitis. If streptococcal infection is secondary, penicillin should not be used, because the probability of a polymorphic rash after use is significantly increased.

In this case, the patient is part of an EBV-susceptible population. Although her contact history is unknown, she presented with a fever and abnormal liver function. After the first ward-round after admission, a physical examination found several enlarged soybean-sized lymph nodes at the front of the neck, back of the neck, and groin. They were movable and painless, and did not adhere to the surrounding tissue. In addition, a routine blood test showed that white blood cells were significantly increased, abnormal lymphocytes were higher than 10%, and antibiotics such as penicillin and cephalosporins were ineffective, so the possibility of infectious mononucleosis should be considered.

Because the hospital virus typing system uses enzyme-linked immunosorbent assay (ELISA), and the sensitivity of reagents is not high enough to judge EBV-infected people with low antibody titers, immunofluorescence can be used to detect heterophile antibodies and EBV-specific antibodies. This is also helpful to diagnose EBV infections with negative heterophile antibodies, and to detect EBV DNA by a polymerase chain reaction. Compared with in situ hybridization, this method has the advantages of sensitivity, rapidity, and high specificity. Continuous blood tests can observe changes to the leukocytes and abnormal lymphocytes, and can clarify whether it affects platelets during the course of the illness. Because the disease is self-limiting, it can also become severe. Early symptomatic treatment should be given for abnormal liver function and increased myocardial enzymes, and drugs should be administered to protect the functions of various organs if necessary, in order to restore organ function and prevent multiple organ failure. Antiviral therapies such as interferon, acyclovir, adenine arabinoside, famciclovir, and ganciclovir may also be tried. The patient's condition will be observed according to the treatment, and further laboratory tests will be required to confirm the diagnosis. Because the patient has used penicillin, attention should be paid to whether she develops a rash in the course of the disease, to inform the diagnosis basis.

V. Ward-round analysis on day seven after admission

After admission, the patient's infectious mononucleosis improved, and the examination results showed that the heterotropic antibody-IgM was negative, the EBV specific antibody-IgM was positive, and the EBV DNA test was positive. On the ninth day of the illness (the second day after admission), red macules and papules appeared on the patient's face, accompanied by itching (excluding drug allergy). A series of rashes began to merge, so the diagnosis of infectious mononucleosis was considered to be valid.

Since admission, compound glycyrrhizin (40 mg once a day) and glutathione (0.6 g once a day) were given intravenously to protect the liver, reduce enzymes, and protect organ function. After three days, the patient's body temperature did not return to normal, peaking at 37.8°C. After seven days, a routine blood test showed that the white blood cells had returned to normal. No abnormal lymphocytes were found, but the liver function showed that transaminase was significantly higher than before, and jaundice was not significantly higher. In view of the poor efficacy of conventional hepatoprotective drugs, there have been reports about cases of liver cell necrosis and even death due to liver failure after EBV infection. Pediatric patients under five years old with EBV infections are mostly suffering from recessive infections, and symptomatic infections mostly occur in adolescents. However, the patient in case is young. If the EBV infection is not controlled, it will cause issues with the liver, kidneys, bone marrow, and nervous system, and the prognosis may be poor. Interferon – a low-molecular-weight protein with broad-spectrum antiviral effect produced by the human body – can enhance the body's immune system, and can be used for the defense and adjuvant treatment of various viral diseases. It exerts a curative effect through antiviral treatment and immunomodulation. A small dose of interferon is safe for children, so interferon α-2B is injected intramuscularly (1 million U) every other day. Interferon can have side effects such as fever, inhibition of the hematopoietic bone marrow system, and liver function fluctuation. Therefore, changes to the body temperature, routine blood work, and liver function should be monitored regularly during treatment.

VI. Condition at discharge (28 days after admission)

On the day of the interferon treatment, the patient's body temperature rose to 38.8°C, without chills and other accompanying symptoms. The next day's routine blood examination showed that the white blood cells were lower than before, but still within the normal range, and the platelets were normal. The original treatment plan was continued. After that, the routine blood examination was conducted once every three days. The white blood cells had dropped below 4.0×10^9/L, and the patient's body temperature gradually decreased, fluctuating from 36.4°C to 37°C. After a week of interferon, liver function was rechecked. ALT was up to 400 U/L, and compound glycyrrhizin dosage was increased. After two weeks of interferon, the patient's body temperature was normal. Her digestive tract symptoms had significantly improved, as had her appetite. The rash had subsided. Her neck and inguinal lymph nodes were still swollen, and her pharynx was free of congestion. Her bilateral tonsils were enlarged to degree I without purulent secretion. After re-examination, her liver function had significantly improved. ALT had recovered to 120 U/L, but had still not returned to normal. Routine blood work returned to normal, and no abnormal lymphocytes were found.

VII. Follow-up

After discharge, compound glycyrrhizin (25 mg) was taken orally twice a day. Because the disease may recur, low fever, fatigue, and enlargement of the lymph nodes may last for weeks or months in some patients. Complications such as hemolytic anemia and thrombocytopenic purpura may occur, so a follow-up of the prognosis should be performed. After discharge, the patient's body temperature remained normal, and she did not experience fatigue, loss of appetite, or yellow urine. Her enlarged lymph nodes gradually reduced. Routine blood work was normal at two weeks, one month, three months, and six months after discharge, without anemia and thrombocytopenia, and her liver function returned to normal after one month.

VIII. Lessons learned

In the early stage of the illness, the first symptoms were fever and digestive tract issues. Without the typical manifestations of infectious mononucleosis and the support of related laboratory tests, the case was easily misdiagnosed as a respiratory tract infection. For diagnosis and treatment, the case should be analyzed in a monistic manner, starting with the common causes of fever, abnormal liver function, and abnormal lymphocyte proliferation. It should focus on the causes of abnormal liver function, taking fever and abnormal hemogram as a breakthrough at first. It should consider the possibility of liver injury caused by infectious diseases first. The successive occurrence of lymphadenopathy and rashes in the course of the illness add to the basis for diagnosis.

In addition to abnormal liver function, the hemogram is obviously abnormal. Abnormal lymphocytes have significantly increased, which is not a characteristic of hepatitis A cytomegalovirus. Mycobacterium tuberculosis, fungal and parasitic infection, and the results of etiological and serological examination do not support the above diagnosis. The insensitivity of conventional reagents is another reason why an early diagnosis cannot be made. Even if the EBV specific antibody is positive, further etiological examination should be carried out, because some autoimmune diseases and viral infections may cause false positives for this antibody. About 90% of patients test positive for heterotropic antibody-IgM, and about 5%–10% do not have an agglutination reaction (perhaps no agglutination antibody existed). The false positive rate is less than 10%, mostly due to technical errors. However, in pediatric patients under 4 years old, the positive rate is only 50% and the titer is low. The final confirmation of the diagnosis of infectious mononucleosis is the determination of EBV DNA by PCR.

As for treatment, cases of fever with obviously elevated white blood cells are easy to misdiagnose as bacterial infections to be treated with antibiotics. Infectious mononucleosis does not respond well to antibiotics, and the appearance of polymorphic rash increases in the course of the illness. Even if it is helpful for future diagnosis, it is not recommended to abuse or use irregular drugs without a clear etiological examination. Organ function protection therapy and timely antiviral therapy can reduce the incidence of liver failure and related complications, but the exact efficacy of interferon in the treatment of infectious mononucleosis has yet to be confirmed.

The cases encountered in clinical work cannot cover the typical manifestations of infectious mononucleosis, such as fever, sore throat, hepatosplenomegaly, rash, and increased abnormal lymphocytes. Therefore, doctors should inquire and check carefully as soon as patients are admitted, as this is easily overlooked by young clinicians. It is very important to check the patient's condition in good time, and understand any changes, so as to collect valuable information for diagnosis and give effective treatment at an early stage.

(Cao Wukui)

Fever and headache for five days, rash for one day

I. Medical history

Patient: Female, 28 years old, from Guangzhou. She was admitted to hospital on 21 September 2007 and stayed until 27 September, suffering from fever, headache for five days, and a rash for one day.

Five days earlier, the patient developed chills and fever, and her body temperature increased rapidly to 40.5°C, accompanied by a headache, nasal congestion, pain in all muscles, eyes, and joints, poor appetite, nausea and vomiting, which were obvious after eating. The vomit consisted of stomach contents, without blood or a coffee-like substance, cough, expectoration, and low back pain. She was treated in two hospitals with ribavirin, lomefloxacin, and loxoprofen, but her condition did not improve. Two days earlier, a densely distributed needle-like rash appeared on her whole body, accompanied by itching. She went to the dermatology department of our hospital for treatment, and was admitted to our department as an outpatient to investigate her fever and rash. Since the onset of her illness, the patient had been in normal spirits and was sleeping as usual, and had no sore throat, cough, expectoration, chest stuffiness, shortness of breath, abdominal pain or diarrhea, and no frequent, urgent or painful urination She displayed no mental and behavioral abnormalities, and her urination and defecation were normal.

Thinking prompts: The main problem with this patient is fever rash. To understand her medical history, we should ask for details about the onset of the fever and rash – whether it was acute or slow, the type of fever, whether it came after pyretolysis (dengue fever is mostly acute onset, but there may be a double-peak fever), and whether there are obvious toxic blood symptoms such as chills, headache, arthralgia, and digestive tract issues. If the rash appeared after the fever, what were its sequence and quantity? Was it accompanied by itching, and what type of rash was it (the typical dengue fever rash usually appears 3–6 days after fever, and can be polymorphic, such as maculopapules, measles-like rash, Scarlatiniform rash, erythematous eruption or subcutaneous hemorrhage)? What was its distribution (the typical dengue fever rash is mostly distributed on trunk, limbs, or head and face, and often does not appear on the palms and soles)? As for medical treatment, questions should focus on whether antibacterials have been used, their effect, and whether the patient's condition has changed (aggravation or improvement), or new symptoms (this case is a viral disease, and the effects of antibacterial treatment are often difficult to perceive, so the anti-dengue virus effect of ribavirin cannot be determined).

Gathering medical history and performing physical examination should also include asking whether there are similar cases in or around the patient's home, to find out whether there is evidence of a phenomenon called aggregation (common with dengue fever). Ask whether the patient has sat or lain in grass, to identify tsutsugamushi disease. Ask whether there are mice in the houses in her neighborhood, and whether there is any change in urine volume to identify hemorrhagic fever with renal syndrome. Ask whether she has had measles or the measles vaccination, and inquire whether she has been in contact with infected water. Check the tenderness of her gastrocnemius muscle to identify leptospirosis. Ask whether she has any allergies to drugs and foods, to distinguish it from a drug rash. Physical examination should also include a capillary fragility test to identify whether there is obvious hair cell vascular damage. This can help with the diagnosis of dengue fever.

II. Physical examination on admission

T 38.5°C, R 18 times/min, P 78 times/min, BP 128/72 mmHg, acute sickly look, mental fatigue, flushed skin on face and chest, densely distributed needle-like papules on the trunk and proximal extremities, color fading under pressure, no bleeding and desquamation, slight congestion of bulbar conjunctiva, no eschar or ulcer anywhere on her skin; multiple enlarged lymph nodes can be touched in the bilateral groin, with a diameter of about 5–10 m., which were hard, movable, and not tender; no abnormality was found in the physical examination of the heart, the breath sounds of both lungs were clear, and no dry and moist rales were heard. The abdomen was flat and soft; the liver and spleen could not be palpated below the costal margin, and shifting dullness was negative. There was no percussion pain in either kidney area. No positive signs were found in the nervous system.

III. Auxiliary examination on admission

Routine blood test: RBC 5.02×10^{12}/L, Hb 152 g/L, WBC 2.61×10^9/L, N 36%, L 30%, M 24%; PLT 75×10^9/L.

Eight biochemical items: AST 60 U/L, ALT 78 U/L, A 38 g/L, K^+ 3.18 mmol/L, Cr 70.8 μmol/L, BUN 2.31 mmol/L, CRP 43.9 mg/L and ESR 25 mm/h.

Chest X-ray: There was no abnormality in either lung.

Thinking prompts: On the basis of acquiring a complete medical history and physical examination, routine blood examination is helpful to distinguish bacterial infections or viral infections. The total number of white blood cells in the former is increased, and is normal or decreased in the latter. However, some cases are exceptional. Viral diseases such as epidemic hemorrhagic fever and Japanese encephalitis may cause an increase in the total number of white blood cells, while bacterial diseases such as typhoid fever and gram-negative septicemia may cause a decrease in the number of white blood cells). Routine blood tests also help to observe the presence of hemoconcentration, increased hematocrit with decreased platelets for early detection, and diagnosis of dengue and hemorrhagic fever. Biochemical blood tests can help us to perceive liver and kidney damage, make a differential diagnosis, and more importantly monitor the severity of the disease. C-reactive protein, the erythrocyte sedimentation rate, a PPD test, and a typhoid lipopolysaccharide antibody (LPS-PHA) test can indicate viral or non-viral infection, or Mycobacterium tuberculosis or Typhoid Bacillus infection, as can a complete set of antinuclear antibodies (ANA), and an anti-neutrophil antibody (ANCA) test, to eliminate the possibility of autoimmune diseases. Bacteria 2 (Widal test and Weil-Felix test) blood culture can eliminate the possibility of bacterial infection. Perform a chest X-ray to identify a lung infection or pneumonia. Leptospirosis antibodies and hemorrhagic fever antibodies should also be tested with a leptospirosis agglutination test, to distinguish them from common febrile diseases in this area.

IV. Ward-round analysis on admission

Initial diagnosis: The patient had a persistent high fever with obvious symptoms of systemic poisoning. After four days of fever, a whole-body rash appeared. The cause was unknown, and the patient was diagnosed with a fever and rash, to be investigated.

> **Thinking prompts:** Clinical diagnosis should focus on the diagnosis and differentiation of acute fever with rash.
>
> **Step 1:** Distinguish between infectious and non-infectious diseases, and identify which kind of non-infectious diseases they should be distinguished from. According to the patient's acute onset, fever, rash, swollen lymph nodes, and systemic poisoning symptoms such as chills and severe digestive tract poisoning symptoms, the first consideration is that she has an infectious disease. In non-infectious diseases, attention should be paid to rashes of rheumatic diseases such as systemic lupus erythematosus, especially if the patient is female. However, rashes in patients with rheumatic diseases generally appear at the same time as fever, and the poisoning symptoms are not serious, but are often accompanied by multiple organ damage such as kidney. In addition, this patient developed a rash after receiving treatment, and had a history of using antipyretics, so we should note the possibility of a drug rash.
>
> **Step 2:** Which common infectious diseases can cause fever and rashes? Viral diseases such as dengue fever, measles, rubella, chickenpox, and epidemic hemorrhagic fever; bacterial diseases such as scarlet fever, typhoid fever, and septicemia; Rickettsia diseases such as epidemic typhus, local endemic typhus, and tsutsugamushi disease. Leptospirosis can also cause fever and often bleeding rashes, but it is mainly caused by kidney damage, with a history of contact with infected water. Parasitic diseases,

such as worm larvae migratory disease, may also cause recurrent fever with a mild and only slightly itchy rash, which may be migratory. This is not the case for the patient in question here.

Step 3: From the epidemiological data (age at onset, season of onset, region), clinical manifestations such as fever, accompanying symptoms, rash characteristics, signs, and preliminary laboratory examination, a careful analysis is made:

1. Bacterial diseases: scarlet fever, epidemic cerebrospinal meningitis, septicemia, and typhoid fever

(1) Scarlet fever: The rash usually appears on the second day of the fever, accompanied by an obvious sore throat, and blood tests will show that the proportion of leukocytes and neutrophils has increased. In this case, the rash appeared four days after the fever, and the ratio of leukocytes to neutrophils decreased. This did not match the clinical manifestation of scarlet fever, so the possibility could be ruled out.

(2) Epidemic cerebrospinal meningitis: It is more common in winter and spring, particularly when there are cases in the local area or a history of contact with patients. The rash is characterized by petechia and ecchymosis of the skin mucosa. The main clinical manifestations are sudden chills, high fever, headache, vomiting, and meningeal irritation. Severe cases include septic shock, convulsions, disturbance of consciousness, rapid-onset coma, and respiratory failure. Laboratory examination will show that white blood cells and neutrophils have increased significantly, and the cerebrospinal fluid will show suppurative changes. A definitive diagnosis can be made from a blood culture and cerebrospinal fluid culture.

(3) Septicemia: Fever with a mostly hemorrhagic rash may also occur (petechiae and ecchymosis are the most common), with many primary lesions. Rashes are common in gram-positive bacterial septicemia, so white blood cells are obviously increased.

(4) Typhoid fever: Fever may be accompanied by leukopenia and liver damage. However, typhoid fever is usually not accompanied by obvious chills, and the rash occurs later, mostly on the 6th to tenth day after the onset of fever. The rash is rosy in character, small in number, and pale in color, and is mainly distributed in the trunk, often accompanied by abdominal distension, constipation, diarrhea, and other symptoms of digestive tract poisoning. The clinical manifestation of this case is inconsistent with typhoid fever.

2. Viral diseases such as chickenpox, measles, rubella, and dengue fever

(1) Varicella: The rash can occur on the first day of the fever, typically with papules, herpes, pustules, and eschar. This is inconsistent with the symptoms of this patient, so it is easy to rule out.

(2) Rubella: The rash occurs on the first or second day after the fever, and the

general symptoms are mild, often accompanied by swollen lymph nodes behind ears, occiput, and neck. It can be ruled out in this case.

(3) Measles: Catarrhal symptoms usually accompanied by respiratory tract issues. When a rash occurs, it comes out in 3–5 days, starting behind ears and then moving to the hairline, forehead, face, neck, chest, back, abdomen, and limbs. The rash varies in shape and size. It stands out from the skin, and mostly occurs in winter and spring. Therefore, measles can be ruled out in this case.

(4) Dengue fever: The epidemic season of dengue fever is summer and autumn in Guangzhou. The virus is transmitted by Aedes mosquitoes. The clinical manifestations are high fever, aversion to cold, chills with obvious poisoning symptoms, headaches, pain in the muscles and joints, and extreme fatigue. The rash appears on the third to sixth day of fever, and may be measles-like or scarlet fever-like, with obvious itching. It subsides in 3–4 days, without pigmentation and desquamation. Bleeding may occur from the fifth to eighth day of the disease, including gingival bleeding, epistaxis, hemoptysis, gastrointestinal bleeding, urinary tract bleeding, abdominal hemorrhage, and visceral hemorrhage. Laboratory examination shows that leukocytes and platelets decrease, which may be accompanied by a slight increase of transaminase. Dengue fever is a viral infection for which antibiotic treatment is ineffective, and general antipyretic and analgesic drugs have a poor reaction.

3. Rickettsial diseases: epidemic typhus, local endemic typhus, and tsutsugamushi disease

(1) Epidemic typhus: It occurs frequently in cold seasons in cold regions, mostly in situations of war, famine, and poor personal hygiene. Most typhus rashes are bright red congestive maculopapular, and exist in isolation and do not fuse. These characteristics, and the fact that there is no epidemic typhus in Guangzhou, mean that this possibility can be ruled out.

(2) Local endemic typhus: Due to the characteristics of the rash and epidemiological data, it can also be ruled out.

(3) Tsutsugamushi disease: Guangzhou is an epidemic area of tsutsugamushi disease. It is characterized by typical eschar, swelling of the lymph nodes at the eschar, rash, and leukopenia. The rash is mostly congestive maculopapular, which is not itchy. This patient is unlikely to be diagnosed with tsutsugamushi disease, as her case lacks the support of typical eschar signs and the Weil-Felix test. There is no simple and definite clinical diagnosis method (mice should be inoculated and isolated), and it is not a self-limiting disease. However, there are specific treatment methods, so we should conduct a detailed physical examination of the patient again, and note the results of the Weil-Felix test examination.

Step 4: After detailed analysis, the diagnosis focuses on which diseases are more likely, and they should be ranked in order of importance. According to the sudden onset of fever, the large number of rashes, the decrease of leukocytes and platelets, and the seasonal coincidence, dengue fever, measles (or measles-like rash), tsutsugamushi disease (fever and rash cases in epidemic areas should be ruled out) and drug rash are the most likely.

This patient's clinical manifestations are consistent with dengue fever, and the diagnostic basis is as follows: ① Epidemiological data: The patient developed this disease in epidemic season, and came from an epidemic area; ② The clinical manifestation was acute fever with obvious toxic blood symptoms, especially bone and joint pain; ③ The rash was measles-like; ④ There were enlarged lymph nodes; ⑤ Other diseases featuring fever and rashes can be ruled out.

According to the above analysis, the patient was examined further to confirm the diagnosis. The examination of serum antibodies is the most commonly used clinical examination method, and a diagnosis can be confirmed when two copies of the serum are positive more than one week apart. Isolation of the dengue virus from vertebrate and mosquito cell strains can be used to make a definitive diagnosis, but it is difficult and dangerous to perform. It requires blood samples at a very early stage (within three days of the onset of the disease), and the amount of the virus in blood drops rapidly after the onset. Therefore, it is mostly used for epidemiological investigation to determine the prevalent serotype, and less for routine clinical examination. PCR nucleic acid and antigen examination is helpful for early diagnosis, but there is a certain false positive rate, so it has not been widely used in clinical diagnosis.

V. Ward-round analysis five days after admission

Because there is no specific treatment for dengue fever, anti-mosquito isolation should be given, antibacterial drugs should be stopped, dengue antibody IgM should be checked, and rehydration, bleeding prevention, and symptomatic support should be given.

On the day of hospitalization, the dengue antibody IgM was positive 1/40, and there was a positive Widal test and Weil-Felix test (OX_K 1/80). Tests for epidemic hemorrhagic fever antibodies and leptospira were negative, and no bacterial growth was found in the two blood cultures. Autoimmune antibody tests were all negative.

On the second day after admission, the patient developed gingival bleeding and epistaxis, and the symptoms of systemic poisoning were still severe. She was given 2,500 ml of rehydration per day. On the second day, she had an obvious headache and severe vomiting. After active dehydration treatment, her symptoms gradually improved. On the third day after admission, the whole-body rash subsided without pigmentation or desquamation.

VI. Condition at discharge (the seventh day after admission)

The patient had no fever, her headache and vomiting disappeared, and her whole-body rash subsided, but there was still some soreness of the muscles, bones, and joints. On the seventh day of hospitalization, routine blood tests showed that WBC 5.61×10^9/L, RBC 5.02×10^{12}/L, Hb 112 g/L, N 62%, L 35%, PLT 175×10^9/L, M 3%.

According to biochemical examination, AST 20 U/L, ALT 18 U/L, K$^+$ 3.5 mmol/L, Cr 76.8 μmol/L, BUN 4.31 mmol/L.

CRP and ESR decreased significantly.

On the sixth day of hospitalization, the positive titer of the dengue antibody IgM was 1/160. The Weil-Felix test was positive (OX$_K$ 1/80), and the patient was diagnosed as severe dengue fever after discharge.

VII. Follow-up

After discharge, she still suffered from osteoarticular pain, weakness, and mild depression. Her body temperature was normal after discharge.

VIII. Lessons learned

This case could be easily misdiagnosed as drug eruption due to the fever and rash. It should be differentiated from infectious diseases according to its late appearance, symmetrical distribution, more obvious compressed part, mild symptoms of infection and poisoning, and no lymph node enlargement. Muscle and osteoarticular pain are the prominent manifestations of this disease, which often appear earlier, with a degree similar to a broken bone. This is different from other infectious diseases, and it can still exist for a period of time after the fever is reduced.

This case could also be misdiagnosed as tsutsugamushi disease due to the fever, rash, lymph node enlargement, and positive Weil-Felix test (OX$_K$ 1/80). Careful physical examination is required to find eschar and ulcers, the titer of positive Weil-Felix test (OX$_K$ 1/80) is low, and the two copies of the serum do not rise, which can help to rule out the possibility of this disease. Therefore, attention should be paid to the intersection of the Widal test and the Weil-Felix test in febrile diseases. The fact that there are two copies of the serum is of great significance for both diagnosis and differential diagnosis. If the titer of the dengue antibody is low at the first examination, as in this case, the examination should be repeated more than five days later to obtain double serum results and make a clear diagnosis. During treatment, care should be taken not to rehydrate excessively. Brain edema may appear during rehydration, which should be noted and treated as quickly as possible.

(Zhao Zhixin & Gao Zhiliang)

Chest pain for three days

I. Medical history

Patient: Male, 37 years old, from Zhejiang. He was admitted to hospital for chest pain for three days, and stayed from 7 March until 9 April 2007.

Three days earlier the patient developed chest pain in the left back, which was a paroxysmal stabbing pain, without fever, cough, expectoration, or hemoptysis. A CT scan showed that there were many nodular lesions in both lungs with cavities. The local hospital gave cefoperazone/sulbactam and meropenem anti-infection treatment, but the effect was not good.

> **Thinking prompts:**
> Problems in the collecting of medical history:
> 1. Find out whether the chest pain is accompanied by symptoms such as fever and night sweats, and whether there is obvious weight loss.
> 2. Find out whether the patient had any specific dietary habits before falling ill, such as eating raw river crabs.
> 3. Find out whether there is a history of contact with tuberculosis patients.
> 4. Find out whether the patient is in normal health, or whether they have any basic diseases.

Follow-up medical history: The patient developed fatigue, loss of appetite, yellow eyes, yellow urine, fever, nausea, and vomiting without obvious inducement three months ago.

Liver function tests were conducted by the local hospital: ALT 1,226 U/L, AST 1,076 U/L, TB/CB 101/45 µmol/L, and HBV DNA 3.12×10^8 copies /ml. The patient was diagnosed with severe chronic hepatitis B, and was given liver protection, jaundice reduction, and nucleoside analogue for antiviral treatment. During the 2-month treatment, the patient suffered fatigue and loss of appetite, and the yellowing of his eyes and urine worsened. TB rose to 300 µmol/L. Local doctors began to treat him with dexamethasone (DXM) (5 mg–3 mg–2 mg, from 8 February to 4 March). The patient had a low fever and no obvious night sweat. He denied eating raw food, and reported no history of contact with tuberculosis patients.

Thinking prompts: This is a very important medical history. With a three-month hospitalization for liver disease in local hospitals, the possibility of parasitic diseases in the lungs can be ruled out. From the perspective of the causal relationship between the occurrence and development of diseases, we should not consider lung tumors first, but find out why there are lung lesions in the treatment of liver diseases. Naturally, attention will be paid to glucocorticoid treatment in the last month. Glucocorticoid is a good inducer of glucuronosyltransferase, which can sometimes make great contributions to the treatment of receding jaundice in liver diseases. However, it is also an immunosuppressant, which can lead to pathogenic bacteria infection. The lung lesions in this patient are nodular with cavities, so viral and general bacterial infections can be ruled out. The focus of investigation is on tuberculosis and fungal infection.

Therefore, the physical examination of this patient should focus on looking, touching, knocking, and listening to the lungs. Note whether other organs (including the heart, brain, and lymph nodes) are involved, and do not ignore the primary liver sign.

II. Physical examination after admission

T 37.3°C, P 100 times/min, R 18 times/min, BP 131/84 mmHg. Chronic liver disease, sickly look, clear consciousness, but low spirits. The skin and sclera are yellow-stained; no petechiae or ecchymosis found, subcutaneous nodules not touched, and superficial lymph nodes not enlarged. There is no liver palm or spider nevus, and no tenderness in the sternum. The border of cardiac dullness was normal, normal heart voice, normal heart rate, 100 beats/min, rhythm, soft systolic murmur of grade 2 audibility at the apex of the heart, and no pathological murmur in other valve areas. The left lung breathes heavily, with moist rales and no pleural fricative sounds. Abdominal distension; Murphy sign negative; no tenderness and rebound pain, no touching mass, positive shifting dullness, unsatisfactory palpation of liver and spleen, normal bowel sounds, no edema in both lower limbs, negative flapping-wing tremor, no obvious percussion pain in both kidney areas. No deformity of the limbs; normal muscle strength and muscle tension; no redness or movement limitation of joints. Meningeal irritation sign and pyramidal tract sign negative.

Thinking prompts: After physical examination, it was found that the signs of liver disease in this patient were obvious, showing jaundice and massive ascites. The infection is mostly in the lungs, so the next auxiliary examination will focus on these two organs.

III. Auxiliary examination at admission

Routine blood test: WBC 8.2×10^9/L, N 0.899, L 0.063, E 0.009, PLT 51×10^9/L, RBC 3.09×10^{12}/L, Hb 98 g/L; CRP 62.50 mg/L.

Liver function: A/G 34.9/20.2 g/L, ALT 31 U/L, AST 34 U/L, TB/CB 107/54 μmol/L.

Electrolytes: K^+ 2.91 mmol/L, Na^+ 135 mmol/L, Cl^- 93 mmol/L.

Routine urine test: Bilirubin (+), urinary bile yuan (++), others normal.

Routine stool, normal renal function, ESR 58 mm/h; PPD skin test negative;

Electrocardiogram normal.

Abdominal B-ultrasound: Indicating liver cirrhosis, large spleen, and massive ascites.

Lung CT: There were multiple nodules in both lungs with cavities, close to the pleura, with crescent-shaped air gaps, and halo signs at the edge of the lesion. The lesion was significantly heightened after CT enhancement. Fungal infection was considered, and there was a small amount of pleural effusion on both sides.

IV. Ward-round analysis on admission

Diagnosis: Pulmonary aspergillosis; severe chronic type-B viral hepatitis.

(1) Tuberculosis: The patient was a middle-aged male, with chest pain and a low fever for three days. He had had hepatitis B before, and had used glucocorticoid. Rough breath sounds in left lung, moist rales could be heard, and auxiliary examination found that ESR increased rapidly. Lung CT showed multiple nodules with cavities in both lungs and a small amount of pleural effusion on both sides, so the possibility of tuberculosis was considered. Although a PPD skin test was negative, tuberculosis infection could not be ruled out. If a patient has no cough or expectoration and sputum cannot be sent for inspection, fiberoptic bronchoscopy can be considered to find lesions. Tissues can be taken for pathological examination, or secretions can be taken to test for tuberculosis, so as to make a clear diagnosis.

(2) Pulmonary aspergillosis: This is a rare fungal infection of the lung, which generally has no obvious systemic symptoms. The common clinical symptoms are hemoptysis, coughing, chest pain, and fever, which often occur in people with low immunity. The patient suddenly developed chest pain with a low fever. He had been using glucocorticoid for one month before, and his neutrophils and C-reactive protein in the hemogram increased. Furthermore, CT showed that the nodule with cavity was close to the pleura, with crescent-shaped air gaps and halo signs at the edge of the lesion. The lesion was significantly heightened after CT enhancement. It is highly likely that the patient was infected with pulmonary aspergillosis.

The golden standard for the diagnosis of these two diseases is etiological diagnosis. In order to establish a basis for diagnosis, the patient underwent a lung biopsy under CT location after admission. The pathology showed fungal granulomatous inflammation (Aspergillus was considered first).

Clinical classification of pulmonary aspergillosis:

1) Allergic aspergillosis: Acute onset, asthma, low fever, itchy throat, coughing, and brown phlegm. Wheezing can be heard in the lungs. X-ray examination shows that the lungs were infiltrated with lesions distributed in leaves and segments, showing migratory changes. After disengagement or treatment, symptoms will disappear quickly.

2) Pulmonary aspergilloma: Aspergilloma parasitizes in the cavity formed by the original pulmonary tuberculosis, bronchial cyst, bronchiectasis, and lung cancer. Symptoms are mild, with cough and repeated hemoptysis. X-ray examination shows round, oval, or sausage-shaped aspergilloma in the original cavity, which moves with the change of body position.

3) Pulmonary aspergillosis: It is mostly secondary to chronic lung disease, and can occur in patients with long-term use of antibiotics, adrenal cortical hormone, or immunosuppressants, as well as immunocompromised patients. Clinical manifestations include high fever, coughing, brown sticky sputum, or purulent sputum and hemoptysis. Invasion of the pleura can cause pleuritis or empyema. X-ray examination shows patchy infiltration and multiple nodular shadows in the lungs, accompanied by increased lung texture.

4) Disseminated aspergillosis: Aspergillosis spreads to the whole body or lungs through blood, with severe illness, such as high fever, chills, coughing, and difficulty breathing. X-ray examination shows limited or multiple infiltrations and nodular shadows in the early stage, and the lesions will rapidly expand and merge into large consolidation or necrosis to form cavities.

V. Treatment

Drugs that are effective against aspergillosis include amphotericin B and its liposomes, itraconazole, voriconazole, caspofungin, and micafungin. Considering the patient's poor liver function, on the basis of liver protection, antivirals such as compound glycyrrhetinic acid, reduced glutathione, ademetionine, and lamivudine were considered. However, caspofungin was selected for anti-aspergillosis treatment due to its relatively few adverse reactions. The first dose was 70 mg/d, reduced the next day to 50 mg/d for maintenance treatment.

After two weeks of treatment, low fever subsided and chest pain eased.

Routine peripheral blood test: WBC 8.3×10^9/L, N 0.633, L 0.25, PLT 106×10^9/L, RBC 2.94×10^{12}/L, Hb 92 g/L; CRP 13.30 mg/L.

One month after the treatment with 50 mg/d of caspofungin, a lung CT scan showed that the lesions had been absorbed and improved.

Routine blood tests: WBC 6.3×10^9/L, N 0.478, L 0.406, PLT 155×10^9/L, RBC 3.46×10^{12}/L and Hb 122 g/L;

Liver function: A/G 45.2/47.8, ALT 18 U/L, AST 38 U/L, TB/CB 44/25 μmol/L.

The treatment was changed to oral voriconazole 200 mg twice a day, and the patient was discharged.

VI. Follow-up

After discharge, the patient continued to take 200 mg of voriconazole orally twice a day, and we observed clinical manifestations such as fever, coughing, and expectoration. Blood, C-reactive protein, and liver function were checked every month, and a lung CT was performed every 1-2 months for six months. During the follow-up, there were no symptoms, and the blood, C-reactive protein, and liver function were normal. After six months, re-examination showed that only the bilateral pleura was slightly thickened.

VII. Lessons learned

Pulmonary aspergillosis is a rare infectious pulmonary disease, and clinical understanding remains insufficient. The clinical symptoms are atypical, and are often manifested as hemoptysis, coughing, chest pain, and low fever, which are frequently misdiagnosed as pulmonary tuberculosis or other respiratory diseases. We should be alert to patients who have been using antibiotics and immunosuppressants for a long time. The rate of detection by CT scan is higher than by chest X-ray. If a CT scan shows pulmonary nodules with cavities close to the pleura, crescent-shaped air gaps, and halo signs at the edge of the lesions, pulmonary aspergillosis should be considered. Repeated sputum smears and positive sputum cultures for Aspergillus are common methods of clinical diagnosis. When sputum samples cannot be obtained, a lung biopsy under CT location is one of the most effective methods of diagnosis.

(Yu Yunsong)

Fever with chest pain for one week

I. Medical history

Patient: Male, 27 years old, Wenzhou native, distributor. Admitted for fever with chest pain for one week.

The patient developed chills and fever (about 38°C) with a dry cough and tearing pain in the right side of his chest one week before treatment, especially when inhaling deeply and coughing, accompanied by chest tightness and shortness of breath. Two days earlier, chest pain occurred on the left side, similar in nature to the right side, accompanied by fatigue, dryness and heat, and night sweats.

> **Thinking prompts:** The patient was a young man, and the course of his illness was one week, mainly manifesting as fever and chest pain. The first thing we suspect is an acute infection, which commonly includes lobar pneumonia and tuberculous pleurisy. Chills, fever, coughing, and chest pain after catching a cold indicate lobar pneumonia. However, if lobar pneumonia is not treated with anti-infection medication, it often causes high fever, reaching 40°C. A temperature of only 38°C does not meet the clinical manifestations of typical lobar pneumonia, so there is also the possibility of tuberculous pleurisy.

II. Physical examination on admission

T 38.3°C, H 98 times/min, R 26 times/min, BP 120/60 mmHg. Acute sickly look, soft neck; jugular vein not distended when lying down. Grade 3 murmurs can be heard in the mitral valve area during systole in the heart. Percussive dullness in both lungs; auscultation breath sound decreased. The abdomen was soft without tenderness. No rashes or subcutaneous nodules were found on the body. No other positive signs were found.

III. Auxiliary examination on admission

Routine blood test: White blood cells 13.7×10^9/L, including neutrophils 30% and eosinophils 46%. ESR was 49 mm/h.

B-ultrasound: Pleural effusion on both sides.

Chest CT: Both lungs can be seen; patchy and cloud-like shadows of increased density can be seen in the posterior segment of the right lung apex and the anterior segment of the left lung, with unclear edges and a small amount of pleural effusion on both sides (more on the right side).

After admission, the patient's pleural effusion specimen was milky yellow and purulent, with white blood cells (++++), including 93% lobulated nucleus and 120,000/μl red blood cells. A large number of neutrophils were found in pleural effusion cytology. No bacteria grew in the pleural effusion culture.

Bone marrow examination showed eosinophilia and negative bone marrow culture.

> **Thinking prompts:** There are not many indications of this patient's positive signs. Both percussion and auscultation of the lower lungs suggest the possibility of pleural effusion. Typical lobar pneumonia also has exudation, but it is mostly unilateral. Tuberculous pleurisy and empyema cannot be ruled out. Pleural effusion caused by neoplastic and connective tissue diseases is uncommon in 27-year-old male patients, and there is no evidence to support it at present, so these possibilities can be temporarily ignored.

IV. Ward-round analysis on admission

An increase in white blood cells is expected in patients, but it is obviously unusual that eosinophils were as high as 46%. Due to the increase of eosinophils, the following diseases should be considered: ① Allergic diseases: Such as bronchial asthma, drug allergy, and urticaria. ② Parasitic infection: Parasites in extraintestinal tissues, such as blood fluke, clonorchis sinensis, lung fluke, filaria, and hydatid worms. Hookworm in the intestinal tract can cause a very obvious increase in eosinophils. ③ Skin diseases: Eczema, exfoliative dermatitis, and pemphigus. ④ Blood diseases. ⑤ Some malignant tumors: Especially with metastasis or necrosis. ⑥ Some infectious diseases: The acute stage of scarlet fever.

Schistosomiasis can be ruled out, as can malignant tumors. More evidence is required, ideally through bone marrow examination. Imaging examination confirmed our speculation that the patient did have pleural effusion, but it required further laboratory examination. The patient was admitted to hospital for further examination.

If the patient has pleural effusion, it should be clear whether it is leakage or exudate. This patient's pleural effusion was yellow and turbid, containing a large number of white blood cells – a typical purulent exudate. Therefore, the common pathogens considered are pyogenic coccus, Escherichia coli, and Bacteroides fragilis. Usually, pathogens can be found in a smear or bacterial culture, but in this case, no bacteria were cultured in pleural effusion. A myelogram still indicated eosinophilia, and empirical anti-infection treatment can be started before the pathogen is identified. In addition, patients with eosinophilia should be asked about their history of contact with parasites, and a whole set of parasite antibodies should be screened at the same time. Of course, the focus is on blood fluke and lung fluke antibodies.

V. Diagnosis and treatment after admission

Imipenem/cilistatin (1 g, twice a day, intravenous drip) and metronidazole (0.5 g, twice a day, intravenous drip) were given on the second day after admission. Blood eosinophils increased significantly, and the direct count was as high as 8,624/µl after re-examination. After follow-up questions, it was discovered that the patient frequently ate raw crabs.

On the fourth day after admission, imipenem/cilistatin and metronidazole were stopped, and praziquantel 600 mg was given twice a day for six days as a course of treatment. Glucocorticoid and prednisone 20 mg/d were added orally for three days. After one week of treatment, the chest CT was re-examined, and showed that the lesions in both lungs had been absorbed, leaving only left pleural thickening. Blood eosinophils were re-examined at 2,728/µl.

Final diagnosis: Lung fluke disease.

> **Thinking prompts:** Lung fluke disease (also known as paragonimiasis) is a chronic lung infection caused by lung fluke. There are two kinds of lung flukes that affect the human body in China, namely P. Westermanii and Paragonimiasis skrjabini. The former is found in Taiwan, Zhejiang, Liaoning, Jilin, and Heilongjiang provinces. The latter is found in Sichuan, Jiangxi, Yunnan, Fujian, Guangdong, Guizhou, and Shaanxi provinces. People and animals (dogs, cats, pigs, and wild animals) are the final hosts of paragonimiasis. The eggs are discharged into water, and develop into cysts in the second intermediate host (stone crab, crayfish) through the first intermediate host (Simisalcospira calculus). People eat raw stone crabs and crayfish, and develop cysts. The cysts break in the stomach and duodenum, and the larvae emerge and enter the abdominal cavity through the intestinal wall. They enter the chest and lungs through the diaphragm, and develop into adults in the lungs. The parasite enters the mediastinum, and can invade the brain along the internal carotid artery. Pathological changes in the lungs show an inflammatory reaction, infiltrated neutrophils and eosinophils, and destroyed lung tissue, resulting in abscesses and cysts, surrounded by fibrous capsules containing cholesterol crystals, Charcot-Leiden's crystals, and eggs. Most of the cysts have only one adult, which forms the cyst, and then moves to another location to form a new one. The cavity of the old focus can be closed, and cured after fibrosis and calcification.
>
> The atypical presentation of this patient lies in the acute onset and lack of typical coughing or peach-like bloody phlegm. This makes misdiagnosis likely at first, possibly as empyema. However, as clinicians in an infectious disease department, we should be very alert to the changes seen in eosinophilia, and must always screen for parasitic diseases.

VI. Lessons learned

Paragonimiasis is a common parasitic disease in China. It is often related to eating raw crabs and crayfish, and its incidence has been on the rise in recent years. Paragonimiasis typically occurs in the lungs, but there are often atypical lesions. Invasion of the intracranial brain tissue is a common element of ectopic damage, but it is often misdiagnosed, and should therefore command vigilance. If paragonimiasis is found in the lungs, we should check whether the patient has intracranial lesions. Conversely, if intracranial lesions are found, we investigate the possibility of parasitic brain diseases.

(Wang Xinyu & Shi Guangfeng)

Repeated fatigue, anorexia, and epigastric distention for more than one month

I. Medical history

Patient: Female, 36 years old, from Shunde in Guangdong Province. She was admitted to hospital for repeated fatigue, lack of appetite, and epigastric distention for more than one month. She was hospitalized from 11 to 17 January 2008.

One month earlier, the patient began to suffer from fatigue and loss of appetite without obvious inducement, accompanied by epigastric distention and slight discomfort, which was obvious mostly after eating. There was no obvious nausea, vomiting, abdominal pain, or diarrhea. Another hospital treated her for chronic gastritis, but the effect was poor. A week earlier, a liver function test showed AST 176 U/L, ALT 188 U/L, TB 21.3 μmol/L, CB 5.3 μmol/L, A 36.2 g/L, HBsAg (−). The patient came to our hospital for further diagnosis and treatment, and was admitted to our department from the outpatient department with liver damage, of which the cause was to be investigated. Since the onset of her illness, she had suffered from poor sleep, frequent palpitations, and dizziness, but no coughing or expectoration; no chest pain, chest tightness, and shortness of breath; no obvious oliguria and swollen feet; no gingival bleeding or epistaxis; soft yellow stool, sometimes unformed, 2–3 times a day, no asphalt-like or white clay-like stool; weight loss of around 2 kg.

The patient had eaten shellfish within one month before the onset of the disease. She had no history of eating raw fish.

II. Physical examination on admission

T 38.5°C, R 18 times/min, P 78 times/min, BP 128/72 mmHg. Moderate nutritional development. There was no yellow stain on the skin and sclera; superficial lymph nodes could not be palpated; no abnormality in the head and facial features; no resistance in the neck; no distension of the jugular vein; the trachea was in the middle, and there was no swelling of the thyroid. Her heart and lungs were normal. Her abdomen was flat and soft; the liver and spleen could not be palpated below the costal margin; there was no obvious percussion pain in the liver area; the xiphoid process was slightly tender, and the Murphy sign was positive. There was no obvious percussion pain in the bilateral kidney area. No shifting dullness. There were no positive signs of the nervous system.

> **Thinking prompts:** This case started slowly, with digestive tract symptoms such as lack of appetite, epigastric distention, and unformed soft stool. Physical examination showed that upper abdominal tenderness and Murphy sign were positive. Laboratory examination showed elevated serum ALT, so diseases that could cause cholecystitis and liver damage were considered. When inquiring about medical history, we should ask whether the patient has a history of contact with people suffering from hepatitis, particularly at home; whether the patient has had a blood transfusion, or has received blood products; whether there is a history of sharing razors, acupuncture needles, and tattoo equipment; whether there is a history of intravenous drug addiction, to rule out viral hepatitis; whether the patient is addicted to alcohol, how much alcohol is consumed, and how long is the history of alcoholism, to distinguish it from alcoholic liver disease, and whether there is a family history of hereditary metabolic diseases; whether there is a long-term medical history, to see whether there is chronic drug-induced liver damage; whether there is joint pain and rash, to see whether there is an autoimmune disease. Physical examination should also investigate signs of chronic liver disease, such as liver palm, spider nevus, dull complexion, and pigmentation, as well as clinical manifestations of liver cirrhosis such as abdominal wall varicose veins, ascites, and edema of the lower limbs.

Gathering medical history: No history of alcohol abuse, no history of drug use before illness.

III. Auxiliary examination on admission

Routine blood test: WBC 5.61×10^9/L, RBC 3.02×10^{12}/L, Hb 102 g/L, N 36%, L 30%, PLT 175×10^9/L, E 24%.

Liver function test: AST 154 U/L, ALT 203 U/L, TB 18.3 μmol/L, CB 5.3 μmol/L, A 36.2 g/L.

Blood biochemical examination: K^+ 3.18 mmol/L, Cr 70.8 μmol/L, BUN 2.31 mmol/L.

Chest X-ray: There was no abnormality in the heart or lungs.

ECG: Approximately normal.

B-ultrasound: The light spots on the liver were dense and thickened, and there were small patches or small lumps of echo. The spleen was slightly enlarged.

IV. Ward-round analysis on admission

Preliminary diagnosis: The case characteristics were analyzed, and the main problems were put forward. The main symptoms were fatigue, loss of appetite, and epigastric distention. Laboratory examination showed liver function damage, which was consistent with the clinical manifestations of hepatitis. However, the cause of liver damage was unknown. The patient was diagnosed with liver damage, the cause of which needed to be investigated.

Thinking prompts:

Step 1: What diseases can cause liver damage? The causes of liver damage include infectious diseases such as viral hepatitis, parasitic infections (liver fluke and blood fluke), infective-toxic hepatitis such as leptospirosis, liver damage associated with typhoid fever, tsutsugamushi disease and hemorrhagic fever with renal syndrome, and various chronic infections (tuberculosis). Non-infectious diseases can lead to liver damage, including alcoholic liver damage, drug and poison liver damage, autoimmune hepatitis, hereditary metabolic diseases (such as hepatolenticular degeneration, fatty liver, and hyperthyroidism), hematological diseases, and malignant tumors. In addition, this case had obvious clinical manifestations of chronic cholecystitis, which should be differentiated from simple chronic cholecystitis and liver damage caused by an acute attack of cholelithiasis.

Step 2: Is this case chronic or acute liver damage? Acute liver damage usually has a more acute onset, and the digestive tract symptoms are more obvious. Liver function tests often show that ALT and AST are obviously increased, usually to more than 500 U/L. Meanwhile, chronic liver damage has a slower onset, and the digestive tract symptoms are mostly mild, but chronic neurasthenia is more prominent. Typical patients may have signs of chronic liver disease. In this case, chronic liver damage was considered. However, the course of the disease was only one month, which means that the possibility of mild liver damage cannot be completely ruled out.

Step 3: What are the common causes of chronic liver damage? Diseases with acute liver damage as a clinical manifestation were excluded. Among the above causes, viral hepatitis (especially hepatitis B and C) is the most common infectious disease, followed by parasitic infections (liver fluke and blood fluke). Tuberculosis can cause chronic liver damage, but it is rare and not a common cause. Toxic liver damage in acute infection is mostly acute, mostly with clinical characteristics of corresponding infectious diseases, so it does not need to be differentiated in this case. Alcoholic liver damage, drug and poison liver damage, autoimmune hepatitis, fatty liver, and hepatolenticular degeneration are common in non-infectious diseases.

Step 4: Remove some diseases excluded by existing evidence: At present, laboratory examination shows HBsAg (−), and B-ultrasound examination shows no obvious fatty change, which can exclude hepatitis B and fatty liver. The patient had no history of alcoholism, so alcoholic liver damage can be ruled out. The patient had no special medication history before the onset of the disease, so drug-induced liver damage could be ruled out.

Step 5: Analyze the common causes of chronic liver damage:

1. First, consider viral hepatitis other than hepatitis B. At present, hepatitis A, C, and E are common.

Hepatitis A: It is transmitted through the fecal-oral route, and most infected people are infants, children, and adolescents. It can be clinically manifested as recessive infection and acute hepatitis of various degrees. HAV IgM (+) can be found in laboratory examination at the early stage of infection, and lasts for 3–6 months. This patient had eaten shellfish within one month before the onset of illness, and should be given an HAV-IgM examination. This case had a slow onset, with no fever and mild elevation of ALT, which is inconsistent with typical hepatitis A.

Hepatitis C: Hepatitis C can be transmitted through blood transfusions, injections, close contact, sexual contact, and damaged skin. Clinical manifestations include varying degrees of acute and chronic hepatitis and liver cirrhosis. Moreover, the onset process is mostly slow, the early clinical manifestations are mild and nonspecific. Most patients have only mild liver function abnormalities, which are found accidentally during physical examination. There is no epidemiological data to support hepatitis C in this patient, but there are still 40% of sporadic infected people who have no history of injections, blood transfusions, or blood products, so it is still necessary to check HCV antibodies and HCV RNA in patients with unexplained liver damage.

Hepatitis E: The transmission route of hepatitis E is the same as that of hepatitis A. It usually occurs in winter and spring, and can be manifested as acute hepatitis or acute severe hepatitis. It is more common in adults. In the early stage of infection, it is often manifested as acute hepatitis with obvious digestive tract symptoms, such as loss of appetite, nausea and vomiting, jaundice, and short-term fever. Serum ALT and AST increased by more than 500 U/L. Therefore, this case does not support acute hepatitis E, and it can be ruled out. However, the proportion of mild liver damage caused by hepatitis E is not clear at present, and chronic hepatitis has been reported in some specific populations, such as long-term immune-suppressed patients. Anti-HEV-IgM IgG mostly disappears in a short time, so if this patient can be diagnosed with anti-HEV-antibodies, especially if they turn from negative to positive, and then turn negative in the recovery period, HEV infection should be considered.

2. Second, consider parasitic diseases. The most common diseases that can cause liver damage are liver fluke disease and schistosomiasis.

Liver fluke disease: Liver fluke disease is usually acquired by eating raw fish. Those who are lightly infected have no symptoms, or only upper abdominal fullness, loss of appetite, or mild abdominal pain. In severe cases, there is a loss of appetite, epigastric fullness, mild diarrhea, and dull pain in the liver area. It can be accompanied by neurasthenia symptoms such as dizziness, insomnia, fatigue, listlessness, palpitations, and hypomnesis. The diagnosis was based on the detection of liver fluke eggs in feces or bile. Eating raw fish is common in Shunde, Guangdong Province, and it is an endemic area for liver fluoriasis. The patient in this case denied eating raw fish, but she should be asked whether she has ever eaten undercooked freshwater fish, such as in hot pot, or whether she fails to separate raw and cooked food. Routine blood and stool samples should be checked for liver fluke eggs and liver fluke antibodies.

Schistosomiasis: Caused by contact with infected water. The clinical manifestations are fever, rash, loss of appetite, epigastric distention, diarrhea, and vomiting. More than 90% of patients may have hepatosplenomegaly. This patient had no obvious history of contact with infected water, and no obvious manifestation of hepatosplenomegaly and fever. The clinical manifestations were inconsistent. A diagnosis can be made through further examination of routine blood, finding eggs in stool, a stool cercariae incubation test, and a COPT (circular ovum precipitation test).

3. Women are more prone to autoimmune diseases. Attention should be paid to the existence of autoimmune hepatitis.

Autoimmune hepatitis: Autoimmune hepatitis is a chronic inflammation of the liver with unknown causes, which is characterized by hyperglobulinemia, and circulating autoantibodies. Histologically, there is interfacial hepatitis and hepatocyte infiltration in the portal areas. In addition to liver damage, there are often extrahepatic manifestations such as arthritis, gingival bleeding, rashes, and Hashimoto thyroiditis. Because autoimmune hepatitis has no specific clinical manifestations and no laboratory method for definitive diagnosis, the diagnosis must exclude viral hepatitis and parasitic diseases, and be established only after the detection of autoantibodies and pathological changes.

4. For liver damage of unknown cause, we should routinely check for hepatolenticular degeneration, so that we can give specific copper-expelling treatment as early as possible.

Hepatolenticular degeneration (Wilson's disease) is an autosomal recessive disorder in which copper is not metabolized. Most patients develop symptoms at 10–25 years old, which can be manifested as liver function damage. Clinically, it is very similar to chronic hepatitis, and can be easily misdiagnosed. Some cases develop into cirrhosis due to mild symptoms, nonspecific clinical manifestations, and lack of early treatment. The diagnosis depends on serum copper, ceruloplasmin, 24-hour urine copper quantification, and K-F ring detection in the cornea. Symptoms related to the nervous system are more helpful for diagnosis. Although the patient in this case was older, this possibility cannot be ruled out. Relevant examinations such as serum copper, ceruloplasmin, and urine copper quantification should be performed.

According to the above analysis, on the basis of completing the patient's medical history and performing a physical examination, hepatitis markers were examined to eliminate the most common viral hepatitis. Liver fluke antibodies were examined, and liver fluke eggs were examined in the stool to confirm the diagnosis of liver fluke disease. Serum copper and ceruloplasmin, and 24-hour urine copper detection were performed to rule out hepatolenticular degeneration. Autoimmune hepatitis-related antibody detection was performed in order to distinguish it from autoimmune diseases.

V. Ward-round analysis on day four of admission

Routine blood test after admission: WBC 6.61×10^9/L, RBC 3.2×10^{12}/L, Hb 98 g/L, E 16.4%, PLT 175×10^9/l.

For three consecutive days, the stool was examined for liver fluke eggs. The examination was negative the first time, but 92/g of liver fluke eggs were found in the second and third stools. Liver fluke antibodies were positive.

Five hepatitis-B tests: HBsAg (−), HBsAb (+), HBeAg (−), HBeAb (−), HBcAb (−), HBV DNA (−); Hepatitis C antibody negative, HCV RNA (−). No positive results were found for hepatitis A and hepatitis E markers.

Serum copper and ceruloplasmin were normal, ANA (−). AFP, CEA, CA199, CA125, and serum ferritin were normal.

After being questioned about her medical history, the patient admitted that she had eaten undercooked freshwater fish, so she was considered as having liver fluke disease. She was given 25 mg/kg of praziquantel on the fourth day of hospitalization, three times a day for two days, and was given symptomatic treatment for liver protection.

VI. Condition at discharge (14 days after admission)

The patient was discharged from hospital two days after taking the medicine, without any obvious discomfort. The symptoms of fatigue, lack of appetite, and epigastric distention disappeared after two weeks of discharge. Liver function was normal after outpatient examination, and the number of liver fluke eggs found in three stools was 0/g.

VII. Lessons learned

Liver fluke disease is usually characterized by mild gastrointestinal symptoms or chronic cholecystitis, and is easily misdiagnosed as chronic gastritis and chronic cholecystitis. Therefore, for patients with chronic gastritis and chronic cholecystitis, especially those with no obvious improvement after treatment, attention should be paid to whether they have eaten raw fish. Due to a lack of typical epidemiological history of eating raw fish, this patient was easy to misdiagnose due to an initial negative stool test for liver fluke eggs. It is very important to inquire about medical history and repeatedly check for liver fluke eggs in the stool. Because liver flukes are small and stool is discharged irregularly, it is common to get a single negative result. After admission, the causes of liver damage were screened for, combined with the fact that the patient came from an epidemic area. Blood eosinophils increased, her stool was examined many times, and she was finally diagnosed with liver fluke disease. The symptoms disappeared after a deworming treatment. Therefore, for patients with liver function damage, we should consider all possible factors, starting with common causes and eliminating them one by one.

(Zhao Zhixin & Gao Zhiliang)

Joint pain for three months, anemia for two months, and fever for one month

I. Medical history

Patient: Female, 31 years old, a nurse at a drug rehabilitation center. She was admitted to hospital because of joint pain for three months, anemia for two months, and fever for one month.

Five months earlier, the patient developed a cough with expectoration, and bright red blood in the sputum. A chest X-ray at the city hospital showed speckled shadows in the lower lung fields, and pleural effusion on the right side, which was considered to be tuberculosis. She was given 2HREZ/7HRZ (H isoniazid, R rifampicin, E ethambutol, Z pyrazinamide) anti-tuberculosis treatment. Three months earlier, she lost her appetite and developed joint pain, which started in both elbows and then spread to the temporomandibular joints and shoulders. Occasionally, there was chest pain on the right side, with no redness, swelling, dyskinesia, symmetry of the large joints, migratory pain, or rash. The patient's liver function was found to be slightly abnormal, and phospholipids were given to protect the liver. Her liver function returned to normal, but her symptoms were not relieved to any great extent. Two months earlier, a routine blood examination revealed anemia, no rash or bleeding, no soy sauce-colored urine, and no fever. Her fever began one month earlier and it was worse in the afternoon. Her body temperature was 38°C–39°C. The patient had no intolerance of cold, chills, and night sweats, and still coughed and expectorated. She continued to receive anti-tuberculosis and anti-inflammatory treatment (penicillin, third-generation cephalosporins, and quinolones), but there was no obvious improvement in her symptoms. However, no other symptoms appeared. She was transferred to our hospital for further treatment.

The patient was in good health. She had no history of contact with infected water, had not eaten raw food, and denied any history of infectious diseases or genetic diseases in her family. She had a history of contact with cats and dogs.

Thinking prompts: The outstanding manifestations of this patient are joint pain, anemia, and fever, so we should focus on the following questions: ① The nature and location of the joint pain, the presence or absence of multiple-location or migratory joint pain, local presence or absence of swelling, heat pain, dyskinesia, joint deformation, and morning stiffness. Special attention should be paid to chest tightness, shortness of breath, sore throat, rashes, erythema, and subcutaneous nodules, which can help differentiate infectious arthritis, rheumatoid arthritis, rheumatic fever, and adult-onset Still's disease. ② Whether there are gastrointestinal issues, bleeding, skin bleeding spots, petechiae, ecchymosis, or purpura, which can help differentiate gastrointestinal diseases from blood system diseases. ③ In case of fever, attention should be paid to the course and type, the frequency, accompanying symptoms, and treatment, especially whether antibiotics, glucocorticoids, and immunosuppressants are used in large quantities to cause double infection. ④ In addition, ask about the patient's history of infectious diseases, visiting epidemic areas, and occupational characteristics, especially whether there is close contact with poultry and mosquitos. There may be important clues for some pathogen infections, especially parasitic infections.

II. Physical examination and related auxiliary examinations

1. Physical examination

T 37.5°C. The patient was conscious, with stable breathing, an anemic appearance, no white spots in the pharynx or oral cavity, no swelling in the tonsils, no palpable swelling in the superficial lymph nodes, no facial butterfly erythema and subcutaneous nodules, no hemorrhagic spot, ecchymosis, purpura, or rashes anywhere on her body, and no redness, swelling, fever, or obstacles to activity in the joints, and no joint deformation. There were low respiratory sounds in the right lower lung, but no rales, no enlargement of the heart border, and no heart murmur. Her abdomen was flat and soft. Her liver was 1 cm below her rib, with medium quality and no tenderness. Her spleen was 2 cm below her rib, with medium quality and shifting dullness (±). There was mild edema of both lower limbs. There was no specific manifestation of the nervous system.

2. Auxiliary examination

Routine blood test: WBC 7.8×10^9/L, N 79.6%, Hb 66.71 g/L, PLT 126×10^9/L.

CRP 211 mg/L, ESR 147 mm/h.

Biochemical parameters: A 25.4 g/L, r-GT 159 U/L. Other results normal.

Urine routine (−).

Chest X-ray: A small amount of pleural effusion on both sides.

Abdominal B-ultrasound: Hepatosplenomegaly, a small number of ascites, and no special manifestations in the uterine appendages.

Echocardiography: Lower to moderate pericardial effusion, slight tricuspid regurgitation.

Thinking prompts: All patients with FUO (fever of unknown origin) should undergo a comprehensive physical examination. For this patient, the doctor should look out for oral leukoplakia after a physical examination, which is helpful for the diagnosis of fungal infection. Doctors should also consider the presence of inflammation in the laryngopharynx, which is helpful for the diagnosis of streptococcal infection;

the existence or non-existence of bleeding spots, ecchymoses, purpura, and rashes; the existence of enlarged superficial lymph nodes (including supratrochlear, retro-auricular, and armpit), the presence of swollen and tender liver and spleen, to diagnose blood system diseases; and the existence of joint deformities, red swelling, thermalgia, or dyskinesia. The presence of heart murmurs is significant for identifying infectious arthritis and autoimmune diseases. Significant characteristic signs such as facial butterfly erythema suggest systemic lupus erythematosus (SLE), and annular erythema is more common in rheumatic fever.

III. Preliminary diagnosis

The patient has a continuous or intermittent fever (T > 38°C, more than three weeks, outpatient visits > two times, or hospitalization for three days), of which the etiology is unclear. This is consistent with FUO.

Thinking prompts:

1. Analyze the causes of FUO: Infectious diseases or non-infectious diseases.

(1) Supporting infectious diseases: ① The patient has a mid-routine fever, and this is more common in infectious diseases, especially when occult focal infection with atypical clinical symptoms of septicemia, or when the course of the disease is prolonged because of factors such as pathogen infection (including tuberculous infection) that reacts poorly to antibiotics. Moreover, with a history of tuberculosis, and long-term treatment with anti-tuberculosis drugs, the patient's immune status was low, which may cause a variety of concurrent infectious diseases. ② The patient had a fever. Peripheral blood neutrophils, CRP, and ESR increased. ③ The presence of hepatosplenomegaly, and multiple serosal cavity effusion.

(2) Supporting non-infectious diseases: ① Female patient, 31 years old, with joint pain, anemia, and fever. ② Malnutrition: Anemia and low albumin. ③ ESR increased significantly. ④ Liver and spleen enlargement, multiple serous cavity effusion, and other multiple organs were involved. ⑤ The effect of antibiotic treatment was not obvious.

2. Further examination is required after the preliminary diagnosis

(1) General etiological examination: Blood culture, bone marrow culture, typhoid antibodies.

(2) Special pathogen examination: ① The patient had a history of contact with cats and dogs, so it is necessary to rule out some parasitic diseases. Further examination needed: Toxoplasma gondii antibodies, blood agglutination test for cat-scratch fever, and the Weil-Felix test. ② The patient had a history of tuberculosis, so it is necessary to rule out tuberculosis progression and miliary tuberculosis. Tuberculosis antibodies, tuberculin test, and chest CT were needed. ③ To exclude autoimmune diseases, it is

necessary to check ANA, AMA, ANCA, antistreptolysin-O test, rheumatoid factor, and thyroid function. ④ To exclude blood system diseases and tumors, it is necessary to check tumor markers and cytological examination: Bone penetration, lymph node biopsy (not done, because the lymph nodes are too small), and looking for exfoliated cells in the chest and abdominal fluid. Coombs test, Ham test, Rous test, reticulocyte count. ⑤ The patient is a nurse at a drug rehabilitation center, and is in a high-risk group for HIV infection, so it is necessary to check HIV antibodies to exclude HIV infection.

IV. Ward-round analysis after one week

On admission, ceftriaxone sodium and levofloxacin were given as anti-inflammatory drugs, and anti-tuberculosis treatment was continued, to observe the changes in the disease.

The results are as follows: HIV antibodies, typhoid antibodies, Widal test, blood culture, bone marrow culture, Weil-Felix test, PPD test, tuberculosis antibodies, and exfoliated cells in the chest and abdominal fluid were all negative. Tumor markers were normal; thyroid function, blood sugar, and uric acid were normal. Coombs test, Ham test (−), Rous (−), and reticulocyte count was normal. Bone marrow routine: Iron utilization decreased, granulocyte proliferation was active, neutrophil alkaline phosphatase (NAP) score increased, indicating the infection phase. Bone marrow biopsy hematopoietic tissue proliferation was active, and Toxoplasma gondii IgM luminescence method (+).

Thinking prompts:

1. Infectious diseases that can be ruled out

(1) Viral infection: Generally, the course of the fever does not exceed 7–14 days. For EB viral infection, this can stretch to one month, but lymphocytes are predominant in peripheral blood, and abnormal lymphocytes are seen. The patient's HIV antibodies (−). The possibility of HIV infection can be ruled out.

(2) Common bacterial infectious diseases, including typhoid fever, paratyphoid fever, and other Salmonella infections: After the patient was admitted to hospital, ceftriaxone sodium and levofloxacin were given as anti-inflammatory drugs for one week; symptoms were not relieved, and typhoid antibodies (−), Widal test (−), blood culture (−) and bone marrow culture (−). This possibility can be ruled out.

(3) Some special pathogen infections: Chlamydia and mycoplasma often cause infections of the respiratory tract and urogenital system; Rickettsial infection often occurs in poor sanitary conditions, with a history of rat flea bites, fever rash, Weil-Felix test (+), and is sensitive to Rifampicin and Quinolone antibiotics. So, the possibility of chlamydia, mycoplasma, and Rickettsia infection can be ruled out.

(4) Fungal infection: This patient's oral leukoplakia (−) and pathogen (−), so it can be ruled out.

(5) Tuberculosis progression: During the anti-tuberculosis treatment this

patient underwent, chest CT showed no indication, PPD test (−), tuberculosis antibody (−), so it can be ruled out.

2. Non-infectious diseases can be ruled out

(1) Autoimmune diseases: In this case, the young female patient had a fever, joint pain, anemia, and a rapid erythrocyte sedimentation rate. SLE, rheumatic fever, and rheumatoid arthritis are the most common autoimmune diseases, but no facial butterfly erythema, annular erythema, carditis, or joint deformity were found during the physical examination. Further examination showed that ANA, AMA, ANCA, antistreptolysin-O test, rheumatoid factor and HLA-B27 were all negative, and this possibility could be ruled out.

(2) Metabolic diseases: The patient's thyroid function, blood sugar, and uric acid were normal, so this can be ruled out.

(3) Blood system diseases: The patient had a fever, anemia, hepatosplenomegaly, and lymphadenopathy, but the peripheral blood test and routine bone marrow test did not indicate leukemia. Coombs test, Ham test (−), Rous (−), reticulocyte count was normal, so the possibility of hemolytic anemia can be ruled out.

(4) Tumor: A CT scan and B-ultrasound of the patient's chest and abdomen did not indicate tumors. Exfoliative cells in the chest and abdominal fluid (−) and tumor markers were normal, so this possibility can be ruled out.

3. Diseases that cannot be ruled out: Lymphoma (bone marrow biopsy did not indicate lymphoma, but multiple bone marrow biopsies in multiple locations are required).

4. Possible diseases

(1) Toxoplasmosis: Toxoplasma gondii IgM luminescence method (+), bone marrow NAP score increased, indicating the infection phase; the third generation cephalosporins and quinolones were ineffective against Toxoplasmosis.

(2) Iron deficiency anemia: The patient had anemia, and bone penetration results showed that the utilization of iron was reduced.

V. Further diagnosis

Based on the above analysis, a further diagnosis can be obtained:

1. Iron-deficiency anemia (clear).
2. Toxoplasmosis possible.
3. The possibility of lymphoma and tumor should be eliminated.

VI. Further treatment measures

Although the diagnosis of iron deficiency anemia is clear, it cannot explain a patient's whole clinical process. Anti-Toxoplasma gondii treatment works well and has few side effects, so further treatment measures were taken:

1. An iron supplement for the anemia.
2. Albumin support therapy.
3. Combined antibiotic treatment was chosen for Anti-Toxoplasma: SMZco – two tablets, twice a day, azithromycin 500 mg/d.
4. Continue to observe changes to the patient's condition, and perform another bone marrow biopsy and lymph node biopsy if necessary.

VII. Ward-round analysis after 14 days of treatment

After seven days of anti-Toxoplasma treatment, the patient's body temperature began to return to normal. After seven days of continuous treatment, another ultrasound was performed, and pleural effusion, ascites, and pericardial effusion were absorbed. The patient was discharged from hospital in a stable condition.

VIII. Lessons learned

The patient – a 31-year-old female nurse – had a history of contact with cats and dogs, and her clinical manifestations included fever, joint pain, anemia, multiple serosa cavity effusion, hepatosplenomegaly, and superficial lymph node enlargement, which was in line with the diagnosis of FUO. After clinical observation and further examination, viruses, common bacterial infections, Salmonella infections, tuberculosis progression, autoimmune diseases, and blood system diseases (except lymphoma and tumors) were excluded.

Because the patient had a history of contact with cats and dogs, some specific pathogen infections cannot be ruled out. Therefore, we were compelled to examine Toxoplasma antibodies, and the basic diagnostic ideas were as follows: ① Toxoplasma gondii was a possibility. ② Lymphoma can be ruled out. According to the effectiveness of clinical anti-Toxoplasma treatment, the final clinical diagnosis was toxoplasmosis.

Reviewing our understanding of toxoplasmosis: Toxoplasmosis is a zoonotic parasitic disease caused by Toxoplasma gondii parasitizing the human body. Most cases are recessive infections, and can occur in healthy people but are more likely to occur in the immune-compromised population. Toxoplasma gondii can invade a variety of organs, so the clinical manifestations are very complex, and it is easy to misdiagnose and miss. Animals and poultry have a high infection rate. Contact history can be used as a diagnostic clue. The pathogen must be found, or the immunological reaction must be positive. Use the recommended treatment scheme according to the proceedings of the Fourth National Symposium on Toxoplasmosis.

(Sheng Jifang)

Recurrent fever for two months, and bilateral calf muscle pain for two weeks

I. Medical history

Patient: Female, aged 58. She was admitted to hospital on 5 May 2005 because of recurrent fever for two months and bilateral calf muscle pain for two weeks.

> **Thinking prompts:** Which diseases should be considered with a patient like this? What conditions should be considered in the gathering of her medical history? What signs should be paid attention to in physical examination, and what laboratory examinations should be given in a targeted manner?
>
> The patient is a middle-aged woman who has suffered a fever for two months. From the perspective of long-term fever, according to the current clinical analysis report, the main causes of FUO (fever of unknown origin) are infectious diseases, connective tissue diseases, malignant tumors and hematological diseases, and various febrile diseases. Therefore, it is necessary to collect comprehensive medical history, perform a physical examination, and run tests from these aspects, which is also the diagnostic thinking for diseases with FUO (fever of unknown origin).
>
> Connective tissue diseases, such as rheumatic fever, polymyositis and dermatomyositis, and adult-onset Still's disease (AOSD), should be considered first in cases of female patients with long-term fever and myalgia. Gastrocnemius pain is most likely to be diagnosed as leptospirosis. It is also necessary to investigate the patient's history of contact with infected water. What should be considered for connective tissue diseases? Except for fever and myalgia of the lower limbs, patients have no other symptoms or discomfort. Rheumatic diseases should be considered. Common examples are as follows: ① Polymyositis and dermatomyositis, mainly manifested as symmetrical proximal myasthenia in varying degrees. The course of disease is generally slow, and can also occur suddenly. There may be swelling and tenderness in the early stage, and muscular atrophy in the late stage. Patients with dermatomyositis may have photosensitive rashes on the face, chest, and hands. Patients with polymyositis and dermatomyositis often have systemic symptoms such as fatigue, weight loss, and fever.

Both polymyositis and dermatomyositis may be accompanied by malignant tumors, which are more common in patients over 50 years old. Dermatomyositis with tumors is more common than polymyositis. The symptoms of myositis can be improved after tumor resection, but there is also the possibility of recurrence after many years. Laboratory examinations include elevated serum zymogram, myogenic damage indicated by electromyography, and positive autoantibodies. Muscle biopsy can be performed to identify pathological changes. Hormone therapy, immunosuppressants, gamma globulin, and immunotherapy are required in treatment. ② Adult-onset Still's disease (AOSD) – an exclusive or clinical diagnosis in the presence of fever, rash, joint symptoms, increased white blood cells and neutrophils, increased erythrocyte sedimentation rate, negative blood culture, ineffective antibiotic treatment, and effective cortical hormone. Pharyngalgia, myalgia, enlargement of the lymph nodes in the liver and spleen, serositis, and liver damage can occur clinically. ③ Mixed connective tissue disease, which has the clinical manifestations of systemic lupus erythematosus, scleroderma, or polymyositis. Serological characteristics are that high titers of extractable nuclear antigen antibodies can be detected in both the active and remission stages of the disease. This disease typically occurs in young women, and usually has special manifestations: Diffuse swelling of the face and fingers, finger sclerosis, Raynaud's phenomenon, joint pain, arthritis, myositis, positive RNP antibodies but negative SM antibodies. The use of low-dose cortical hormone treatment is advocated.

The patient developed a fever without obvious inducement, and her body temperature fluctuated at 38.5°C, without chills, sore throat, or other discomforts. The treatment effect of cefradine at local hospitals was not good, and her body temperature rose again after returning to normal just once. She developed a fever two weeks earlier with pain in her gastrocnemius (calf), and was treated at county hospitals with ceftazidime and fluconazole. The effect of the treatment was poor, and the posterior myalgia was gradually aggravated, most obviously when walking and pressing, accompanied by mild edema in the calf and back of the foot. Routine blood examination showed that leukocytes were $7.7 \times 10^9/L$, hemoglobin was 98 g/L, and platelets were $186 \times 10^9/L$, ANA (+), dsDNA (–), SM (–). She was transferred to our hospital for fever and myalgia of unknown origin.

The patient had schistosomiasis at the age of 30, cholecystitis 12 years earlier and breast cancer resection one year ago. She had no history of contact with contaminated water, and no family history of disease.

Thinking prompts: What should be considered in the diagnosis of patients after admission: Fever and myalgia of unknown origin? Connective tissue disease? Parasites? Bacterial infection? Postoperative metastasis of breast cancer?

The patient was admitted to hospital with a fever that had lasted two months, with two weeks of myalgia as the main complaint. The main symptoms were long-term fever and leg pain in both lower limbs. The diagnosis should start from these two aspects. Fever of unknown origin includes four major diseases: Infectious diseases, tumors, connective tissue diseases, and other fever diseases. The patient had been feverish for two months before admission, and had been treated with antibiotics as an outpatient for a long time, but they were ineffective. At present, general bacterial infection can temporarily be ignored. The diagnosis is still unclear when combined with examinations at other hospitals.

II. Physical examination at admission

Positive results of physical examination in hospital: T 38.3°C, mild dorsal foot edema, tenderness of the bilateral gastrocnemius, obvious percussion pain, grade 5 muscle strength of both lower limbs, no muscle atrophy, mild pharyngeal congestion, operation scar about 20 cm long on the right chest, swelling of superficial lymph nodes, negative physical examination of heart and lungs, slightly hard palpation of abdomen, unsatisfactory palpation of liver and spleen, no nodules anywhere on the skin, no redness or tenderness of joints.

III. Preliminary diagnosis

On the second day after admission, the attending physician made rounds and analyzed the patient's medical history: The patient, female, aged 58, was admitted to hospital because of recurrent fever for two months and bilateral calf muscle pain for two weeks. Cefradine, ceftazidime, and fluconazole were given at another hospital, with a poor curative effect. The patient had a history of schistosomiasis and breast cancer resection. The physical examination in hospital showed a temperature of 38.3°C, with slight edema on the back of the foot, tenderness of the bilateral gastrocnemius muscles, and obvious percussion pain. One loxoprofen (Loxonin) tablet was taken when her body temperature was high on the first night after admission. Her body temperature dropped obviously, and the myalgia was relieved. The diagnosis is unknown at present.

Diagnosis:

1. The patient had a long-term moderate fever, and had been taking antibiotics for a long time, but the effect was not good. Therefore, it is necessary to eliminate the possibility of a tumor, and consider the possibility of breast cancer metastasis.
2. For patients with fever of unknown origin, the possibility of infectious diseases should still be considered as a cause of long-term fever. The poor effectiveness of antibiotics may be due to a failure to cover certain pathogenic microorganisms.
3. The causes of gastrocnemius pain could be epidemic hemorrhagic fever or leptospirosis, but corresponding epidemic history was lacking in this case.

IV. Auxiliary inspection

Routine blood: WBC 6.9×10^9/L, neutrophil 82.1%, eosinophil 7.4%, hemoglobin 85 g/L.

ESR 96 mm/h; the rheumatoid factor was 176 U/ml, and the c-reactive protein was 61.5 mg/L.

Serum albumin 22.1 g/L, cholinesterase 1,161 U/L, total cholesterol 2.76 mmol/L.

Urinary routine: Occult blood (++++), 1–3 red blood cells /HP, 0–2 white blood cells /HP.

Myocardial enzyme spectrum: AST 63 U/L, CK and others were negative.

Blood sugar normal, HIV, syphilis, HBV, HCV, and PPD were negative.

Chest radiograph showed no obvious abnormality.

B-ultrasound: Chronic schistosomiasis liver disease, multiple gallstones.

Tumor markers: CA199 58.1 U/ml, ferritin 419.7 ng/ml.

Routine stool negative, blood culture negative.

AMA negative, ANNA (+), ANA 1:80 (+), anticardiolipin antibody negative, lactate dehydrogenase normal.

V. Further diagnosis and treatment

On the fourth day after admission, the chief physician made rounds: The patient's body temperature remained high, especially at night. IgG+C3+C4 examination showed that IgG 1,950 ng/dl, C3, and C4 decreased slightly. Because gastrocnemius pain is a major sign of leptospirosis, penicillin can be used if the cause of fever is unknown. In order to avoid the Herxheimer reaction, a small dose of penicillin can be used first and then gradually increased. In addition, patients with fever and myalgia can be treated with NSAIDs, such as Loxonin. At the same time, supportive treatment should be strengthened.

After the above treatment, Loxonin had a positive effect on the patient's fever and myalgia. On examination, it was found that her throat was slightly congested, and there were a lot of white spots in her mouth. Therefore, a secondary local fungal infection caused by broad-spectrum antibiotics before admission should be considered. The throat swab culture suggested a small amount of Candida albicans, and fluconazol was given intravenously at 0.2 g. The first dose was doubled, and the patient's sore throat was relieved. Her throat swab culture showed a small amount of Candida albicans. Penicillin and fluconazole were continued, but the diagnosis was still unclear. Diagnostic treatment with penicillin was ineffective.

After eliminating rheumatic diseases, we consulted with the infectious diseases department, and asked about the presence of cats in the patient's home, considering toxoplasmosis as a diagnosis. We checked that the IgM of Toxoplasma gondii antibody was strongly positive and the diagnosis was clear, and gave her sulfamethoxazole (SMZ).

VI. Lessons learned

Toxoplasmosis is a systemic infectious disease caused by Toxoplasma gondii, of which cats are the most common intermediate hosts. Toxoplasma gondii parasitizes the intestinal mucosa, and the oocysts that are discharged can survive in the soil for a year and a half. People who have cats at home or have close contact with cats, those who have eaten uncooked animal meat and drunk contaminated unboiled water, and babies born to mothers infected with Toxoplasma gondii during pregnancy are susceptible to this disease. Its clinical manifestations are extremely complicated, ranging from simple lymph node enlargement to fatal acute fulminant pneumonia and cerebrospinal meningitis, and may have mental, nervous, eye, heart and respiratory symptoms. Some patients may have a rash, muscular arthropathy, and hepatomegaly. Patients suspected of this disease can be examined by lymph node biopsy or animal inoculation of blood and cerebrospinal fluid to find pathogens, and can also be diagnosed by serological tests.

Leptospirosis is an acute infectious disease caused by various types of pathogenic Leptospira. Rats and pigs are the main sources of infection. Leptospira is excreted with the urine of infected animals, which pollutes water sources. When people come into contact with contaminated water, they become infected through the skin and mucous membranes. The disease usually occurs in the summer and autumn rice cutting season, or after heavy rain and flooding. Typical patients have rapid onset with high fever, lassitude, general aches, conjunctival congestion, tenderness of peroneal muscles, and swelling of the superficial lymph nodes. In the middle stage, it may be accompanied by diffuse pulmonary hemorrhage, and obvious damage to the liver, kidneys, and central nervous system; most patients recover in the late stage, and some may have post-fever, ocular uveitis, and occlusive inflammation of the cerebral artery. Diffuse pulmonary hemorrhage, and liver and renal failure are often the causes of death.

This patient's diagnosis is clear, based on keeping a cat at home, and strong positive IgM in Toxoplasma gondii antibodies. Chronic fever and bilateral gastrocnemius pain are typical signs of leptospirosis, but the diagnosis of leptospirosis and toxoplasmosis generally has its own epidemiological history. Through the diagnosis of this disease, we notice that we can still encounter uncommon infectious diseases on the ward of the non-infectious department, and we cannot ignore the gathering of medical history, especially in patients with fever of unknown origin.

(Sheng Jifang)

Chills, fever, and fatigue for 14 days, yellowness of urine and eyes for six days, and no urine for two days

I. Medical history

Patient: Male, 32 years old, a farmer from Nanchuan County in Chongqing. He was admitted to hospital for chills, fever, and fatigue for 14 days, yellow urine and eyes for six days, and no urine for two days. He was hospitalized from 11 to 12 August 2002.

The patient started to show intolerance of cold and fever with a temperature of 40.2°C, accompanied by fatigue, soreness, and pain in the extremities, and a headache after working in the paddy field 14 days before admission (28 July 2002). Diagnosis and treatment at a local health center were ineffective (the diagnosis and course of treatment were unclear), and the patient still developed fever, especially in the afternoon and at night. His body temperature dropped after the antipyretic medication was given, but was still abnormal. After eight days (5 August 2002), excessively yellow urine began to appear, like strong tea. Soon, yellow staining of the skin and bilateral sclera appeared, and the urine volume decreased. There was no itching, and no gray or dark stool.

The patient then went to the county hospital, and was admitted with fever and jaundice of unknown origin – possibly leptospirosis. After being treated with anti-infection penicillin and symptomatic support, the symptoms became worse. His jaundice deepened, and his urine volume gradually decreased. After 12 days (9 August 2002), there was no urine, no edema of the lower limbs, convulsion, or coma. For further diagnosis and treatment, the patient came to our department for treatment on 11 August 2002, and was admitted to the outpatient department with fever and jaundice of unknown origin. Since the onset, he had suffered from poor spirit, poor diet and sleep, no vomiting and diarrhea, normal stool, and no obvious weight loss.

The patient had no previous health issues, with no history of infectious diseases such as hepatitis, tuberculosis, and typhoid fever. He denied a history of operations and injuries, blood transfusions and blood products application, and drug and food allergies, and had no clinical history of issues with his respiratory, circulatory, digestive, and urinary systems.

The patient was born and raised in his original domicile, and had no history of contact with sources of epidemics. He worked in paddy fields, but had not come into contact with poison or contamination from radioactive substances. He had no history of alcohol and tobacco, and had no unhealthy habits. His parents, wife, and children were in good health. There was no history of genetic diseases in the family or similar diseases around them recently.

II. Physical examination on admission

T 39.9°C, P 118 times/min, R 36 times/min, BP 111/49 mmHg. Normal development, moderate nutrition, carried into the ward, active body position, conscious and cooperative during physical examination. Appearance of acute severe illness, severe yellow staining of skin on his whole body, with interspersed petechia, especially in chest and abdomen, without liver palm or spider nevus. No palpable superficial lymph node enlargement all over the body. No deformity in the head and facial features. No eyelid edema or ptosis. The sclerae of both eyes were severely yellow stained; the bulbar conjunctiva was congested; the cornea was transparent; the eyeball moved freely PERRLA (pupils are equal, round and reactive to light and accommodation); the diameters were about 0.3 cm.

There were no pale lips, no bleeding ulcers in oral mucosa, midline protrusion of the tongue, without tremors, no congestion in the pharynx, and no swelling in the bilateral tonsils. Soft and symmetrical neck, no deviation of trachea, no jugular vein distention, hepatic jugular vein reflux sign (−), no bilateral thyroid enlargement.

During auscultation, the breath sounds of both lungs were thick; dry and moist rales were not heard. There was no uplift in the precordial area; percussion showed that the heart border was not widened; the heart rate was 118 beats/min, and the rhythm was uniform, and no pathological murmur was heard in each valve area. The abdomen was flat, with no intestinal type and peristalsis waves, and with no varicose veins in the abdominal wall. Soft abdomen, tenderness in the middle and upper abdomen, no rebound pain and muscle tension, 4 cm below the liver rib, 6 cm below the xiphoid process, medium quality, dull edge and slight pain to touch. The spleen was not palpable below the costal margin; no percussion pain in liver, spleen and kidneys, negative shifting dullness in abdomen, and no edema in the lower limbs. Bilateral gastrocnemius tenderness was obvious, and no positive signs were found in the nervous system.

III. Auxiliary examination at admission

1. County hospital inspection (6 August 2002)

Liver function: ALT 207 IU/L, AST 303 IU/L and TB 106.4 μmol/L.

Renal function: BUN 15.26 mmol/L, Cr 184.6 μmol/L and uric acid (UA) 204.0 mmol/L.

Chest X-ray film: ① Double lower lung infection, pulmonary interstitial, and pulmonary parenchyma are involved; ② Proliferation and fibrosis of the right upper lung.

Abdominal Color Doppler ultrasound: ① The liver is large, and the echo in the liver is increased and enhanced; ② Thickening and coarseness of gallbladder wall; ③ Splenomegaly.

2. Examination after transfer to hospital (11 August 2002)

Liver function: ALT 171 IU/L, AST 1290 IU/L, GGT 225 IU/L, ALP 383 IU/L, TP 41.1 g/L, A 22.6 g/L, TB 252.8 μmol/L and CB 143.8 μmol/L.

Renal function: K^+ 4.68 mmol/L, Na^+ 122.1 mmol/L, Cl^- 96.4 mmol/l, GLU 3.49 mmol/L, BUN 31.19 mmol/L, Cr 497.9 μmol/L, Ca^{2+} 1.9 mmol/L, P^{3+} 2.02 mmol/L, UA 743 mmol/L;

Enzyme spectrum of myocardium: LDH 4,184 IU/L, α-HBDH 3,902 IU/L, CK 2,221 IU/L, CK-MB 120 IU/L;

Three items of coagulation: PT 26.9 seconds, APTT (activated partial thromboplastin time) 97.9 seconds, PTA (prothrombin activity) 28.7%;

Routine blood: WBC 2.3×10^9/L, N 49%, L 30%, classification of rod nucleus 10%, monocyte 3%, abnormal lymphocyte 7%, E 0%, RBC 2.74×10^{12}/L, Hb 80 g/L, PLT 34×10^9/L; ESR 9 mm/h;

Urine routine: Urine protein (+), RBC (++), WBC 2–3/HP;

The markers of hepatitis A, hepatitis C, hepatitis D, and hepatitis E were all negative. Serological markers of hepatitis B: HBsAb, HBeAb, and HBcAb were positive; AFP negative; blood culture was carried out three consecutive times, and the results of the culture for five days were all negative. HIV antibodies were negative; TP negative; Widal test (H, O, A, B, C) was negative.

ECG: ST-T changes; chest X-ray in the frontal and lateral position: Pleural thickening with fibrous lesions in the tip area of double upper lungs, and previous tuberculosis suspected.

Abdominal CT: ① Liver and spleen were slightly larger, and liver density was slightly lower, which should be used for diagnosis combined with clinical symptoms. There was suspected low density of shadows in the left outer lobe of the liver, so contrast CT should be applied if necessary; ② Stellate calcification in the left lateral lobe of the liver; ③ The gallbladder wall was slightly thick and fuzzy, and edema is suspected; ④ A little pleural effusion on the left side.

IV. Preliminary diagnosis

The patient suffered from chills, fever, and fatigue for 14 days, accompanied by jaundice for six days and anuria for two days, with acute fever. The reason was still unclear. It was considered to be fever with jaundice of unknown origin: ① Leptospirosis? ② Typhoid fever? ③ Hemolytic anemia?

> **Thinking prompts:** Acute fever with jaundice can be caused by either infectious or non-infectious diseases according to their etiological classification. The most common infectious diseases are viral hepatitis, suppurative obstructive cholangitis, infectious mononucleosis, leptospirosis, hemorrhagic fever with renal syndrome, typhoid hepatitis, and cytomegalovirus (CMV) infection (hepatitis type). Common non-infectious diseases include acute hemolysis, acute alcoholism, cholelithiasis,

calculous cholecystitis, drug fever, autoimmune hepatitis, liver cancer, metastatic cancer, and malignant histiocytosis.

The following section offers more details about the above-mentioned diseases:

1. Infectious diseases

(1) Viral hepatitis: Acute icteric hepatitis, the most common in clinics, consists of acute viral hepatitis A and acute viral hepatitis E. Jaundice appears when the fever is relieved, that is, fever often occurs before jaundice, and is mostly relieved when jaundice appears.

(2) Infectious mononucleosis: Angina, enlarged lymph nodes, pleomorphic rash, increased abnormal lymphocytes in blood (which can be foam type, irregular type, and infantile type according to their cell morphology), and positive heterophile agglutination test results.

(3) Hemorrhagic fever with renal syndrome: Fever, hemorrhage, impairment of renal function and five stages (fever, hypotension, oliguria, polyuria, and recovery) are the characteristics of hemorrhagic fever with renal syndrome. This case should be distinguished from hemorrhagic fever with renal syndrome. If necessary, a serological test can be helpful for diagnosis.

(4) Dengue hemorrhagic fever: Similar to dengue fever, but with severe bleeding, sometimes accompanied by shock. Dengue fever is characterized by pain in the muscles, bones, and joints; a rash appears after 4–5 days of fever, which is often prevalent and can be diagnosed by serological examination.

(5) Typhoid hepatitis: Because there are more atypical cases of typhoid fever, and more complications and complex types, the misdiagnosis rate is about 25%, which deserves attention. The diagnosis should be based on relevant epidemiological data, with fever rising gradually, persistent high fever, rash for 7–13 days, few rashes, rose rash, indifferent expression, hard of hearing, relatively slow pulse, hepatosplenomegaly, decreased white blood cell count, decreased or disappeared eosinophil count, positive blood Widal test, and Salmonella typhi isolated from blood culture or bone marrow culture. For patients with typhoid hepatitis, hepatomegaly is more obvious than splenomegaly, and there is obvious liver function damage, which is manifested as increased alanine aminotransferase (ALT) and jaundice in some cases.

(6) CMV infection (hepatitis type): Its clinical features are obvious digestive tract symptoms, hepatosplenomegaly, and abnormal liver function. Cases with jaundice and obvious liver function damage can be diagnosed as CMV hepatitis. The possibility of CMV infection should be considered in patients with the following conditions: ① Fever with pneumonia and hepatitis for unknown reasons in adults, and persistent high fever in immunocompromised patients with basic diseases; ② Adult fever of unknown cause, lymphocyte ratio > 50%, atypical lymphocyte ratio > 10%, Paul-Bunnell test negative; ③ The diagnosis depends on serological and histopathological examination.

(7) Suppurative obstructive cholangitis: Chills, high fever, systemic poisoning, deep

jaundice, pain in the right upper abdomen, abdominal muscle tension, and obviously increased white blood cell count.

2. Non-infectious diseases

(1) Autoimmune hepatitis (AIH): Its clinical manifestations are fatigue and digestive tract symptoms, which are often nonspecific. However, if it is accompanied by an irregular fever of unknown origin, it has a certain differential significance from other types of hepatitis. Its clinical features include great variation to the results of liver function examination, which can be manifested as acute and chronic liver damage, cholestasis, and the levels of transaminase and bilirubin just exceeding the normal upper limit or being 30–50 times higher than normal. Autoantibody detection is of great significance to the diagnosis of AIH: ANA positive and anti-SMA positive suggest type I autoimmune hepatitis; anti-LKM1 positive indicates type II a AIH; anti-LKM1 positive and anti-GOR positive indicate type II b AIH; anti-SLA positive indicates type III AIH; anti-SMA positive indicates type IV AIH. Liver histopathology is often characterized by three major features: Interfacial hepatitis, i.e., clastic necrosis, rosette hepatocytes, plasma cell infiltration, and no cholestasis, copper deposition, or other characteristic lesions that can deny AIH.

(2) Malignant histiocytosis: In cases that have the following clinical manifestations, clinicians should be highly alert to the possibility of malignant histiocytosis: ① Long-term fever, pancytopenia with bleeding; ② The liver, spleen, and lymph nodes are obviously enlarged; ③ Special manifestations such as jaundice, pleural effusion, joint pain, skin damage, and intestinal symptoms; ④ Antibiotic treatment is ineffective, while glucocorticoid is temporarily effective or ineffective. Clinical manifestations may be similar to severe hepatitis, with 85% of patients having hepatomegaly and 75% having splenomegaly. Because hepatosplenomegaly is caused by infiltration of malignant tissue cells, the liver and spleen are full and firm when touched.

(3) Primary liver cancer (HCC): Typical HCC is not difficult to diagnose, so we should note the identification of early and atypical HCC. The possibility of HCC should be considered in the following cases: ① Those who have a history of hepatitis B or C and have recent unexplained wasting or digestive tract symptoms; ② Patients with a high risk of liver cancer and fever of unknown origin, acute abdominal swelling, diarrhea, hypoglycemic coma, polycythemia or anemia, and a leukemia-like reaction; ③ Sudden appearance of obstructive jaundice with unknown causes; ④ Patients with liver pain of unknown origin.

Its clinical features are as follows: About 95% of patients have hepatomegaly, hard texture, uneven surface, and obvious tenderness. About 85% of HCC patients have jaundice in the middle and late stages of the disease, most of which are obstructive and a few are hepatocellular.

(4) Cholangiocarcinoma (common bile duct or hepatic cholangiocarcinoma): Cholangiocarcinoma is difficult to diagnose. For middle-aged patients (especially men) with progressive obstructive jaundice that can be temporarily relieved, there is hepatomegaly with

no obvious tenderness, jaundice is deep, and other indexes of liver function are not seriously damaged. In patients with normal duodenal function after repeated examination with a barium meal in the upper digestive tract, the possibility of cholangiocarcinoma is highly doubtful. Pay close attention to further examination. If cholangiocarcinoma is accompanied by secondary infection, then chills, high fever, and increased white blood cell count may occur. Its clinical features are obstructive jaundice with white clay stool, bilirubin urine, and hepatomegaly can occur in the early stage of the disease. Jaundice can be temporarily decreased in the course of disease due to the rupture of cancer tissue and the improvement of bile drainage.

(5) Cholelithiasis and calculous cholecystitis: Upper right abdominal pain, high fever and jaundice, and a possible history of previous attacks. Murphy's sign is positive, sometimes showing obstructive jaundice (the proportion of combined bilirubin is obviously increased, > 60%), skin itching, clay-colored stool; imaging such as B-ultrasound suggests that biliary calculi can support the diagnosis.

(6) Acute hemolysis: Its clinical features are firstly chills, fever, and hemoglobinuria (soy sauce-like urine), then jaundice and lumbago.

(7) Acute alcoholism: A history of heavy drinking, which can be ruled out in this case.

(8) Drug fever: A history of drug use, often with polymorphic drug eruption. Sometimes there will be toxic hepatitis at the same time, and attention should be paid to identification.

(9) Leptospirosis: Diagnostic points are as follows: ① Relevant epidemiological data: Epidemic season, occupation as a farmer, pig raising, working in paddy fields, history of contact with contaminated water; ② Acute onset, fever, congestion of the bulbar conjunctiva, general pain, gastrocnemius pain and tenderness, inguinal lymph node enlargement and tenderness; complicated with jaundice, pulmonary hemorrhage, kidney damage, or meningoencephalitis; ③ A slight increase in the white blood cell count and neutrophil ratio in the peripheral blood, and positive serological examination and/or pathogen isolation.

Liver damage from leptospirosis is mainly seen in bleeding-type jaundice. Jaundice usually occurs 3–7 days after illness, and 80% of cases are accompanied by bleeding of different degrees, such as the epistaxis, petechiae of the skin and mucous membrane, ecchymosis, purpura, hemoptysis, hematuria, and vaginal bleeding. Severe cases include gastrointestinal bleeding, shock, and even death. The total serum bilirubin can be more than five times normal, while ALT and AST rarely exceed five times (but transaminase in this case was much higher than five times).

In the process of diagnosis and treatment in county hospitals, the illness worsened after penicillin was administered, of which the dosage and course of treatment were unknown. If it was treated with a large dose of penicillin, and worsened, then considering the Herxheimer reaction (which is unique to the treatment of leptospirosis with penicillin), this would support the diagnosis of leptospirosis.

V. Further diagnosis and treatment

After being admitted to hospital on 11 August 2002, the patient suffered from a high fever, and his body temperature fluctuated between 39.6°C and 39.9°C. He did not urinate after admission, and his kidney function was seriously damaged. His liver function was also seriously damaged; UN, Cr, and AST were obviously increased, and he suffered from severe jaundice and hepatomegaly. He proceeded to the next level of care, and was reported as critically ill.

Physical cooling, continuous low-flow oxygen inhalation, and ECG monitoring were performed, and the patient was treated with liver protection, enzyme reduction, jaundice reduction, diuresis, and symptomatic support. From 22:30 on 11 August 2002 to 05:00 the next day, dark watery stool was dissolved three times, with a total volume of 400 ml, without hematemesis. Routine stool: Occult blood (++++), 0–2 pus cells/HPF.

In consideration of upper gastrointestinal bleeding, the patient was treated with acid suppression, stomach protection, a blood transfusion (red blood cell suspension and whole blood), hemostasis (vitamin K_1, Etamsylate, aminomethylbenzoic, Hemopexin, lyophilizing thrombin powder and somatostatin), albumin supplementation, boosting pressure, diuresis enhancement, and meropenem anti-infection. However, the patient still failed to urinate, and his condition gradually worsened. At 05:30 on 12 August 2002, he appeared delirious and unresponsive, in a shallow coma with dysphoria, shortness of breath, shallow and fast breathing, P 132 times/min, R 30 times/min, BP 94/50 mmHg. Both pupils were equal, round with a diameter of 0.1 cm, insensitive to light reflection; thick breathing sounds on both sides, and no wet and dry rales.

Due to unconsciousness and miosis, cerebral hemorrhage was considered likely. Because of kidney damage and anuria, mannitol dehydration was avoided to aggravate kidney damage. Dopamine and furosemide were used to strengthen diuresis. Due to respiratory failure, coramine and lobeline were used for repeated intravenous injection.

At 09:00 on 12 August, the patient was conscious, and still had shortness of breath – shallow and fast, with T 39.0°C, P 126 times/min, R 29 times/min, BP 95/49 mmHg. PERRLA (pupils are equal, round and reactive to light and accommodation). The rest was the same as before. We continued to protect his liver with blood transfusions, hemostasis, diuresis, and symptomatic support, and carried out active hemodialysis.

The results of a leptospirosis serum antibody test at the municipal health and epidemic prevention station reported positive, and the patient was diagnosed with leptospirosis (bleeding-type jaundice) after considering his medical history, clinical manifestations, physical signs, and laboratory examination. However, due to financial reasons, the patient's family strongly requested that he leave hospital, so he was automatically discharged.

VI. Follow-up (the next day after discharge, that is, the sixteenth day of the course of the disease)

The patient died at home due to sudden respiratory and cardiac arrest. Follow-up showed that he had no urine in his body, and still had dark bloody stool. It was speculated that the direct causes of death might be hyperkalemia, hemorrhagic shock, intracranial hemorrhage, cerebral edema, and cerebral hernia.

VII. Lessons learned

1. Early diagnosis of leptospirosis: Leptospirosis is a natural-focus acute infectious disease caused by leptospira. Most provinces, municipalities, and autonomous regions in China are infected with the disease, especially the southern provinces and cities. Pigs and mice are the main sources of infection. Spirochetes in their urine pollute soil or food, and people can get sick through skin or digestive tract infection. The morbidity of farmers working in paddy fields is high, and the peak of the epidemic is from July to September. The incubation period is around ten days, but can be as short as several days or as long as one month.

According to the type, virulence, and immune function of leptospira, it shows different clinical types, such as infection poisoning type (also called influenza typhoid type), bleeding-jaundice type, pulmonary hemorrhage type, renal failure type, meningoencephalitis type, and gastroenteritis type. The patient in this case had a rapid onset, chills, high fever, congestion and edema of the bulbar conjunctiva, obvious abnormal urine, serious damage to renal function, and negative serological examination of viral hepatitis, so leptospirosis could be considered.

Fever, general aches, fatigue, weakness, conjunctival congestion, gastrocnemius pain and tenderness, and swelling and pain of the lymph nodes are considered as the three main symptoms and signs of this disease. During the epidemic season, if a patient has been in contact with contaminated water, and there is a main symptom and main sign, a primary diagnosis of leptospirosis should be considered and made. However, the white blood cells and neutrophils in this case were not high. In 570 cases of leptospirosisin in Guilin, Guangxi, only 1.25% of them have white blood cells < 4.0×10^9/L, and 2.5% have white blood cells > 20.0×10^9/L. For cases with no white blood cells and a slightly increased neutrophil ratio, diagnosis should be especially circumspect. In addition, be sure to distinguish it from other diseases that can cause fever, jaundice, hemorrhage, and kidney damage, such as hemorrhagic fever with renal syndrome, which ultimately needs serological diagnosis.

2. Herxheimer reaction: Penicillin is the first choice for leptospirosis, but the first dose should not be too large. It is safer to apply gradual increments to prevent a large number of leptospira from being killed and releasing toxins that induce the Herxheimer (contradictory) reaction). The Herxheimer reaction should be considered if chills and high fever suddenly occur within a few hours of penicillin administration, and if the blood pressure drops, with cold limbs and shock-like symptoms.

Studies have shown that the incidence of the Herxheimer reaction is obviously increased in patients with positive blood culture. However, it is not known whether this patient was diagnosed and treated at the local county hospital with the Herxheimer reaction after penicillin was administered, or whether his condition worsened. It is speculated that the Herxheimer reaction is likely. Therefore, if we do not understand the Herxheimer reaction, we could mistake it for a general drug reaction and miss its guiding role in the diagnosis of leptospirosis.

The patient in this case was hospitalized for one day in total. When the positive results of his leptospira serum antibody test were reported at the municipal health and epidemic prevention station, the patient's family had given up treatment, and he remained in a critical condition. Before a definitive diagnosis was made, it was possible to choose the carbapenem broad-spectrum antibiotic meropenem to fight infection, in order to control a possible serious infection and its progression as quickly as possible. However, after a diagnosis of leptospirosis, penicillin should be the first treatment. Because the prognosis in this case was extremely poor, even if small doses of penicillin are gradually increased, it cannot change the outcome for the patient due to multiple organ dysfunction (MODS).

3. Leptospirosis complicated with acute hemolysis: Besides hemorrhagic leptospirosis jaundice, leptospirosis complicated with acute hemolysis should also be considered. If it is known whether there is soy-sauce urine, progressive Hb decrease, progressive jaundice aggravation (hyperbilirubinemia), increased reticulocyte, and lumbearlier, tests should be carried out to check the coagulation function, as well as the sugar-water test, acid hemolysis test (Ham test), and antihumanglobulin antibody test (Coombs test), to check for hemolysis.

(Wang Yuming)

Intermittent fever for more than two months

I. Medical history

Patient: Male, 28 years old, from Xuancheng in Anhui Province. He was admitted to hospital with intermittent fever for more than two months, and was hospitalized between 21 October and 13 November 2004.

In mid-August 2004, the patient developed fever without obvious inducement, reaching temperatures of up to 39.5°C, without obvious aversion to cold and chills, accompanied by mild headache, dizziness, and fatigue. Slight cough, no expectoration, no nasal congestion, runny nose, chest pain, night sweat and hemoptysis; no obvious chest tightness, palpitations, and shortness of breath; no frequent, urgent, or painful micturition; no abdominal pain, diarrhea, nausea, or vomiting; no rash, joint swelling or pain, gingival bleeding, or epistaxis. After his illness, the patient was given anti-infection treatment in the form of penicillin, cefuroxime, cefoperazone, amikacin, and fosfomycin, with intermittent use of acetaminophen (Bufferin) and dexamethasone for symptomatic and supportive treatment at a local hospital. His body temperature dropped to normal, and then rose to about 39.2°C a week later. He came to our hospital for treatment after repeated attacks for two months.

The patient was generally healthy, with no history of chronic hepatitis and tuberculosis, contaminated diet, and drug and food allergies. He had been working in Guangdong for the past two years. Before that, he lived in the rural area of Xuancheng, and had a history of canine contact. He had no history of working in the fields in recent years, and denied any contact with contaminated water.

> **Thinking prompts:** Problems encountered in the gathering of medical history.
>
> 1. The clinical symptoms, especially the regularity of the fever, were not inquired about carefully enough. The acute onset, degree of fever, and accompanying symptoms were clearly described in the patient's comprehensive medical history, but the type and course of the fever lacked detail. Some diseases have a characteristic type and course of fever. For example, continued fever can be seen in typhoid, tsutsugamushi disease, camp fever, and lobar pneumonia. Remittent fever can be seen in influenza, sepsis, pyogenic infections, infectious endocarditis, severe tuberculosis, and malignant histocytosis. Intermittent fever can be seen in malaria, pyelonephritis, lymphoma, and

brucellosis. Relapsing fever can be seen in Hodgkin's disease. Undulant fever can be seen in brucellosis. Saddle fever can be seen in dengue fever. In this case, the evolution of the fever type, duration, antipyretic condition, and the interval for recurrence after subsiding were not described, and the effect of specific medication on the fever was not described in any detail. The changes of accompanying symptoms since the onset of the disease (such as whether the symptoms persisted, were aggravated, or were relieved), and whether other new symptoms appeared, were not provided. This would have been helpful for differential diagnosis.

2. Incomplete epidemiological data. Apart from the information already provided, the patient's working and living environment, and whether he was in contact with domestic animals, birds, and rats were unclear. Contact with birds may be related to psittacosis and cryptococcus infection. Contact with domestic animals such as sheep, cattle, and pigs may be related to brucellosis. Contact with rodents may be related to hemorrhagic fever with renal syndrome, leptospirosis, and relapsing fever. Contact with dogs may be related to kala-azar.

3. Information about diagnosis and treatment from the external hospital was incomplete. Any hospital's diagnosis and treatment data should be taken seriously, and the symptoms and signs at the onset, the examination results from the external hospital, and the changes in the disease after treatment should be queried and recorded clearly. The process of diagnosis and treatment at other hospitals has guiding significance for the current differential diagnosis and treatment selection. The detailed records of the use of antibiotics and adrenocortical hormones in a patient's medical history should be complete, and the dosage, usage, and course of treatment should be fully recorded, because in cases of infectious disease, the selection, dosage, and course of treatment of anti-infective drugs are closely related to the effectiveness of treatment, and may affect follow-up treatment. Similarly, the use of adrenocortical hormones and immunosuppressants will also affect the outcome of the disease, and may even cause complications.

Follow-up medical history: During his time working in Guangdong, the patient lived on the urban-rural fringe. The surrounding environment was very poor, and was infested with rats. Two days after the onset of his illness, the patient took Bufferin. His fever was slightly relieved, but his body temperature did not return to normal. On the third day, he went to a local hospital for treatment. Except for a slight enlargement of his liver and spleen, he had no other positive signs during physical examination. His routine blood and liver function were normal, and he was treated with penicillin (usage: 4.8 million U, intravenous drip, once). Three hours later, he developed chills and a fever. The local hospital considered this as a transfusion reaction. 10 mg of dexamethasone was given. After an intravenous injection, the patient's symptoms eased and his body temperature returned to normal. However, he still developed a fever the next day, and was given cefuroxime (usage: 3.0 g, IV, twice a day). Since there was no remission of symptoms after two days, the patient was given cefoperazone (usage: 2.0 g, intravenous drip, twice a day), amikacin (usage: 0.2 g, intramuscular injection, twice a day), and dexamethasone (usage: 5 mg, intravenous injection, once a day). After two days, the symptoms were relieved. His fever subsided, accompanied by sweating.

The patient stopped taking hormones and continued anti-infection treatment for three days. After one week, he developed a fever and other symptoms again, and went to a local hospital for treatment. The anti-infection treatment with cefoperazone combined with amikacin continued, but hormones were not given. After three days, the symptoms were not obviously relieved, so fosfomycin (usage: 2.0 g, intravenous drip, three times a day) was used instead. After two days, the symptoms were relieved. His fever subsided, accompanied by sweating, and the anti-infection treatment continued for three days. After two weeks, the illness recurred once again. After treatment with fosfomycin to fight infection for three days, the fever subsided, accompanied by sweating, and the treatment stopped after one continuous week. After 20 days, the patient fell ill again when returning to his hometown to visit relatives, and was hospitalized for diagnosis and treatment.

II. Physical examination after admission

T 39.5°C, P 103 times/min, R 17 times/min, BP 110/75 mmHg, clear consciousness, poor spirit, no yellow stain on the skin and mucous membrane anywhere on the body; no petechiae, ecchymosis, macula, papule, rose rash and other rashes; no eschars or ulcers. Superficial lymph nodes were not enlarged. No yellow staining of the sclera; no edema of the bulbar conjunctiva. No tenderness in the sternum. Heart rate was 103 beats/min, which was regular, and murmurs and abnormal heart sounds were not heard in either valve area. Respiratory movements were normal, and there were no abnormalities in chest tapping and no abnormal findings on auscultation. The abdomen was flat and soft, and there were no tenderness or rebound pain anywhere. The mass was not palpated. The liver was 1.5 cm below the right rib, soft and without tenderness. The spleen was just palpated under the rib, and it was soft without obvious tenderness. There was no percussion pain in the liver, spleen, and kidney regions, and shifting dullness was negative. No limb deformity; muscle strength and tension were normal. The meningeal irritation sign and pyramidal tract sign were negative.

> **Thinking prompts:** The patient was a young male with recurrent relapsing fever. Physical examinations at other hospitals identified hepatosplenomegaly. The patient had worked in the south for a long time, and lived in a poor environment. Clinically, the diseases that need to be considered include infectious diseases such as malaria, typhus, relapsing fever, septicemia, tuberculosis, and infection with focus, as well as non-infectious diseases such as leukemia and lymphoma. Therefore, physical examination must be comprehensive and careful. Attention should be paid to signs such as rash, lymph nodes, the size and texture of the liver and spleen, tenderness of the sternum, and possible focus of infection.

III. Auxiliary examination on admission

Routine blood test: WBC 4.9×10^9/L, N 0.6, L 0.4, PLT 180×10^9/L, RBC 4.4×10^{12}/L and Hb 116 g/L.

Urine routine, stool routine, occult blood, liver function, electrolytes, and blood sugar were all normal.

Mycoplasma pneumoniae antibody was negative.

CRP was normal, ESR was 51 mm/h.

Antistreptolysin O, rheumatoid factor, and urinary protein were all negative.

ECG and chest radiograph normal. No abnormal masses or enlarged lymph nodes were found in the abdominal B-ultrasound.

> **Thinking prompts:** On the basis of gaining a complete medical history and physical examination, peripheral blood smear, bone marrow imaging, and histochemical cell staining should be performed to exclude the possibility of leukemia; the B-scan ultrasonography of the abdomen should investigate whether the deep lymph nodes are enlarged, and histological examination of the liver and spleen puncture and bone marrow puncture can also be considered to exclude the possibility of lymphoma. Autoimmune antibodies such as ESR, C-reactive protein, and antinuclear antibodies were tested to eliminate the possibility of autoimmune diseases. A smear of the peripheral blood and bone marrow should be performed to identify malarial parasites, spirochete, and L. donovani, to exclude the possibility of malaria, relapsing fever, and kala-azar. Blood culture and bone marrow culture can exclude the possibility of bacterial infection. The Weil-Felix test can exclude the possibility of typhus. A chest X-ray and B-ultrasound of the liver were performed to determine whether there was any focus of infection. A PPD skin test, anti-tuberculosis antibodies, and other tests can indicate viral or non-viral infection or tubercle bacillus infection.

IV. Diagnosis and treatment

The patient's body temperature exceeded 39°C for more than two weeks, but the cause is still unclear, meaning that it is FUO. To further clarify the etiology, we should start from two aspects: Recurrent fever and hepatosplenomegaly.

> **Thinking prompts:** The etiology of fever of unknown origin can be infectious diseases and non-infectious diseases, the latter commonly being malignant tumors and autoimmune diseases. The patient was a young male with recurrent relapsing fever. Both anti-infection treatment and corticosteroid treatment had certain effects. Physical examination found hepatosplenomegaly, so both diseases should be considered. The patient had been working in the south for a long time, living in a poor environment, so some rare infectious diseases such as malaria, typhus, and relapsing fever should also be considered.

1. Diagnostic thinking

(1) Infectious diseases

1) Viral infectious diseases: Viral diseases may be accompanied by chills, and may also have symptoms in the digestive system and respiratory system at the same time, such as fatigue, lack of appetite, malignancy, vomiting, coughing, and expectoration. Some viral infections may also cause systemic symptoms and signs such as rashes, and the duration of the fever is generally not more than one week, and rarely more than two weeks. A few viruses, such as EB virus and cytomegalovirus infection, can have a long course, and can also show hepatosplenomegaly. White blood cells in the peripheral blood generally do not increase, but there can be increased elevated lymphocytes and abnormal lymphocytes. In the diagnosis of CMV infection, anti-CMV-IgM can be detected, and the cytomegalovirus gene can also be detected with gene diagnosis technology such as PCR technology. EB virus infection can be diagnosed by detecting virus-related antibodies, such as virocapsid antibody (VCA), early antibody (EA), nuclear antibody (EBNA), complement fixing antibody (CF/S), and neutralizing antibody (S). A heterophilic agglutination test can also be performed. For this patient, we should re-examine the hemogram, note the abnormal lymphocytes, and carry out the detection of related antibodies, so as to exclude the possibility of infection from these two viruses.

China is a country with a large incidence of viral hepatitis. If the patient has hepatosplenomegaly, we should consider whether there is the possibility of chronic and viral hepatitis. Fever and hepatosplenomegaly suggest the possibility of both diseases. Serological and virological indicators related to HBV and HCV infection should be checked. However, in this case, non-hepatophilic viral infection could not be ruled out because of the high body temperature and long duration of fever, which did not conform to the general manifestations of hepatophilic viral hepatitis. A liver puncture can be performed for histological examination if necessary.

2) Bacterial infection: The patient had recurrent fever that was relieved after antibiotic treatment. The possibility of bacterial infection should be considered. However, after bacterial infection, fever is usually accompanied by obvious toxic blood symptoms, such as intolerance of cold and chills. A peripheral hemogram is generally characterized by increased neutrophils, and a normal hemogram is rare, so the clinical manifestations of the patient did not fully support bacterial infection. Of course, some infections with a focus cannot be completely excluded, because the previous anti-infection treatment was not enough, and it was possible that the local infected focus intermittently released bacteria and/or toxins, resulting in recurrent fever. Therefore, it is necessary to perform repeated blood and bone marrow cultures before using antibiotics. The serum endotoxin level can also be detected to help diagnosis. At the same time, according to the specific situation, some necessary auxiliary examinations can be repeated, including chest X-ray and B-ultrasound, to find the focus of infection in good time.

Although the clinical manifestation does not support the diagnosis of tuberculosis, it needs to be included in the scope of differential diagnosis. A simple PPD skin test can provide some clues, and the detection of serum tuberculosis antibody has some value. Chest radiographs should be re-examined. If there are suspicious lesions, a chest CT can be considered, which is very helpful for the diagnosis of early pulmonary tuberculosis.

3) Malaria: The patient had been working in tropical areas for a long time, with recurrent fever, swollen spleen, and sweating when the fever receded, so the possibility of malaria cannot be completely ruled out. However, there were no obvious chills before fever, and the regularity of recurrent attacks and anemia were not obvious. Moreover, the patient's hepatomegaly could not be explained by malaria, so the clinical symptoms did not support it. Of course, we should also note the possibility of excluding atypical malaria and falciparum malaria. When fever occurs, we should note making thick and thin smears of blood to find Plasmodium. If necessary, we can use PCR to detect specific genes.

4) Typhus: There were rats in the patient's working and living environment, and he had a recurrent fever and spleen enlargement, so the possibility of typhus should be considered. However, toxic blood symptoms were not obvious, and there was no rash or central nervous system symptoms. The liver enlargement cannot be explained, so the clinical manifestations are not supported. A Weil-Felix test can be done to definitively exclude the disease.

5) Kala-azar: The patient lived in rural areas for a long time, and had a history of contact with dogs; he had a recurrent fever for a long time, had no obvious toxic blood symptoms, and had hepatosplenomegaly. However, hepatosplenomegaly in kala-azar is more obvious, so Leishmania or antibodies can be examined by serum immunology. L. donovani can also be found by a puncture of the spleen, liver, and bone marrow, or a smear of peripheral blood, so as to definitively diagnose or exclude this disease.

6) Relapsing fever: Rats are the transmission medium of relapsing fever, and the patient often comes into contact with them in his working and living environment. Judging by the type, course, and other accompanying characteristics of fever, such as relapsing fever type, sweating when the fever recedes, and hepatosplenomegaly, the possibility of relapsing fever should be strongly considered. However, this basis is not enough to support the diagnosis: The patient's headache was not severe, and there was no pain in joints and muscles of the limbs, no rash, and no tenderness in the gastrocnemius. Further diagnosis should be made by finding spirochetes in peripheral blood and bone marrow smears, detecting serum specific antibodies, and performing the Weil-Felix test.

(2) Non-infectious diseases

1) Lymphoma: The patient had a recurrent fever for a long time, and his body temperature was relatively high, with sweating after the fever, accompanied by hepatosplenomegaly. Therefore, the possibility of lymphoma cannot be completely excluded. Although neither his superficial nor deep lymph nodes were enlarged, this is not enough to exclude infiltration of other lymphoid organs. Histological examination of the liver and spleen puncture may be considered, and if necessary, whole body image scanning, such as PET-CT, may be performed to make a definitive diagnosis.

2) Leukemia: There was no anemia or bleeding, and no tenderness in the sternum; the peripheral blood cell count was normal, and no immature cells or other abnormal cells were found, so the likelihood of leukemia is not high. However, bone marrow puncture and even bone marrow biopsy are necessary.

3) Autoimmune diseases: In this group of diseases (many similar diseases can occur at the same time), the basic pathological change is vasculitis, and the most common clinical symptoms are chronic and moderate-low fever. At the same time, there may be rashes, joint redness, pain, and even deformity. Due to abnormal immune function, there may be hepatosplenomegaly, with a higher incidence rate in females. However, this case was characterized by a high fever that lasted for a long time and had no definite signs. In order to rule out a diagnosis, a variety of autoantibodies can be detected.

2. Diagnosis and treatment

According to the above analysis, after the patient was admitted to hospital, blood was collected for bacterial culture, and then levofloxacin was given to fight infection. At the same time, symptomatic supportive treatment was given. After two days of treatment, the high fever was relieved, accompanied by sweating, and the patient still had a low fever of 37.8°C. At the same time, the PPD skin test was (+); there were no obvious changes in the peripheral hemogram, and no abnormal lymphocytes were found. The anti-CMV-IgM, EB virus capsid antibodies (VCA), early antibodies (EA), tuberculosis antibodies, and antinuclear antibodies were all negative, as were the serological and virological indexes related to HBV and HCV infection. Bone marrow cytology showed no abnormality and no abnormal cells. Plasmodium, L. donovani, and spirochete were not found in the peripheral blood and bone marrow smears. Four consecutive blood cultures and bone marrow cultures were also negative, and no abnormality was found in chest radiograph or chest CT examination. Therefore, considering the possibility of relapsing fever, the results of the Weil-Felix test are shown in Table 21-1.

Table 21-1 Weil-Felix test results

	1:40	1:80	1:160	1:320	1:640
OX_2	–	–	–	–	–
OX_k	+++	++	+	+	+
OX_{19}	–	–	–	–	–

At this point, the diagnosis of relapsing fever was clear, and it was considered as the tick-borne variety. Only tetracycline tablets were given orally – 0.5 g, once every six hours, for four days. The patient's body temperature dropped to normal, and symptoms such as headache, dizziness, and fatigue disappeared. After taking the medicine for another week, the patient's body temperature remained normal, and he was discharged without conscious discomfort. ESR was re-examined at discharge, and it returned to normal.

Thinking prompts: The spirochetes of tick-borne relapsing fever often invade the brain, where they are protected by the blood-brain barrier and remain in situ. Once the antibiotic level in the blood drops, the spirochetes can invade again, so single-dose therapy is not used. Tetracycline (0.5 g or 12.5 mg/kg, once every 6 hours and taken orally for ten days) is generally the first choice of treatment for adults. Alternatively, 0.1 g of doxycycline can be taken orally twice a day, for ten days. If there is a contraindication to using tetracycline, erythromycin (0.2 g or 12.5 mg/kg, once every six hours) can be taken orally for ten days. If it is confirmed or suspected that the central nervous system has been invaded, penicillin G (Benzylpenicillin) should be injected intravenously at a dose of 3 million U once every four hours, or ceftriaxone sodium 2.0 g, once a day, or divided into two injections for 10–14 days.

Check for the Herxheimer reaction when using antibiotics during the high fever period, and bear in mind that it can also occur when a high fever suddenly drops. The severity of this reaction is related to the quantity and speed of elimination of the spirochetes in blood, so the first dose should not be too large. In order to reduce this reaction, adrenocortical hormone can be used at the beginning of the course of medication. Anaphylactic shock may occur alongside the reaction, so symptomatic treatment such as dexamethasone, cardiotonic therapy, and anti-shock should be given immediately. Tetracycline was chosen for treatment because this patient had chills and fever when using penicillin at the other hospital, which may not have been an infusion reaction but a Herxheimer reaction caused by penicillin. During use, the patient was closely observed, and the Herxheimer reaction was not found.

V. Follow-up

Two weeks after discharge, the patient's body temperature was normal during follow-up. See Table 21-2 for the re-examination of the Weil-Felix test results.

Table 21-2 Re-examination of Weil-Felix test results

	1:40	1:80	1:160	1:320	1:640
OX_2	−	−	−	−	−
OX_k	++	+	±	−	−
OX_{19}	−	−	−	−	−

Follow-up one year after discharge showed normal body temperature and no specific discomfort.

Thinking prompts: Because antibiotic treatment has special effects on this disease, there are generally no sequelae. The main purpose of the follow-up is to measure body temperature regularly to prevent recurrence. At the same time, because the borrelia recurrentis antigen mutates easily, the immune period after the disease is short – about one year. Therefore, we should work on education: Encourage the patient to note personal hygiene, and cooperate with rat prevention, rat killing, and tick killing to prevent re-infection.

VI. Lessons learned

This case was difficult to diagnose as relapsing fever on admission because of the lack of typical symptoms such as severe headache, soreness of limbs and muscles, pain in the joints, and no history of tick bites, not to mention the corresponding typical skin manifestations left after tick bites, and no typical signs such as tenderness of gastrocnemius. In addition, relapsing fever is rare in China at present, so it is very easy to miss and misdiagnose. On admission, we analyzed and judged the two main symptoms of the patient's recurrent fever and hepatosplenomegaly, and carried out various examinations. Finally, he was definitively diagnosed as having a relapsing fever.

The chills and fever experienced by the patient when using penicillin at the other hospital may not be a complete infusion reaction, but may be a Herxheimer reaction caused by the penicillin, which may be an important clinical clue in diagnosis. The decrease in body temperature during treatment with antibiotics at the other hospital may be part of the disease's own development, not just the result of antibiotic treatment, because the antibiotics selected at that time were not specific for borrelia recurrentis. When the patient was first admitted to hospital, this also misled us, and we spent a long time considering common and regular infectious diseases in error.

On admission, levofloxacin was used once after blood culture. After treatment, the patient's body temperature dropped significantly, but did not return to normal. At that time, it was considered that the infection was not completely controlled, so the drug was used until a definitive diagnosis was made. There was no spirochete in the patient's peripheral blood and bone marrow smear, which may be related to the small number of spirochetes in the blood. The positive rate may be increased if a thick blood smear or centrifugation and concentration are performed. In recent years, it has been reported that centrifugation with high-quality buffy coat (QBC) and detection of borrelia recurrentis with a fluorescence microscope can significantly improve its sensitivity.

Animal inoculation can also be adopted to improve the detection rate. The possibility of leptospirosis and tsutsugamushi disease must be ruled out if the Weil-Felix test is positive. The diagnosis of this patient was based on clinical manifestations and a positive Weil-Felix test result, and the outcome of treatment confirmed that the diagnosis was correct. The diagnosis and treatment of such rare diseases should be meticulous and comprehensive, and a process of understanding should be allowed. It cannot be considered a failure on the part of the other hospital to have made a misdiagnosis in a short time, because the disease itself has too many particularities.

Through the diagnosis and treatment of this case, we learn firstly that epidemiological history is still an important aspect of diagnosing infectious diseases, and cannot be ignored. Secondly, for the etiological diagnosis of fever of unknown origin, we must grasp the main existing symptoms and signs, and carry out relatively targeted examinations around them. Thirdly, the idea of differential diagnosis must be open. Diseases that cannot be ruled out must be included in further differential diagnosis, and diseases that can be ruled out should be temporarily shelved. Fourthly, rare diseases should be considered only after the common diseases are completely excluded. Fifthly, subtle phenomena should be noted, such as the Herxheimer reaction in this case, which was initially considered as infusion reaction. Finally, difficult diseases can be complicated, making the process of differential diagnosis is complex and relatively time-consuming. It should not be rushed.

(Zhang Ruiqi & Miao Xiaohui)

References

Lu, Hongzhou, and Shi Yaozhong. "Relapsing Fever." *World Journal of Infectious Diseases* 5, no. 2 (2005): 96.

Ma, Yilin. *Epidemiology*. 4th ed. Shanghai: Shanghai Science and Technology Press, 2005.

Half a day of diarrhea
with two instances of convulsions

I. Medical history

Patient: Male, 54 years old, a farm worker from Wuhan in Hubei Province. He was hospitalized after half a day of diarrhea and two instances of convulsions, between 30 May and 13 June 2005.

After eating frogs and squid at a wedding banquet for 17 hours, the patient had six bouts of diarrhea from 05:00 to 06:00 on 30 May 2005. The stool was yellow and watery, with a total volume of about 2,000 ml. There was no abdominal pain, no tenesmus, and no symptoms such as vomiting and fever. The patient fainted with convulsions and obnubilation at 06:00 when using the toilet, without symptoms such as distortion of commissure, sursumversion, or foaming at the mouth. He recovered consciousness a few minutes later. The patient had had another ten episodes of diarrhea by 10:00, which was still yellow and watery, with a total volume of about 4,000 ml, and he developed convulsions and consciousness disorders again. The patient was taken to the local hospital by his family, where examination showed BP 80/40 mmHg; H 124 times/min. An ECG showed sinus tachycardia and right atrial hypertrophy. Blood biochemistry results: Glu 8.47 mmol/L, BUN 14.7 mmol/L, Cr 264.9 µmol/L, ALT 69 U/L, AST 56 U/L. His condition did not improve after rehydration, acidosis correction, volume expansion, anti-infection treatment with sodium bicarbonate, low-molecular dextran, and levofloxacin.

He was transferred to our hospital at 17:00 that day. Outpatient examination showed: WBC 17.36×10^9/L, N 88.9%, RBC 6.09×10^{12}/L, Hb 193 g/L, PLT 287×10^9/L; stool routine: Watery, mucus (+), WBC 3–4/HP, occult blood OB (±); stool microscopic examination (−); blood chemistry parameters: ALT 66 U/L, K^+ 5.75 mmol/L, Na^+ 145.6 mmol/L, BUN 13.8 mmol/L, Cr 259.1 µmol/L; a brain CT performed in the emergency department showed encephalatrophy. After high potassium correction treatment, the outpatient admitted him with infectious diarrhea caused by either: ① Toxic bacillary dysentery; ② Cholera.

Since the onset of illness, the patient had had a poor appetite and sleep quality, and was in low spirits. His urine volume, strength, and weight had also decreased significantly.

Medical history: Subtotal gastrectomy for gastric ulcer bleeding in 1996. He denied a history of hypertension or heart disease; 30 years of smoking (an average of 20 cigarettes/day).

Thinking prompts: The patient had an acute onset of a dangerous condition with rapid progress. We can initially summarize his clinical characteristics as large amounts of painless watery diarrhea, and convulsions appearing early. The following points should be noted when gathering further medical history:

1. Prevalence

Epidemiological investigation needs to be made for patients with diarrhea, to identify whether the same symptom has occurred successively in a group or family members. Food poisoning originates from contaminated water or food, accompanied by watery diarrhea and/or symptoms except gastrointestinal ones. However, this case was seemingly random; the patient's family and other co-diners did not develop diarrhea. Epidemic seasons have important significance for the diagnosis of infectious diarrhea. The onset of the patient's illness was at the end of May, which was the high incidence season for infectious intestinal diseases such as bacillary dysentery and cholera.

2. Predisposing factors

Diarrhea patients often have a history of eating a contaminated diet before the onset. This patient ate frogs and squid at noon the day before his onset, and sprayed an organophosphorus pesticide with high-efficiency and low-toxicity called Nongda two days before. Therefore, the possibility of infectious diarrhea and acute organophosphorus pesticide poisoning should be considered.

3. Onset

Consider whether there was aura or prodromal symptom before the convulsion attack, whether the patient maintained consciousness during attack, and whether it was accompanied by autonomic nerve symptoms such as sweating, palpitations, facial pallor, or flushing. If the patient falls unconscious, we should note the sequential order of the symptoms. This patient had diarrhea first, rather than fecal incontinence due to losing consciousness, which suggests a severe bowel disease with impairment of the central nervous system.

4. Medical history

The patient had undergone a subtotal gastrectomy, suggesting that his gastric acid secretion was reduced, and the inactivation ability of harmful bacteria was relatively poor, which is more likely to cause infectious diarrhea. If a patient has convulsions, we should also investigate whether it is accompanied by hypertension, diabetes, hyperthyroidism, or heart disease. At the same time, we need to know whether there is any family history of similar onset.

5. Quantity and properties of stool

Acute diarrhea can be watery and dysentery varieties. The mucous membrane of the bowel with watery diarrhea shows mild inflammation or only non-specific infiltration without blood or pus, which might not be accompanied by tenesmus or abdominal pain. Dysentery diarrhea involves the destruction of the intestinal mucosa, and bloody purulent stool, often accompanied by acute abdominal pain and cramping. The two can coexist. Watery diarrhea is usually caused by enterotoxins of bacterial toxins such as vibrio cholerae, while dysentery diarrhea can be seen in bacillary dysentery, amoebic bowel disease, and acute ulcerative colitis. Stool changes in toxic dysentery are not always obvious, but poisoning symptoms such as convulsions are severe.

II. Physical examination on admission

T 37.9°C, P 112 times/min, R 26 times/min, BP 90/60 mmHg. The patient's condition developed normally, with moderate nourishment and drowsiness. He was carried onto the ward in a supine position with cyanosis of the lips. There was no petechia ecchymosis on the skin anywhere on his body. His skin was dry and had poor elasticity, without superficial lymph node enlargement. Both pupils were equal and round (diameter: 4.5 mm) and reflex response to light was slow. There was pharyngeal congestion with a supple neck. Bilateral lung breathing sound was thick, without dry or moist rales. No pathological noise could be heard in the heart sound auscultation. His abdomen was flat and soft; the liver and spleen could not be palpated below the costal margin. No tenderness or rebound pain. Active borborygmus; physiological reflexes present; pathologic reflexes not elicited.

Thinking prompts: For patients admitted with acute diarrhea and convulsions, the following four aspects should be considered during physical examination: ① Systemic conditions: Including vital signs, especially blood pressure and pulse, presence of anemia, cachexia, lymph node and thyroid enlargement, skin elasticity, presence of icteric, exophthalmos. ② Abdominal examination: Check for the presence of abdominal distension, abdominal mass, tenderness, rebound pain, hyperactive/hypoactive bowel sounds, and intestinal peristalsis. Routine digital rectal examination (DRE) should be performed. ③ Nervous system examination: Since the patient had nervous system symptoms such as convulsions and drowsiness, specialized examination of the nervous system is essential. Close attention should be paid to the symmetry of the limbs and the positive signs of focal nervous system injury, which can be a reference for locating and qualifying the convulsion. ④ Specialized cardiological examination: The patient had manifestations such as low blood pressure, high heart rate, and shock, and the ECG showed sinus tachycardia and right atrial hypertrophy. Thus, excluding heart diseases should be considered.

Examination is mandatory for every case of diarrhea, and is a routine diagnosis and treatment in intestinal outpatient department, aiming to prevent missed diagnoses of cholera. Patients with diarrhea should undergo routine blood tests, stool tests, cultures, and drug sensitivity tests as well as giving their complete medical history and undergoing physical examination. This is to distinguish infectious diarrhea from non-infectious diarrhea.

The patient in this case suffered from convulsions and transient disturbance of consciousness, so lumbar puncture and cerebrospinal fluid examination should be considered after the vital signs are stable. If patients have diarrhea, shock, and convulsions, we should consider the possibility of systemic disease accompanied by manifestations of intestinal diseases such as Gram-negative bacilli septicemia, and hyperthyroidism. Therefore, blood culture and thyroid function should be examined even if the patients have no symptoms of fever. This patient's heart rate was high. He was in shock, and his ECG was abnormal. His myocardial enzymes and Doppler echocardiography could give clues about cardiovascular diseases. The patient had liver and kidney dysfunction, so we need to monitor liver function and renal function in good time. An abdominal liver and kidney B-ultrasound should also be included as part of the routine examination.

III. Auxiliary examination on admission

Routine blood test: WBC 18.46×10^9/L, N 86.51%, Hb 194 g/L, PLT 287×10^9/L.

Routine stool: WBC 3–4/HP.

Liver function: ALT 41 U/L, AST 100 U/L, TP 99.6 g/L, cholinesterase 18,320 U/L.

Renal function: BUN 17.62 mmol/L, Cr 491.8 μmol/L, Glu 8.22 mmol/L, HCO_3^- 17.2 mmol/L.

Electrolytes: K^+ 6.64 mmol/L, Na^+ 123.2 mmol/L, Cl^- 92.9 mmol/L, Ca^{2+} 2.94 mmol/L.

IV. Diagnosis

1. Initial Diagnosis:

Infectious diarrhea caused by ① cholera and ② bacillary dysentery (toxic type) waiting to be ruled out.

The patient had a history of eating a contaminated diet, with a rapid onset and a dangerous condition. He had clinical manifestations such as large amounts of painless watery diarrhea, shock, convulsions, renal impairment, and blood concentration, which was initially diagnosed as cholera. However, his hemogram was elevated and his routine stool was WBC 3–4/HP, so other types of infectious diarrhea (such as toxic bacillary dysentery) could not be ruled out.

> **Thinking prompts:** After noting the characteristics of the patient's clinical manifestations, his condition can be summarized as large amounts of painless watery diarrhea, convulsions, shock, and renal failure. Based on his medical history, physical examination, and auxiliary examinations, we can analyze these clinical manifestations thus: A contaminated diet may be the cause; copious painless diarrhea is the main sign; insufficient blood volume and an electrolyte disorder lead to convulsions and shock; and renal failure occurred due to severe dehydration.

2. Diagnostic thinking

Generally, diarrhea is either infectious or non-infectious. The etiology of infectious diarrhea accompanied by convulsions is classified into the following six categories: ① Acute bacterial food poisoning, including Salmonella, Staphylococcus aureus, Proteus, Botulinum, Vibrio parahaemolyticus, Pathogenic Escherichia coli, Pseudomonas aeruginosa, heat-resistant B.welchii (B.perfringens), and fungi; ② Acute bacterial enteric infection, including acute toxic-type bacillary dysentery, cholera, Escherichia coli enteritis, Yersinia enteritis, Campylobacter jejuni enteritis, and acute vibrio parahaemolyticus enteritis; ③ Acute viral enteric infection, including rotavirus enteritis, enteroadenovirus enteritis, and Norwalk virus enteritis; ④ Acute parasitic diseases, including acute schistosomiasis, acute amoebic enteropathy, and cryptosporidiosis; ⑤ Systemic acute infectious diseases such as sepsis, encephalitis B, acute severe viral hepatitis, leptospirosis, and poliomyelitis; ⑥ Candida albicans enteritis.

The etiology of non-infectious diarrhea accompanied by convulsions is classified into the following two categories: ① Acute poisoning, including from plants (such as fermented-corn flour, sprouted potato food, ginkgo seeds, hemp seeds, and toadstools), acute poisoning caused by animal based agents (such as tetrodotoxin, animal liver, and fish gall), and acute poisoning by chemical agents (such as acute organophosphorus pesticides, zinc, and arsenic); ② Systemic non-infectious diseases such as allergic gastroenteropathy, uremia, hyperthyroid crisis, and anaphylactoid purpura (hemorrhagic capillary poisoning).

Question: Is this patient suffering from infectious diarrhea or non-infectious diarrhea? Based on clinical data and the clinical characteristics of non-infectious diarrhea diseases, non-infectious diarrhea can be ruled out: ① Acute diarrhea caused by anaphylactoid purpura (hemorrhagic capillary poisoning) is not rare, but it is generally accompanied by skin purpura. ② Patients with severe allergic gastrointestinal diseases may have symptoms such as anaphylactic shock and renal failure, but they generally present with gastrointestinal symptoms soon after eating (within 2 hours), accompanied by colic, conjunctival congestion, and urticaria. ③ Patients with uremia and hyperthyroid crisis may also have clinical manifestations of diarrhea and convulsions, but generally have medical history of kidney problems or hyperthyroidism. This patient did not have uremia or hyperthyroidism. ④ Acute organophosphorus pesticide poisoning generally occurs within 12 hours of the organophosphorus pesticide entering the human body. At the initial stage, non-specific symptoms such as fatigue, headache, and vertigo appear first, followed by symptoms of muscarinic poisoning such as hyperhidrosis, salivation, nausea, vomiting, diarrhea, blurred vision, and miosis. This patient had been in contact with a pesticide called Nongda before the onset of illness, but this is a high-efficiency and low-toxic organophosphorus pesticide with a long interval (two days before onset). Considering the fact that the patient's pupils were equal and round (diameter: 4.5 mm) and the serum cholinesterase activity was not low, the possibility of acute organophosphorus pesticide poisoning was ruled out. Because the patient had no history of exposure to other toxins, toxin poisoning was completely ruled out.

Non-infectious diarrhea was ruled out, so what kind of infectious diarrhea did the patient have? Below are the characteristics of infectious diarrhea based on the patient's clinical data:

(1) Acute parasitic diseases: Gastrointestinal malaria accompanied by abdominal pain is rare. Fulminant amoebic dysentery is very dangerous. Patients show severe poisoning symptoms and severe diarrhea. The stools are soupy or even bloody/watery, and are often mixed with flaky exfoliated mucosa, with a fetid odor, accompanied by significant abdominal colic and tenesmus. Cryptosporidiosis is generally seen with watery diarrhea in patients younger than five years old, people from rural areas, or immunocompromised individuals such as AIDS patients. Our patient had painless diarrhea, so acute parasitic disease was not considered.

(2) Viral diarrhea: Rotavirus Group A mainly affects infants and young children; group C mainly affects children sporadically, and group B mainly affects adults. Generally, it involves mild to moderate self-limited diarrhea. Poisoning symptoms such as convulsions, renal failure, and shock are rare. Adenovirus enteritis is often accompanied by respiratory symptoms; poisoning symptoms are also rare. Norovirus enteritis has a winter onset, and is more common in adults. It is often accompanied by abdominal cramps and mild diarrhea without mucus, blood, or pus. Viral diarrhea was also not considered in this case.

(3) Pseudomembranous enteritis: Antibiotic-associated diarrhea includes simple diarrhea, colitis, and pseudomembranous enteritis according to the severity of the infection. Pseudomembranous enteritis is a serious illness with a high mortality rate, and is often accompanied by toxemia, toxic intestinal tympanites, and intestinal bleeding or perforation. However, this patient had no history of antibiotic use, so a diagnosis of pseudomembranous enteritis could not be established.

(4) Candida albicans enteritis: Candida albicans is an opportunistic pathogen that is more common in malnourished and immunocompromised patients, and patients with long-term heavy use of antibiotics, steroid hormones, and immunosuppressive agents. This patient was a manual worker in strong physical health before the onset of illness, so Candida albicans enteritis was not considered.

(5) Acute bacterial food poisoning: This is a major toxic disease caused by eating common food contaminated by bacteria or their toxins. Although it manifests as abdominal pain, diarrhea, and even convulsions or renal failure in severe cases, none of the people who dined with this patient at the wedding banquet had symptoms of abdominal pain or diarrhea, so acute bacterial food poisoning was not considered.

(6) Acute bacterial enteric infection: Cholera is characterized by diarrhea first and vomiting later. The initial diarrhea is painless with a large amount of stool with the consistency of rice water. It is often accompanied by muscle cramps and projectile vomiting. Dehydration, shock, and renal failure occur rapidly. Toxic-type acute bacillary dysentery is more common in children with better constitutions. For adults, toxic bacillary dysentery is more common in elderly people with weak constitutions and poor nourishment. Shock occurs earlier and more severely due to toxemia, vomiting, and diarrhea. CNS symptoms such as convulsions are not uncommon. In this case, acute bacterial enteric infection should be considered.

Based on a comprehensive analysis of the characteristics of the above acute bacterial intestinal infections, we can summarize the clinical manifestations of this patient as follows: He had a history of subtotal gastrectomy; he had eaten frogs and squid (high-risk foods) the day before the onset of illness; he passed large amounts of painless watery diarrhea; there was a rapid onset of convulsions, dehydration, circulatory failure, and renal failure. Therefore, cholera should be ranked first in the diagnosis, and toxic bacillary dysentery should be ruled out.

V. Treatment

Because cholera is considered as the initial diagnosis, comprehensive emergency measures should be taken as quickly as possible, especially fluid replacement therapy. The patient should be disinfected and put into isolation, as it is an infectious enteric disease. As the patient suffered from shock and renal failure, anti-shock treatment was urgently needed: Rapid infusion was carried out in the early stage, and low-molecular dextran 10–15 ml/kg and 5% sodium bicarbonate 5 ml/kg were given immediately by intravenous injection within 0.5–1 hour to rapidly correct acidosis and expand volume, followed by rapid infusion with 1/2 sodium-containing solution later. Vasoactive drugs should be used to relieve vasospasm.

1. Ward-round analysis two days after admission

After the previous night's treatment, the patient's diarrhea had not significantly improved, and he developed frequent projectile vomiting. The vomit was yellowish liquid, and the patient's whole body was dry and cold, with a fast but weakening pulse rate. The acidosis was corrected and expanded in volume, BP 90/56 mmHg, H 140 times/min, and urine volume was only 60 ml after admission. Blood gas analysis indicated metabolic acidosis, and routine blood tests included WBC 18.46×10^9/L, N 86.51%, Hb 194 g/L, and PLT 287×10^9/L, suggesting infectious disease. The patient had hemoconcentration with further aggravation of renal impairment. Pupils were equal in size and rounded, with a dull reflex reaction to light. The above situation indicated that the volume of fluid supplement was insufficient, so further fluid supplement, volume expansion, and acidosis correction were required. The patient was quickly given fluid containing 5 g of sodium chloride and 4 g of sodium bicarbonate per liter of solution. Two venous channels were opened, and infusion was started at the speed of 40–80 ml/min. Later, the solution was infused at the speed of 20–30 ml/min. The 24-hour plan for fluid infusion was 8,000 mL. Close attention to the patient's vital signs and urine volume was required while monitoring the acid-base balance and electrolyte disorders and preventing pulmonary edema. Strict isolation was also needed. A large number of Gram-negative vibrios were detected in the patient's excreta, and the municipal CDC identified a Vibrio cholerae infection of O_{139}, which was reported to the hospital leaders immediately, and then to the district and municipal CDC. The following measures were taken immediately: ① The patient was isolated with a Class A infectious disease (implemented at the time of admission). ② The patient's excreta was thoroughly sterilized. ③ The patient's excreta was cultured every other day. ④ The feces of the patient's family members, patients in adjacent beds, and medical staff who had been exposed to them were examined separately and given norfloxacin

200 mg three times a day for two consecutive days. ⑤ The patient continued to rehydrate with 2,000–2,500 ml, and the treatment was adjusted according to his condition. ⑥ Changes to his condition were closely observed.

2. Ward-round analysis three days after admission

The patient recovered consciousness, but his spirit was poor, and he had a dry mouth and flushed face. The humidity and temperature of his skin and limbs had increased compared with before, and he was still vomiting. The vomit was dominated by gastric contents. His blood pressure increased to 140/85 mmHg, H 84 times/min, and he had diarrhea eight times a day with liquid stools of a volume of about 3,000 ml. His urine volume was about 380 ml, and the total WBC and neutrophil count decreased compared with the previous day. The same day, we received a phone call from the municipal CDC. The excreta culture sent by the patient's initial diagnosing medical unit was also vibrio cholerae O_{139} Current treatment included fluid infusion, correction of an electrolyte disorder, maintenance of internal environment stability, and anti-infection and symptomatic support treatment.

3. Ward-round analysis on the sixth day after admission

There was an improvement in the patient's mental state. He could sit up, and his physical strength was recovering. He had facial flushing, BP 126/84 mmHg, H 74 times/min. The day before, he had diarrhea twice with yellowish-green stool; the volume of urine was 1,970 ml; he was no longer vomiting. The patient's facial flushing was due to the systemic poisoning symptoms caused by the toxin.

Laboratory tests: Blood biochemistry showed ALT 206 U/L, AST 459 U/L, BUN 29.31 mmol/L, Cr 941.6 μmol/L; routine blood WBC was 16.74×10^9/L, N 87.7%. No Vibrio cholerae was found in microscopic stool examination, nor in vomit smear staining, and no obvious abnormality was found in the re-examination of electrolytes. Fluid infusion, kidney protection, and liver protection treatments were continued.

4. Morning ward-round analysis on the eighth day after admission

The patient was no longer having diarrhea and vomiting, and excreted soft yellow stools once. He was conscious, and his skin was warm and flexible, with T 36.5°C, R 20 times/min, P 80 times/min, and BP 132/80 mmHg. His urine volume was 3,280 ml/24h, and the combination of stool culture and drug sensitivity did not detect Vibrio cholerae, Salmonella, or Shigella.

5. Morning ward-round analysis on the fifteenth day after admission

The patient was generally well, and had no abdominal pain, diarrhea, vomiting, nausea, or convulsions. His daily urine volume in recent days was 1,500–2,000 ml, and stools were soft and yellow with frequency of once every 1–2 days. Vibrio cholerae was not detected in multiple stool cultures, and we reported it to the municipal CDC. The CDC's response was that the patient could be released from quarantine. His renal function, electrolytes, routine blood test, and liver function were re-examined, and were completely normal. He was discharged the same day.

VI. Follow-up

The patient and his township were followed up for six months, and there were no cases of new-onset cholera.

VII. Lessons learned

This case was sudden in onset, rapid in development, and dangerous. The patient's initial symptoms – diarrhea, convulsions, loss of consciousness, shock, and acute renal failure – were initially misdiagnosed as meningitis and sepsis at a local hospital. Attention must be paid to the sequential order in which the main symptoms appear. In this case, the diarrhea was the former, and convulsions and loss of consciousness were the latter, thus suggesting a severe intestinal disease accompanied by central nervous system damage, rather than fecal incontinence due to loss of consciousness.

China's cholera epidemic area is closer to the coast, and the epidemic season is from July to October. Hubei Province is located in central China, and the onset of this case was at the end of May. The microscopic stool examination was negative, and the routine stool WBC was 3–4/HP. Toxic bacillary dysentery – a more common disease – could easily be considered as the first diagnosis by a doctor. Although it was not the time of high incidence of cholera, the characteristics of early summer and the high temperatures in Wuhan should be taken into account during the diagnostic process. In addition, although the microscopic stool examination was negative, it was necessary to consider that the amount of Vibrio cholerae excreted at the beginning of the onset might be low, resulting in a negative examination result. This requires repeatedly sending the patient's feces for examination, and finally finding Vibrio cholerae before making a definitive diagnosis. Moreover, in the process of treatment, we should promptly and carefully observe the dynamic changes of the condition and the effect of treatment, and quickly reflect, correct, and adjust the treatment strategy for maximum chance of recovery. This case is ultimately a successful experience that is worth summarizing.

Although the local hospital made a misdiagnosis, they did not forget the principle of mandatory examination for every case of diarrhea, which helped to make an earlier and more timely diagnosis for the patient.

In the rehydration therapy for this case of cholera, the "541 solution" was not directly or mechanically applied. Because the patient presented with renal failure combined with high potassium early in this case, unlike most cholera patients who had low potassium, there was no potassium supplement at the beginning of rehydration. Instead, the patient's electrolytes were closely monitored, and at the later stage of rehydration, urination was observed to determine whether potassium supplementation was required, suggesting that an individualized treatment plan should be formulated for treatment.

(Tian Deying)

Vomiting with a severe headache for five days

I. Medical history

Patient: Female, 52 years old. She was hospitalized for vomiting with a severe headache for five days.

The patient started to vomit without any obvious inducements five days earlier. The vomit was a small amount of gastric content, accompanied by a severe total headache without fever, convulsions, limb numbness, or weakness. She was sent to the local hospital, and the WBC in her peripheral blood was 8.7×10^9/L, N 88.3%. A CT scan of her head showed a lacunar infarction in the left corona radiata, and suspicious bleeding in the left internal capsule area. After admission, she underwent dehydration and anti-infection treatment (details unclear). No improvement was noticed, so she was admitted to our hospital. In the course of her illness, there was no cough or expectoration; no frequent micturition, urgent urination, or pain in urination; no abdominal pain or diarrhea, and no obvious emaciation or night sweats.

The patient had suffered from rheumatoid arthritis for more than 20 years, and took prednisone 15 mg once daily and diclofenac 75 mg once daily all year round.

> **Thinking prompts:** The patient was a middle-aged woman presenting with an acute onset characterized by vomiting and headache. Despite the absence of fever, central nervous system infection should be considered. During the gathering of her medical history, attention should be paid to differential diagnosis of central infection, such as if the onset was acute (acute onset is more common for purulent meningitis and viral meningitis, while tuberculous meningitis and fungal meningitis have a subacute or chronic onset), the season (for example, epidemic cerebrospinal meningitis is more common in winter and spring, and epidemic encephalitis B is more common in July to September), accompanying symptoms (fever, skin mucosal petechia, and ecchymosis). Before the onset of the illness, was there an upper respiratory tract infection, otitis media, sinusitis, or craniocerebral trauma? If so, was it combined with cerebrospinal fluid leakage? Ask whether the patient had a splenectomy, chronic liver disease, diabetes, malignant tumor, rheumatic disease, or other immunodeficiencies. Ask whether she had a history of tuberculosis or contact with the disease before the onset and in the course of

her illness disease. To find evidence of extrapulmonary tuberculosis, investigate symptoms of tuberculosis poisoning such as low-graded fever, wasting, night sweats, respiratory infection symptoms such as cough, expectoration, hemoptysis, and symptoms of irritation to the urinary tract and system or digestive system symptoms. This is helpful for identifying the pathogenesis of central infection. Inquire whether the patient has symptoms of cranial nerve palsy, such as vision disorders, dysphagia, hoarse voice, and hearing disorders, and if there was limb paralysis and aphasia (inflammation involving intracranial vessels or brain parenchyma). The patient was vomiting accompanied by a headache, which was thought to be caused by intracranial hypertension. The possible causes were central infection (meningitis, encephalitis, or a brain abscess), intracranial vascular disease, an intracranial tumor, or a parasite.

II. Physical examination

T 38.2°C, P 84/min, R 18/min, BP 105/70 mmHg. She was conscious and slightly agitated, and her answers to the questions were relevant. She had a stiff neck, no swelling of the superficial lymph nodes throughout her body, and her skin and mucosa were not icteric. There were clear respiratory sounds in both lungs, and no dry or moist rales were heard. Her heart rate was 84 beats/min, and the rhythm was regular. Her abdomen was smooth and soft, with no tenderness or rebound pain; her liver and spleen could not be palpated below the costal margin. The fingers of both hands showed swan-neck deformity. Her knees were flexed and could not be extended. Brudzinski's sign was positive, and Kernig's sign was positive.

> **Thinking prompts:** During physical examination, check for signs of meningeal irritation: Nuchal rigidity, Kernig's sign, and Brudzinski's sign. As chronic meningitis is often a part of systemic disease, which can provide clues for diagnosis, physical examination requires attention to the presence of focal lesions, such as abscesses or skin lesions, subcutaneous nodules, the presence of clear nasal discharge (suggesting cerebrospinal fluid rhinorrhea), purulence in the external auditory canal (suggesting cerebrospinal fluid otorrhea and otitis media), and the presence of cranial nerve paralysis (usually the III, IV, VI, and VIII cranial nerves), which is manifested as decreased vision, hearing loss, diplopia, and eyeball movement disorder, suggesting chronic meningitis.

III. Auxiliary examination

Routine blood test: WBC 16.9×10^9/L, N 88.1%, Hb 138 g/L, PLT 358×10^9/L.

Cerebrospinal fluid: LDH 46 U/L, ADA 5 U/L (reference volume 4–44 U/L, the same below), ANA, ENA, and dsDNA were negative. Anti-cyclic citrulline polypeptide antibodies, CCP (+), RfIgG 683 U/L (0–110 U/L), RF IgA > 3,200 U/L (0–120 U/L), and RF IgM > 1,280 U/L (0–40 U/L).

Liver and kidney functions and electrolytes were normal.

Whole chest radiograph and abdominal B-ultrasound scan were negative. ECG showed sinus tachycardia.

Cerebrospinal fluid fungal smear (−), Cryptococcus latex agglutination test (−). Routine CSF and biochemical results are shown in Table 23-1.

> **Thinking prompts:** Patients with suspected tuberculous meningitis should undergo immediate biochemical, routine, and etiologic examination of the cerebrospinal fluid. The simplest and fastest examination is microscopic examination of the cerebrospinal fluid. Before microscopic examination, centrifuging the cerebrospinal fluid and then taking precipitate for examination can greatly improve the positive rate. Gram staining, acid-fast staining, and ink staining can distinguish bacteria, mycobacteria, and cryptococcus. Mycobacterium tuberculosis culture grows slowly, so it cannot provide a diagnosis in time. At present, the Bactec 460 rapid culture system has been widely employed in clinical practice, and can be used for the rapid isolation and identification of mycobacterium tuberculosis. As it is relatively difficult to obtain the pathogen of tuberculosis, immunological diagnosis can be taken as a supplementary measure. At present, the newly launched ELISPOT examination is used for the diagnosis of tuberculosis with high specificity. In particular, it will not cause a cross-over immune reaction with BCG. The differential diagnosis of fungal meningitis can be made with a latex agglutination test for fungal diagnosis, G test (detection of fungal cell wall β-D-glucan), and GM test for Aspergillus (detection of galactomannan). Considering infections of the central nervous system, a routine blood test, chest radiograph, PPD, and erythrocyte sedimentation rate are required, together with cranial CT, MRI, and autoantibody examinations, so as to exclude other central infectious diseases such as brain abscesses and brain parasitic disease, as well as non-infectious central nervous system diseases such as multiple sclerosis, thrombophlebitis, and nervous system vasculitis complicated with connective tissue diseases.

Table 23-1 The patient's CSF on admission

Day after admission	Cell count (/mm³)	Sugar (mmol/L)	Chlorine (mmol/L)	Protein (mg/L)	Bacterial culture	Acid-fast stain	Fungal smear
Day 1	Normal	2.5	113	1,251	Negative	Negative	Negative
Day 4	92 (Multinuclear cell 72)	1.7	111	1,967	Negative	Negative	Negative
Day 14	102 (Multinuclear cell 70)	1.7	106	2,141	Negative	Negative	Negative
Day 21	Normal	3.0	129	1,960	Negative	Negative	Negative

IV. Diagnosis

Initial diagnosis: The patient was a middle-aged female with an acute onset and headache with vomiting, the cause of which remained to be investigated. Due to her headache, vomiting, nuchal rigidity, and increased intracranial pressure, central nervous system diseases should be considered.

Thinking prompts:

(1) Infection of the central nervous system

The patient had a fever with headache and vomiting, and had signs of meningeal irritation such as neck stiffness, positive Kernig's sign, and positive Brudzinski's sign. Combined with the acute onset and high hemogram, and considering that it is probably purulent meningitis, it is recommended to give an anti-infection treatment.

(2) Intracranial vasculopathy

The cranial CT showed lacunar infarction in the left corona radiata, and suspicious bleeding in the left internal capsule area. However, this cannot explain the whole condition. It may be combined with subarachnoid hemorrhage, which can be identified by cerebrospinal fluid examination and can be ruled out.

(3) Connective tissue diseases

The patient had suffered from rheumatoid arthritis for 20 years, but the possibility of intracranial manifestations of rheumatoid arthritis is low. Autoantibodies can be checked to exclude other connective tissue diseases.

(4) Intracranial space occupation

Many of these diseases have a slow onset and a chronic course, which can oppress functional areas and cause sensory and motor disorders such as numbness, weakness, and limb paralysis, which are not supported by CT results.

(5) Rheumatoid arthritis

The patient had many years of medical issues, a typical deformity of the hands and fingers, and positive CCP and RF, which is a clear diagnosis.

V. Treatment

After admission, mannitol dehydration, treatment to decrease intracranial pressure, and 7.2 million U of penicillin (twice a day) + ceftriaxone sodium 2.0 g (twice a day) anti-infection treatment were given, while still giving MTX (methotrexate) + SASP (sulfasalazine) + prednisone for the treatment of rheumatoid arthritis. After more than a week of treatment, the patient showed no significant improvement in her headache symptoms. She still had a fever, with a temperature fluctuation of 38.5°C–39°C. No improvement was noticed in the cerebrospinal fluid after re-examination. The infectious disease department was asked for a consultation to perform the T SPOT-TB test. The result was strongly positive, and combined with the patient's clinical presentation and laboratory tests, led to suspicions of tuberculous meningitis. The patient was given a quadruple diagnostic treatment of isoniazid, rifampin, ethambutol, and pyrazinamide.

After one week of anti-tuberculosis treatment, her temperature returned to normal, and her headache symptoms eased. The cell count of the cerebrospinal fluid returned to normal, sugar and chloride increased, and protein showed a downward trend. Her condition is improving. Anti-tuberculosis therapy was maintained upon discharge, while treatment for rheumatoid arthritis remained unchanged.

VI. Lessons learned

The traditional diagnostic methods for tuberculosis include a mycobacterium tuberculosis skin test (TST), chest radiograph, and bacterial smear and culture, of which a positive bacterial culture is the gold standard for diagnosis. TST is widely used in clinical practice due to its simple operation. However, it is vulnerable to interference from various factors, such as the BCG vaccination, overlapping immunodeficiency, malnutrition, and the application of immunosuppressive agents, in which high false-positive and false-negative results are produced. As the patient in this case had suffered from rheumatoid arthritis for more than 20 years and had taken cortisol hormones for a long time, a false-negative result of a PPD skin test was likely. The sensitivity of the bacterial smear and culture was too low to obtain a valuable clinical specimen, especially for extrapulmonary tuberculosis, which is not conducive to early diagnosis and treatment. The ELISPOT method – a new enzyme immunoassay – has recently been put into use for the detection of mycobacterium tuberculosis infection in Britain and the United States, also known as the T-cell spot test for tuberculosis infection (T SPOT-TB). It has high sensitivity and strong specificity, and is simple and quick to use. This method is derived from a stretch of gene sequences present in M. tuberculosis named RD1, discovered in 1996 by Mahairs et al., while RD1 sequences are lacking in BCG strains and most of the mycobacterial genes in the environment. ESAT-6 and CFP-10 (culture filtrate protein) produced by RD1 coding can be used as specific antigens to stimulate T lymphocytes in the body to produce the specific cytokine INF-γ. The method is to diagnose the presence of tuberculosis infection by detecting INF-γ, and does not cross-immunize with bacillus Calmette Guerin and mycobacterium in the environment. It is not affected by the immune environment of the body, and the false positive rate and the false negative rate are significantly lower than those of TST.

In summary, as a new enzyme immunology method for the detection of tuberculosis infection, ELISPOT has significantly higher sensitivity and specificity than traditional TST, and requires a short application time, which is of great significance for the early diagnosis and treatment of latent tuberculosis and tuberculosis. Currently, ELISPOT is expected to be used as an auxiliary diagnosis method in suspected tuberculosis patients with atypical clinical symptoms, unclear PPD diagnosis, and negative smear and culture. The ELISPOT method can be used to help confirm the diagnosis of tuberculosis infection.

(Jin Jialin & Weng Xinhua)

Headache and fever with intermittent vomiting for 50 days

I. Medical history

Patient: Female, 42 years old, from Jiangsu Province. She was hospitalized on 28 June 2004 because of a headache and fever with intermittent vomiting for 50 days.

The patient suffered headache, dizziness, and fatigue on 5 May. Her headache worsened a few days later, and she developed chills and a fever. Her body temperature fluctuated around 38.7°C, and would not defervesce on its own. When there was vomiting, it was projectile, and the vomitus was gastric contents. When she was sent to the local hospital for examination, abnormal cerebrospinal fluid was found, with white blood cells 160×10^6/L, mononuclear 88%, protein 260 mg/L, chloride 120.7 mmol/L, and sugar 2.02 mmol/L. After being treated with mannitol, dexamethasone, acyclovir, penicillin, and piperacillin for a week, the symptoms were not relieved, and the patient's temperature increased to 40°C.

On 28 May, she was transferred to the neurology department at a Grade A tertiary hospital. On 2 June, she was examined for cerebrospinal fluid leukocytes (135×10^6/L, monocytes 90%, protein 780 mg/L, chloride 108.8 mmol/L, and sugar 1.44 mmol/L). No cryptococcal spores were found. She was diagnosed with tuberculous meningoencephalitis at first, and anti-tuberculosis treatment was used for a week, but the symptoms did not improve. Re-examination on 9 June showed that the cerebrospinal fluid contained white blood cells of 420×10^6/L, polynuclear 68%, protein of 1,380 mg/L, chloride of 103.8 mmol/L and sugar of 1.12 mmol/L. Hence, tuberculous meningitis combined with purulent meningitis was considered. At the same time as continuing the anti-tuberculosis treatment, ceftriaxone sodium and norvancomycin were added to fight infection, but the patient's condition still did not improve. On 24 June, thick capsular bacteria were found in her cerebrospinal fluid, which were suspected to be cryptococcus. Therefore, anti-tuberculosis and anti-infectious drugs were stopped, and anti-fungal treatment with 5-fluorocytosine and itraconazole was begun. Four days later, her headache was obviously relieved, and her fever subsided. No vomiting occurred. For further diagnosis and treatment, the patient was transferred to our hospital. Two weeks before the onset of illness, the patient had experienced overwork, weight loss, and dieting. In the previous 40 days, she had excessive sweating, blurred vision in both eyes, no cough or expectoration, no sore throat or shortness of breath, no abdominal pain or diarrhea, moderate stools, and sometimes yellow urine, no frequent micturition, urgent urination or painful urination, poor appetite, and poor spirit. The patient had previously been healthy, with no history of hepatitis and infectious diseases. She reported no history of penicillin or drug allergies.

> **Thinking prompts:** The patient was a middle-aged woman with chronic onset and a headache with fever and vomiting as the main symptoms. An infection of the central nervous system infection was most likely. Results of tests of her cerebrospinal fluid confirmed this inference. However, it was difficult to identify the nature of the chronic meningitis based on the cerebrospinal fluid results alone, i.e., whether it was purulent meningitis, tuberculous meningitis, or fungal meningitis that had not been cured after treatment.
>
> The features of her medical history had to be combined. Therefore, when gathering medical history, ask for clues about the differential diagnosis of central infection, such as acute or slow onset, season, accompanying symptoms (skin mucosal petechia and ecchymosis); whether there was a history of upper respiratory tract infection, otitis media, or sinusitis before the onset; whether there was craniocerebral trauma; whether there was concomitant cerebrospinal fluid leakage and the like, or whether there was splenectomy, chronic liver disease, diabetes, malignant tumor, rheumatic disease, or other immunodeficiencies and whether there was a history of tuberculosis or contact with tuberculosis. Before the onset and in the course of the disease, ask if there was low fever, weight loss, night sweats, or other symptoms of tuberculosis poisoning; ask if there were symptoms of respiratory infection such as cough, expectoration, hemoptysis, and urinary tract irritation or digestive system symptoms, in order to find evidence of extrapulmonary tuberculosis or fungal infection, which the pathogenic diagnosis of central infection has suggested. Ask if there were symptoms of cranial nerve paralysis, such as vision disorders, dysphagia, hoarseness, hearing disorders, limb paralysis, and aphasia (when inflammation involves intracranial vessels or brain parenchyma); if there were tremors of the hands and feet, or athetosis, dance-like movements (suggesting brain parenchyma damage); and if there were symptoms of spinal cord damage such as incontinence. Tuberculous meningitis often involves intracranial vessels, and ischemic cerebral infarction is a characteristic manifestation of tuberculous arteritis (the middle cerebral artery and external striatal artery flowing through the skull base are the most frequently involved vessels).

II. Physical examination

T 37.5°C, R 20 times/min, P 84 times/min, BP 115/80 mmHg. She was conscious, and her skin and mucosa were free from obvious ecchymosis. Her eyes were bloodshot from the conjunctiva and sclera, her pupils were equal and round (diameter: 3 mm), and the light reflex was sensitive. She had binocular diploma. There were many oral secretions. Her tongue coating was slippery, and there was pharyngeal congestion, tonsil I° swelling, no swelling of the superficial lymph nodes. She had a supple neck, clear respiratory sounds in both lungs, heart rate of 84 times/min, neat rhythm, flat and soft abdomen, and no tenderness. Her liver was 1 cm below the rib, unsatisfactory spleen palpation, free movement of limbs, and no deformity. Kernig's sign (−), Brudzinski's sign (−), and no pathological reflection.

> **Thinking prompts:** During the physical examination, check for the presence and severity of meningeal irritation signs (nuchal rigidity and Brudzinski's sign). As chronic meningitis is often a part of systemic disease, which can provide clues for diagnosis, physical examination should also investigate whether there are focal lesions, such as abscesses or skin lesions, subcutaneous nodules; whether there is clear nasal discharge and external auditory canal purulence (suggesting cerebrospinal fluid rhinorrhea, otorrhea, or otitis media); and whether there is cranial nerve paralysis (usually III, IV, VI, VIII cranial nerves), manifested as decreased vision, hearing loss, diplopia, and eye movement disorders, which is common in chronic meningitis, especially fungal meningitis.

III. Auxiliary examination on admission

Routine blood: WBC 11.33×10^9/L, N 73.5%, L 19.9%, Hb119 g/L, PLT 256×10^{12}/L.

Chest positive radiograph (29 June): Bilateral lung markings increased.

CT of the chest (plain scan on 1 July): Bilateral lung markings increased. CT and MRI scans of her head upon admission showed no obvious abnormalities.

> **Thinking prompts:** Patients with suspected meningitis should undergo immediate biochemical, routine, and etiological examinations of the cerebrospinal fluid. The isolation and identification of pathogens in the cerebrospinal fluid as well as drug sensitivity tests are of great significance for diagnosis, treatment, and prognosis. The simplest and fastest method is microscopic examination of the cerebrospinal fluid. Centrifugation of the cerebrospinal fluid and the taking of precipitate for examination before microscopic examination can greatly improve the positive rate. Gram staining, acid-fast staining, and ink staining can distinguish bacteria, mycobacteria, and cryptococcus. Routine bacterial and mycobacterial cultures are time-consuming but reliable, and can provide drug susceptibility results. Mycobacterium tuberculosis grows slowly in culture, and cannot provide a quick enough diagnosis.
>
> At present, the Bactec 460 system has been widely used in clinical practice, and can be employed for the rapid isolation and identification of mycobacterium tuberculosis. As it is relatively difficult to obtain the pathogen of tuberculosis and fungi, immunological diagnosis measures can be supplemented. There are currently ELISPOT tests for tuberculosis diagnosis, latex agglutination tests for cryptococcus

neoformans diagnosis, G tests for most fungi (detection of fungal cell wall β-D-glucan component), and GM tests for Aspergillus (detection of galactomannan). ELISPOT examines the ESAT-6 and CFP-10 produced by coding with the RD1 gene sequence (the RD1 sequence is absent in the Bacillus Calmette–Guérin strain and the mycobacterium gene in most environments) as specific antigens to stimulate T lymphocytes in the body to produce the specific cytokine INF-γ. It diagnoses the presence of tuberculosis infection by detecting INF-γ, without cross-immunity with Bacillus Calmette–Guérin and the mycobacterium in the environment. At the same time, it is not affected by the immune environment of the body, and its false-positive rate and false-negative rate are significantly lower than those of TST.

Patients suspected of central nervous system infection also need to undergo routine blood tests, chest radiographs, PPD, and erythrocyte sedimentation rate, as well as cranial CT scans, MRI, and autoantibody examinations to exclude other central infectious diseases such as brain abscesses and parasitic brain diseases, and non-infectious central nervous system diseases such as multiple sclerosis, thrombophlebitis, and nervous system vasculitis complicated with connective tissue diseases.

IV. Diagnosis and treatment after admission

Initial diagnosis: The patient had a headache, fever, vomiting, binocular diploma, and abnormal cerebrospinal fluid during the course of the illness, so a diagnosis of central nervous system infection was established.

Thinking prompts:

(1) Cryptococcal meningitis

The patient had a slow onset, including headache, fever, and vomiting; the number of cerebrospinal fluid cells was < 500, and most of them were mononuclear; her sugar and chloride levels dropped; and suspected cryptococcus was found in cerebrospinal fluid, so a diagnosis was established.

(2) Tuberculous meningitis

The patient's social circle was wide, and China has a high incidence of tuberculosis; she had a slow onset, and the cerebrospinal fluid was purulent, so tuberculous meningitis had to be considered. However, the patient did not have tuberculosis lesions or symptoms of tuberculosis blood poisoning. Regular anti-tuberculosis treatment (isoniazid, rifampin, and pyrazinamide) for one month was invalid, so it was not considered temporary.

(3) Viral meningitis

Viral meningitis has either acute or subacute onset, with a headache as the first symptom. It is often accompanied by fever, and can involve damage to the brain parenchyma and consciousness disorders. In this case, the sugar and chloride in the cerebrospinal fluid were normal, so viral meningitis can be ruled out.

(4) Purulent meningitis

The patient had a slow onset, with a headache and fever. Her cerebrospinal fluid was purulent. After receiving strong anti-infection treatment (intermittent penicillin, piperacillin, levofloxacin, cefotaxime, norvancomycin, and ceftriaxone sodium for 40 days), there was no significant relief, so purulent meningitis is less likely.

(5) Intracranial tumor

Two intracranial CT scans outside the hospital and one intracranial NMR showed no abnormality, so intracranial tumors can be ruled out.

(6) Systemic lupus erythematosus

This disease can present similar changes in the cerebrospinal fluid as in this case, but the patient had no arthralgia or rash, and no damage to other systems, so there was no basis for the time being. Further examination was required.

Anti-fungal therapy with amphotericin B combined with 5-fluorocytosine was continued on admission. However, after admission, the latex agglutination test was repeatedly checked. The ink stain and fungal smear were negative.

On 10 July, a cerebrospinal fluid test at a tuberculosis hospital was culture positive for mycobacterium tuberculosis, but given that the condition was temporarily stable on anti-fungal treatment after admission, and the previous anti-tuberculosis treatment was ineffective, anti-fungal treatment was continued. On 17 July, low fever began to appear with obvious and bearable headache, numbness and trembling of the left hand, as well as an inability to hold things. From 22 July onwards, the patient's headache worsened. She became delirious and unresponsive. Her eyes were fixed to the left, with projectile vomiting, limb rigidity, and convulsions. Encephaledema caused by increased intracranial pressure was considered as secondary to epileptic seizures. Dehydration and reducing intracranial pressure were performed, and the symptoms were relieved.

Thinking prompts: When the experimental anti-tuberculosis treatment failed after three weeks, the anti-fungal treatment worked well, and the patient's symptoms resolved quickly. However, laboratory tests were negative for all fungi, which did not correspond to clinical practices. The patient's condition rebounded while continuing treatment, with a positive result for cerebrospinal fluid mycobacterium tuberculosis culture, which had a very low positive rate. In this case, we had to honor the results of the auxiliary examination and restart the anti-tuberculosis treatment.

On 22 July, the patient's cerebrospinal fluid fungal culture was negative at a dermatology institute, and cryptococcus was seen once in the smear, while mycobacterium tuberculosis was seen in the cerebrospinal fluid culture at the tuberculosis hospital. Therefore, tuberculous meningitis had to be considered. Starting that day, four regular diagnostic anti-tuberculosis agents – isoniazid (0.9 g intravenous drip, once a day), rifampicin (0.6 g, once a day), pyrazinamide (0.5 g, three times a day), and ethambutol (0.75 g, once a day) – were added. Following a consult's opinion at the tuberculosis hospital two days later, pyrazinamide and ethambutol were stopped and isoniazid and rifampicin were used continuously, plus p-aminosalicylic acid (8.0 g intravenous drip once a day) + amikacin (0.6 g intravenous drip once a day) combined with a low-dose hormone treatment. The anti-fungal treatment was stopped because it had a poor effect, and because amphotericin B, 5-fluorocytosine, and anti-tuberculosis drugs were harmful to the liver and kidneys.

In the process of treatment for tuberculosis, the patient still had repeated headaches with a high fever of 39°C. A re-examination of her head CT showed no enlargement of the cerebral ventricles. Dehydration drugs mannitol, glycerol fructose, albumin, and furosemide were given to reduce intracranial pressure, and sodium valproate (Depakine) was given to prevent secondary epilepsy. At the same time, a catheter-related bloodstream infection was suspected, and anti-infective therapy with meropenem (Mepem) was added.

Because the patient suffered from repeated epileptic seizures, irritability, disturbance of consciousness, and cognitive issues, we urgently requested a brain surgery consultation to investigate parenchymal brain lesions, cranial hypertension, and cerebral edema. On the afternoon of 28 July, we performed Ommaya external ventricular drainage under general anesthetic.

The patient's headache was alleviated after the operation, but she still had a high fever with a temperature of 38.5°C–39°C. This remained unchanged after the deep venous indwelling catheter was removed and broad-spectrum antibacterial drugs meropenem, ceftriaxone, norvancomycin, and teicoplanin were administered. A cranial MRI on 6 August showed obvious irregular linear enhancement in the basal cistern, and sulcus consistent with changes in tuberculous meningitis.

> **Thinking prompts:** The efficacy of our patient's tuberculosis treatment was not significant. As cerebrospinal fluid tuberculosis cultures were already positive, and the imaging findings were consistent with changes in tuberculous meningitis, it was necessary to exclude the presence of other infections. As the patient had a deep venous indwelling catheter during hospitalization, the first consideration was whether there was a catheter-related bloodstream infection, but her condition remained unchanged after the catheter was removed and various broad-spectrum antibiotics were administered. In view of the excellent effect of the anti-fungal therapy, the possibility of fungal infection cannot be ruled out, although it is not supported by the auxiliary examinations.

Since 7 August, itraconazole combined with 5-fluorocytosine anti-fungal therapy was added. The patient's body temperature decreased significantly, staying at around 37°C. On 16 August, her cerebrospinal fluid was normal again, with protein 383 mg/L, sugar 4.3 mmol/L, and chloride 123 mmol/L. The dose of hormones was reduced. On 17 August, due to pain in the muscles and joints of both lower limbs, the patient stopped using p-aminosalicylic acid, and ethambutol added for anti-tuberculosis treatment, considering that it might have been related to the allergic side effects caused by p-aminosalicylic acid. Anti-tuberculosis therapy was discontinued on 22 August, and anti-fungal therapy was continued for three weeks with a re-examination of normal cerebrospinal fluid. A cranial MRI on 27 September showed an ischemic lesion in the right frontal lobe. On 29 September, the patient was given itraconazole + 5-fluorocytosine orally.

> **Thinking prompts:** The effect of the anti-fungal therapy was very satisfactory, and the diagnosis of tuberculosis was still suspected because the anti-tuberculosis therapy was ineffective, despite the strong support of culture positivity. Therefore, after the symptoms disappeared and the patient's cerebrospinal fluid returned to normal, anti-tuberculosis treatment was stopped and anti-fungal maintenance treatment was used alone. The patient's condition stabilized.

Since 16 October, without stopping the oral anti-fungal medication, the patient developed a fever again, with a temperature of 37.8°C. There were no night sweats, but the fever was accompanied by a headache and a seizure. Re-examination of the cerebrospinal fluid showed that the total protein was 1,494 mg/L, sugar was 2.2 mmol/L, chloride was 112 mmol/L, and white blood cells were 43×10^6/L. She was given isoniazid (0.6 g, administered intravenously once daily), p-aminosalicylic acid (12 g, administered intravenously once daily), amikacin (0.8 g, administered intravenously once daily), and ethambutol (0.75 g, administered orally once daily). The effect was not obvious, and the fever and headache did not subside. A re-examination of the cranial CT on 20 October revealed a mild enlargement of the ventricles. Considering the possibility of fungal infection combined with the patient's medical history, anti-fungal therapy of itraconazole plus 5-fluorocytosine was given for tuberculosis on 27 October. To strengthen the anti-fungal properties of the treatment, amphotericin B was increased at a small dose from 2 November, and the anti-tuberculosis scheme was adjusted: Amikacin was changed to levofloxacin, and the dose of isoniazid was increased to 0.9 g once daily; ethambutol was retained, and pyrazinamide was added (the drug was stopped on 21 December). The patient's body temperature gradually decreased, and her headache was significantly relieved. The cerebrospinal fluid was improved. M. tuberculosis was again culture positive on 21 October.

In January 2005, the patient had a recurrent fever. On 11 January, her cerebrospinal fluid was re-examined and showed white blood cells of 47×10^6/L, sugar of 3.1 mmol/L, chloride of 105 mmol/L, protein of 1,359 mg/L and pressure > 300 mmH$_2$O. Considering that the total amount of amphotericin B had reached 2 g, amphotericin B + 5-fluorocytosine was stopped on 12 January, and itraconazole was taken orally along with rifampin + pyrazinamide for intensive anti-tuberculosis treatment, which improved her condition.

Conditions at the time of discharge: The chief complaint of a headache was obviously improved, and the patient's temperature was stable. However, she developed blurred vision and diplopia. Isoniazid, rifampicin, ethambutol, pyrazinamide, and para-aminosalicylic acid were combined for anti-tuberculosis treatment, and anti-fungal itraconazole was taken orally. The patient's condition was relatively stable, but there were adverse gastrointestinal reactions and appetite deficiency.

Two cerebrospinal fluid mycobacterium cultures were positive, so the diagnosis of tuberculous meningitis was established. However, in the process of several anti-tuberculosis treatments, the patient developed a fever, and her condition was aggravated. The use of

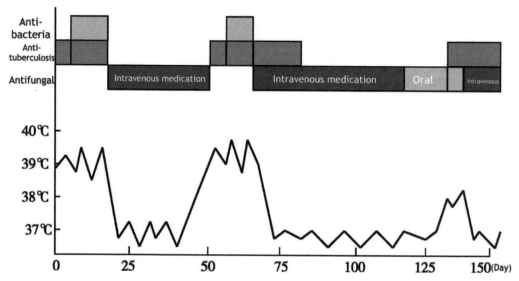

Figure 24-1 Treatment plan and efficacy (the timeline was set as Day 0 from the start of regular treatment on 2 June 2004)

anti-fungal treatment was effective (treatment plan and efficacy shown in Figure 24-1), so a diagnosis of fungal meningitis was also made.

V. Follow-up

A re-examination of the head CT on 16 January revealed lesions in the left frontal lobe, the right deep temporal lobe, and the right annular pool, consistent with tuberculous meningitis with granulomatous formation. Anti-tuberculosis treatment had been given for more than two months, but the CT scan showed that the skull-base lesions in the brain were more obvious than those before. Therefore, we recommended performing brain surgery, and the patient was transferred on 21 January. Part of the lesion had adhered to the optic nerve and inferior colliculus, and it was not completely removed. As a result, the postoperative pathology showed inflammatory tissue, and acid-fast bacilli were found by bacteriology (tuberculosis infection was confirmed again). Anti-tuberculosis treatment was continued after surgery, and was adjusted as five-combination continuous treatment of isoniazid, rifampin, pyrazinamide, streptomycin, and levofloxacin. Several intrathecal injections of amikacin + dexamethasone were given. Re-examination of the cerebrospinal fluid on 15 April revealed a pressure of 95 mmH$_2$O, 12×10^6/L white blood cells, 1,560 mg/L protein, 2.3 mmol/L sugar, and 125 mmol/L chloride. Later, due to hearing impairment, streptomycin was stopped and quadruple anti-tuberculosis therapy was used until December 2005, when the cerebrospinal fluid was re-examined and found to be normal.

VI. Lessons learned

Mixed meningitis, in which two or more pathogens can be isolated from the initial cerebrospinal fluid specimen of a patient with meningitis, is sometimes reported in the literature, although it is considered to be rare. Mixed meningitis has been reported as follows: Mixed infection of two types of bacteria; mixed infection of bacteria and a virus; mixed infection of bacteria and fungi. Very few cases involved infection by three pathogenic bacteria.

Before 1950, community-acquired infection was the most common cause, and the most common pathogenic bacteria were Streptococcus pneumoniae, meningitis, and Haemophilus influenzae. It mainly occurred in infants. After 1950, hospital-acquired infection was the most common cause, and the common pathogen was Gram-negative bacilli, which mainly occurred in adults. Among them, a mixed infection of anaerobic bacteria and aerobic bacteria was the most common.

The foci that can cause a mixed infection of anaerobes and gram-negative bacilli are usually chronic otitis media and/or mastoiditis, chronic paranasal sinusitis, craniocerebral or vertebral plate surgery, head and neck tumors, and craniocerebral trauma combined with infection. Unusual pathogens such as mycobacteria also occur occasionally. With the increasing incidence of AIDS in recent years, opportunistic infections have become common, and the occurrence of mixed meningitis of fungi and tuberculosis in immunodeficient patients has also been reported. In this case, the patient had no definite history of immunodeficiency, and had transient hypo-immunity only before onset, so the development of a mixed infection of tuberculous meningitis and fungal meningitis was unlikely.

Tuberculous meningitis and fungal meningitis are both forms of chronic meningitis. In the absence of other diagnostic clues, cerebrospinal fluid analysis alone shows similar manifestations, making it difficult to distinguish them. The co-infection of the two is rare, making diagnosis more difficult. In our case, despite the positive culture of mycobacterium tuberculosis in the cerebrospinal fluid, several anti-tuberculosis treatments failed. The patient still had a high fever, and her condition worsened. Auxiliary laboratory examinations for fungi were mostly negative, but the effect of clinical treatment was very good. In this case, the clinician used the diagnostic treatment to confirm the diagnosis. Anti-fungal treatment alone had an effect, but could not maintain it. Only when the two treatments are applied simultaneously can the condition be controlled. Combined with the laboratory results, a combined infection of tuberculosis and fungi was finally confirmed. This clinical thinking seems practical and reliable in practice. When relying on medical history, symptoms, signs, and laboratory tests cannot provide a sufficient and complete basis for diagnosis. Diagnosis is clarified in the treatment.

(Jin Jialin & Weng Xinhua)

Sore throat for more than 40 days; intermittent fever for two months; cough and dyspnea after exercise for more than two weeks

I. Medical history

Patient: Female, 38 years old, from Changzhi in Shanxi Province, a cadre of a company in the city of Jincheng. She was hospitalized from 10 to 19 July 2008 because of a sore throat lasting for more than 40 days, intermittent fever for two months, and cough and dyspnea after exercise for more than two weeks.

According to the patient, pharyngeal tingling had presented two months earlier without obvious inducements, followed by fever with a body temperature of up to 41°C. She occasionally felt chilly, but did not experience chills. A doctor at the local hospital found that the patient's pharynx was congested, and diagnosed an upper respiratory tract infection. After hospitalization, she was given cefoperazone and ribavirin, and her body temperature decreased slightly (to about 39°C) without significant relief of her sore throat. She was also given nebulization, Yinhuang Hanhuapian tablets (TCM), Caoshan Huhanpian tablets (TCM), and regular application of ceftriaxone sodium, azithromycin, levofloxacin, and tinidazole for nearly one month. Her body temperature was not stabilized, but her sore throat was alleviated. After more than 40 days, her sore throat disappeared, but her body temperature kept fluctuating at 38°C-39.5°C with no chills. The above treatment was continued in the local hospital, and dexamethasone 10 mg/d was used for a total period of two days. Her body temperature did not decrease significantly. She had developed a dry cough two weeks earlier without sputum, which did not respond to the above antimicrobial therapy. She developed an aggravated cough with thin, whitish sputum, accompanied by dyspnea after exercise.

She was transferred to our hospital for further diagnosis and treatment. She reported that since the onset of her illness, she had suffered no abdominal pain, diarrhea, nausea, or vomiting; no frequent urination, urgency or pain, no joint pain, no rash; poor spirit, decreased appetite; sleep was relatively good; weight loss of about 2 kg; urine and stool were normal.

The patient had also received a blood transfusion (amount unknown) 14 years earlier due to postpartum hemorrhage. She denied any history of hypertension, diabetes, infectious diseases, allergies to drugs and food, or addiction to tobacco and alcohol. She was dutiful and honest, and had a happy marriage with no history of visiting prostitutes. Her husband and children were in good health. The patient had always lived in the city of Jincheng in Shanxi Province, and had no long-term history of travel outside the region. She did not keep any animals in her home. She denied any history of contact with contaminated water, genetic diseases, or infectious diseases in her family, or similar diseases among the surrounding population recently.

II. Physical examination on admission

T 37.5°C. The patient's general condition was fair with moderate nourishment. She was conscious, and was moving freely. She cooperated with the physical examination. No rash, no palpable mass, and no subcutaneous nodules were found on the skin anywhere on her body, and no pathological swelling was noticed in the superficial lymph nodes. There was no congestion in the conjunctiva, no icteric sclera, no ulcers or white secretion in oral cavity, and no congestion in the pharynx and small tonsils. Both lungs had thick respiratory sounds; no dry or moist rales were heard, and no abnormal signs were seen in the heart. Her abdomen was flat and soft, and there was no tenderness or rebound pain in the whole abdomen; the liver and spleen could not be palpated below the costal margin. The ascites sign was negative. There was no percussion pain in the kidney area. Pathological reflections such as Kernig's sign and Brudzinski's sign were all negative, and no positive signs were found in other examinations.

III. Auxiliary examination on admission

Routine blood: WBC 1.4×10^9/L, neutrophil 67%, lymphocyte 33%, eosinophil count 0.02×10^9/L, platelet 126×10^9/L, hemoglobin 89 g/L, erythrocyte 3.16×10^{12}/L.

Urine routine and liver function were normal; stool occult blood was negative. C-reactive protein 36 g/L, ESR 57 mm/h.

Two PPD tests, tuberculosis antibodies, multiple blood cultures, and bone marrow cultures were negative.

ANA, ENA polypeptide zymogram, RF, Brucella agglutination test, WR, and repeated sputum smear for hypha were all negative.

Chest radiograph: The lung markings were thickened.

Color ultrasound examination of abdomen and pelvis showed no abnormality.

Myelogram: The nucleated cells proliferated actively, and the cell morphology of each strain was normal. No parasites were found.

IV. Further diagnosis and treatment

1. **Initial diagnosis:** The patient was a 38-year-old woman whose body temperature had exceeded 38°C for more than two months. A definitive diagnosis had not yet been made, so it was classified as a fever of unknown origin (FUO).

Thinking prompts: The causes of FUO are either infectious diseases or non-infectious diseases. All pathogenic microorganisms, protozoa, and helminth infections in infectious diseases can cause fever. Non-infectious diseases that can cause fever are mainly found in tumors and connective tissue diseases.

2. Diagnostic thinking and treatment

(1) Tumors: The patient was a young female, and the chest radiograph showed no abnormalities except for thickened lung markings. No space-occupying lesions were found in the abdominal and pelvic color ultrasound examinations, and no positive signs were found in the nervous system examinations, so solid tumors could be ruled out. The patient had a fever for two months, and no liver, spleen, or lymph nodes were palpably enlarged. No abnormal cells were found in the peripheral blood and bone marrow images, and there was no bleeding tendency or progressive anemia. Blood system diseases could be ruled out. In conclusion, tumors could also be ruled out.

(2) Connective tissue diseases: The patient had a fever for two months, with an erythrocyte sedimentation rate of 57 mm/h, accompanied by respiratory symptoms, but no joint pain or muscle weakness, and no damage to the skin and other organs and systems. At the same time, laboratory tests were negative for autoantibodies. Dexamethasone 10 mg/d was given at another hospital for two days in total. The patient's body temperature did not decrease significantly, so connective tissue diseases could be ruled out.

(3) Considering infectious fever:

1) Bacterial infectious diseases: The patient had a fever for two months, with a temperature of 38°C–41°C and obvious respiratory symptoms, so bacterial infection of the respiratory system could not be completely excluded. Long-term fever can be a symptom of infectious diseases such as typhoid fever, brucellosis, and tuberculosis, but the patient had been given the antibacterial drugs azithromycin, cefoperazone, and levofloxacin at the local county hospital to regulate the treatment. The above antibacterial drugs have a good effect on most bacteria (including Salmonella and Brucella), and multiple blood cultures and bone marrow cultures were negative. The patient had a high fever that persisted throughout the day without symptoms such as night sweats, and tested negative twice for PPD tests and tuberculosis antibody tests. No signs of tuberculosis were found in chest radiography or B-ultrasonography of the abdomen and pelvis. Therefore, bacterial diseases, including mycobacterium tuberculosis infection, were not considered.

2) Spirochete infection: Spirochete infection is sensitive to most antibiotics such as cefoperazone, and the standard use of antibiotics outside the hospital was ineffective, so spirochete infection could be ruled out.

3) Chlamydia and mycoplasma infectious diseases: Chlamydia and mycoplasma infections are more common in respiratory tract and urogenital tract infections, and antibacterial drugs such as macrolides have good curative effects. Antibiotic therapy was ineffective in this case, so chlamydia and mycoplasma infections could be ruled out.

4) Fungal infections: Fungal infections should be considered, since the patient had a long period of antimicrobial use in combination. However, the body temperature in cases of double fungal infection is often around 38°C, and oral Candida albicans infection is more common. The patient's body temperature was higher. No white secretion was seen in the oral cavity, and there was no diarrhea. The chest X-ray had thick markings, and repeated sputum smear tests showed negative hyphae. Therefore, fungal infection could be ruled out.

5) General viral infectious diseases can be ruled out: The duration of fever in viral infectious diseases is generally not more than 7–10 days, and herpes viruses such as EB viral infection can last for more than two weeks up to a few months. However, patients often suffer from liver, spleen, and lymph node enlargement, and abnormal lymphocytes are visible in the peripheral blood. Early treatment with ribavirin was ineffective. In combination with the patient's medical history, general viral infectious diseases were not considered.

6) Considering AIDS complicated with Pneumocystis carinii pneumonia: The patient had a blood transfusion 14 years ago (in 1994, the blood transfusion law was not implemented in China, and the sourcing of blood was unregulated). She had a long-term fever in clinical manifestations, coughing with dyspnea after exercise, and weight loss. Non-infectious fever and other infectious fevers could be ruled out, so AIDS was the most likely diagnosis. 70%–80% of patients with AIDS can experience one or more episodes of Pneumocystis carinii pneumonia. Its clinical manifestations are mainly chronic cough and fever, tachypnea, and cyanosis. In a few patients, lung rales can be heard, and the X-ray film of the lung is non-specific.

In this case, anti-HIV and T cell subsets were detected after admission, and the results reported on the same day were anti-HIV-positive. The absolute T cell count was decreased, the CD4$^+$ T lymphocyte count was 0.16×10^9/L, and CD4/CD8 = 0.4. The patient was clinically diagnosed with AIDS. Further, her samples were sent to the Provincial Disease Control Center for confirmation tests, and the patient was given a bronchoscopy. Alveolar exudate was taken and stained with hexamethylenetetramine silver for microscopic examination. Black dots were found, and Pneumocystis carinii was considered, which led to the diagnosis of Pneumocystis carinii pneumonia. Two compound sulfamethoxazole (SMZ-TMP) tablets were given orally three times a day, with α1 thymosin 1.6 mg once a day as a subcutaneous injection to the medial upper arm. A week later, the patient's cough, shortness of breath, and breathing difficulties significantly reduced, and her body temperature fell to 37.5°C or so. After a positive anti-HIV confirmation test report, the patient was diagnosed with AIDS combined with Pneumocystis carinii pneumonia. She was transferred to a designated AIDS hospital that day, where she continued treatment.

V. Follow-up

The patient was followed up by telephone for ten days after leaving our hospital. After she was transferred to another hospital, she continued to take 2 SMZ-TMP tablets orally three times a day, with α1 thymosin 1.6 mg once a day as a subcutaneous injection in the medial upper arm. Meanwhile, symptomatic and supportive treatment was given. As a result, the patient's cough, shortness of breath, and dyspnea disappeared, and her body temperature was around 37°C.

VI. Lessons learned

There is still a low incidence rate of AIDS in China, and awareness needs to be improved among healthcare practitioners. HIV infection is followed by a long asymptomatic period, which can be clinically devoid of any symptoms and signs other than positive HIV antibodies in the blood. AIDS itself is characterized by various infections caused by immunodeficiency, especially opportunistic infections, of which the clinical manifestations are non-specific. The main routes of HIV transmission are sexual contact, intravenous drug use, and blood transmission. However, the first two high-risk behaviors are hidden in daily life. It is difficult to obtain reliable epidemiological data, and blood transmission is often ignored, which sometimes causes missed diagnoses. Therefore, in clinical work, we should be vigilant, deepening our understanding of AIDS, and paying attention to the most common opportunistic infections and tumors. Detailed history should be gathered, and careful physical examination combined with laboratory tests should be performed in order to make a timely and correct diagnosis.

(Zhao Longfeng)

Left hand numbness, fatigue; lack of appetite for three days; irritability and refusal to eat for half a day

I. Medical history

Patient: Male, 36 years old, from Fengtai District in Beijing. He was hospitalized between 7 and 10 March 2004 for left hand numbness and fatigue, lack of appetite for three days, and irritability and refusal to eat for half a day.

The patient had been bitten by a domestic dog on the index finger of his left hand six days earlier. The wound was shallow, and there was a small amount of blood flowing out. He had washed it with soapy water for about ten minutes without disinfection using alcohol or iodine. No rabies vaccine and anti-rabies immunoglobulin were administered. Three days earlier, the patient developed numbness in his left hand, with marked fatigue and appetite deficiency, for which he did not seek medical treatment. Recently, in the morning, the patient has shown obvious irritability, nausea, and rejection of food. Soon after admission, he developed hallucinations, mania, fear and disturbance, difficulty drinking water, fear of the wind, fear of light, excessive sweating, salivation, and generalized convulsions. However, he could think clearly.

The patient had previously been healthy, and denied any history of drug or food allergies, mental illness, or contact with contaminated water. There was no genetic history in his family. Epidemiological investigation found that the domestic dog that had bitten the patient also bit 3 chicks, all of which died soon after.

> **Thinking prompts:** There are many diseases that can cause numbness of the limbs, gastrointestinal symptoms, and mental symptoms. Identifying how to link these seemingly unrelated symptoms is something that young doctors need to learn. For this case, gathering medical history requires a detailed understanding of the symptom characteristics, emergence sequence, and disease evolution. Making inquiries about epidemiological history is particularly important, but is often ignored by doctors. In this case, all of the chicks that were bitten by the dog died soon after, indicating that

the dog probably harbored zoonotic pathogenic microorganisms, most likely the rabies virus. During physical examination, special attention should be paid to the nervous system to rule out nervous system diseases.

II. Physical examination on admission

T 37.8°C, H 90 times/min, BP 135/80 mmHg. Conscious, salivating, sweating. Neurological examination: Both pupils equal and round, responsive to light; the neck was supple, no meningeal irritation sign, and no pathological reflection. Tenderness was evident in the wound on the left index finger. Stimulation by sound, light, and water caused paroxysmal convulsions of the muscles throughout the body. There were no positive signs in the heart and lungs. Abdomen was soft; liver and spleen could not be palpated; shifting dullness was negative.

III. Auxiliary examination on admission

Routine blood: WBC 9.5×10^9/L, N 81.9%, L 7.9%, RBC 4.12×10^{12}/L, Hb 125 g/L, PLT 280×10^9/L.

Routine urine and stool results were normal.

Thinking prompts: Routine blood tests performed on the basis of completing medical history and physical examination have no obvious specificity, but they can suggest viral or bacterial infection. A serum neutralization antibody test can be used to detect rabies antibodies. The method is rapid, and has high specificity and sensitivity. A diagnosis can be made by measuring antibodies in the cerebrospinal fluid when the positive neutralizing antibodies in the serum are not enough, but this has not been carried out in China. The detection of rabies virus nucleic acid by PCR is an etiological examination, and a definitive diagnosis can be made when it is positive. It is also possible to detect viral antigens in corneal imprints and hairy root skin tissue using the immunofluorescence antibody technique. However, these methods are difficult to carry out in most hospitals, and have no practical significance. Therefore, a clear epidemiological history and typical clinical symptoms are the keys to making a diagnosis.

IV. Further diagnosis and treatment
1. Initial diagnosis

The patient had a clear history of dog bites, with typical symptoms of fearing water and wind, so the diagnosis was highly likely to be rabies. However, meningoencephalitis caused by psychosis, rabies phobia, tetanus, and other pathogens should be ruled out.

Thinking prompts: Rabies in China is mostly the manic type, which is easily misdiagnosed as mental illness and viral encephalitis due to mania and fear. Analysis can be made according to the patient's current symptoms and signs.

2. Diagnostic thinking

(1) Mental illness: Psychosis usually has a family history, and is preceded by major mental stimulation or long-term mental depression. Psychosis will not cause whole-body paroxysmal convulsions of the muscles due to stimulation from sound, light, or water. It can therefore be ruled out in combination with the patient's medical history, family history, course of onset, clinical symptoms, and laboratory tests.

(2) Hysterical pseudorabies: Also known as rabies phobia, this is hysteria that develops after being bitten by a dog due to an extreme fear of rabies, imagining oneself with the disease. By implication, patients often show exaggerated symptoms, such as aggressive behavior, biting, yelling, and even hydrophobia. Pseudo-hydrophobia is an exaggerated manifestation that does not accurately produce reflex characteristics and lacks fever, special prodromal symptoms, and specific laboratory tests. The patient's condition does not develop progressively, and can recover by itself. Moreover, there are only a few hours or 1–2 days from the time of animal bite to the time of clinical symptoms. However, the incubation period of rabies is generally not so short. Knowing the patient's previous personality is helpful for diagnosis. This case did not meet these conditions.

(3) Tetanus: An early symptom of tetanus is trismus, followed by a "wry smile" and opisthotonos. Patients with tetanus may have painful muscle spasms if they try to swallow, but they do not have hydrophobia. A rare form of localized tetanus – hydrophobia tetanus caused by only involving the cervical nerves that dominate the swallowing muscle group – is easily confused with rabies in a clinical setting. The muscle groups affected by tetanus maintain high muscle tension during the intermission between spasms, and some patients can recover with treatment. In this case, the presence of hydrophobia was typical, and the muscle groups were completely relaxed during the intermissions after convulsions, which was completely different from tetanus. This was the focus of differentiation, so tetanus could be ruled out.

(4) Viral meningoencephalitis: Viral meningoencephalitis has obvious intracranial hypertension and meningeal irritation signs, and consciousness disorders can appear in the early stage. Common viruses include Japanese encephalitis, measles, parotitis, enterovirus, and herpes simplex. Except for rabies encephalitis, brain infections with any of these viruses do not cause hydrophobia. Therefore, this disease was not considered.

(5) Poliomyelitis: Poliomyelitis is prevented by immunization, and the incidence is now very low. Paralytic poliomyelitis is easily confused with paralytic rabies. The former has a double-phase fever onset, and besides the asymmetric flaccid paralysis of bilateral limbs, it is often accompanied by hypersensitization. Affected cerebrospinal fluid shows the phenomenon of cellular protein separation, which is mainly classified as multinucleated granulocytes, while the lymphocytes dominate the whole course of rabies. More importantly, poliovirus can be isolated from the cerebrospinal fluid, pharynx, and feces. The presence of positive complement fixation antibodies and positive specific IgM antibodies can lead to a definitive diagnosis.

(6) Rabies: The patient had been bitten by a sick dog, with the typical symptoms of hydrophobia, fear of wind, excessive sweating, salivation, and numbness at the site of the bite,

as well as paresthesia. The clinical diagnosis of rabies was considered, but there was a lack of confirmation by laboratory tests. Further investigations of viral neutralizing antibodies were needed to confirm the diagnosis. In many primary hospitals, further virus antibody tests cannot be performed, so only clinical diagnosis can be made. Rabies should be considered in this case.

3. Ward-round analysis on the second day after admission

The patient's manic and convulsive symptoms gradually subsided, and his muscle spasms stopped. He entered a coma, and deep and shallow reflexes disappeared. The presence of rabies neutralizing antibodies 4.8 U/L confirmed the diagnosis of rabies. Giving fluid replacement and symptomatic treatment had poor results.

V. Outcome

On the third day after admission, the patient went into a coma. He eventually died of respiratory and circulatory failure.

VI. Lessons learned

The epidemiological history and clinical symptoms of this case were typical, and the clinical diagnosis was easy. The emphasis is on differentiation from other diseases.

(Hou Wei & Meng Qinghua)

Nausea and vomiting for six days; mental dysfunction for three days

I. Medical history

Patient: Male, 17 years old, from Guangxi Province. He was hospitalized between 5 and 10 April 2006 because of nausea and vomiting for six days, and mental dysfunction for three days.

Six days earlier, the patient had nausea without an obvious cause, and vomiting of gastric contents after drinking water. He took Domperidone, but it had little effect. Three days earlier, he suffered sluggishness, delirium, irrelevant answers to questions, and urinary incontinence, and his body temperature rose to 38°C. He was sent to the psychiatric department of the local hospital, where psychiatric diseases were excluded. Because of suspicions of encephalitis, he was transferred to the internal medicine department at our hospital. Through physical examination, meningeal irritation signs were negative. His swallowing reflex was weakened, neurophysiological reflexes present, and pathological reflexes were not elicited.

Auxiliary examination showed that WBC in the routine blood test was 17.8×10^9/L, N 83.7%, and other blood cell counts were normal. Anti-infection penicillin treatment was given for two days, but the patient's condition did not improve. On further follow-up of his medical history, it was discovered that patient had been bitten by a neighbor's dog on his left leg 30 days earlier. Suturing was performed after debridement at the local health clinic, and he was given four doses of rabies inoculations. After being bitten, he did not suffer from hydrophobia, but there was slight skin numbness and formication with wind stimulation. The patient was transferred to our hospital with suspected rabies. He had previously been healthy, and denied any history of drug or food allergies, mental illness, or contact with contaminated water. He denied any genetic history in the family.

> **Thinking prompts:** Since the patient had a definite history of dog bites but no typical rabies symptoms, the possibility of paralytic rabies was considered, and special attention was paid to the nervous system during the physical examination, including swallowing reflex and muscle response to stimulation.

II. Physical examination on admission

T 38.1°C, H 98 times/min, R 20 times/min, BP 98/60 mmHg. Neck resistance check was failed because of non-cooperation; both pupils were equal and round; pharyngeal congestion, diminished swallowing reflex, no abnormality in cardiopulmonary and abdominal examination; neurophysiological reflexes present, and no pathological reflexes elicited. No hydrophobia or anemophobia; no salivation, and no fear of light or sound stimulation. On percussion, there was muscle bulge and erect hair in the area that could be seen and percussed.

III. Auxiliary examination on admission

Routine blood: WBC 11.6×10^9/L, N 89.3%, L 7.3%, RBC 4.35×10^{12}/L, Hb 128 g/L, PLT 215×10^9/L.

Liver and kidney function normal; blood glucose 6.8 mmol/L, and electrolytes, potassium, sodium, and chloride were normal.

Urine, routine stool, chest radiograph, and B-ultrasonography of the abdomen were normal.

Cerebrospinal fluid: Normal pressure, clear appearance, normal cell count and classification.

> **Thinking prompts:** Routine blood tests and blood culture tests performed on the basis of completing medical history and physical examination have no obvious specificity, but they can suggest viral or bacterial infection. Liver and kidney function, biochemistry, electrolytes, and blood glucose are helpful in judging a patient's past disease status and current lifestyle. Routine urine and stool examinations, chest radiographs, and B-ultrasonography of the abdomen are routine examinations that can help determine the conditions of other systems. A serum neutralization antibody test can be used to detect rabies virus antibodies. The method is rapid, and has high specificity and sensitivity. Examination of the cerebrospinal fluid can confirm intracranial infection, and a cranial CT can help to find intracranial space-occupying lesions.

IV. Diagnosis and treatment

1. Initial diagnosis

The patient's medical history was complicated. Although he had a definite history of dog bites, he did not have the typical symptoms of hydrophobia or anemophobia. He was given the rabies vaccine after the bite, so there were still doubts about a diagnosis of rabies. In addition, the patient had a fever, vomiting, and mental dysfunction, so a diagnosis of meningoencephalitis could not be ruled out. An initial diagnosis of fever, mental dysfunction of unknown origin, suspected rabies, and meningoencephalitis cannot be ruled out.

> **Thinking prompts:** There are many diseases that can cause fever and mental dysfunction, including infectious and non-infectious diseases. The former includes infections of the central nervous system caused by bacteria and viruses, such as encephalitis and meningitis; infectious diseases that specifically cause nerve damage, such as rabies, tetanus, and polio; toxic encephalopathy caused by infection in other parts, such as toxic dysentery and sepsis. In addition, there are parasitic infections, such as cerebral malaria and diffuse cerebral cysticercosis. Non-infectious diseases can be seen in hepatic encephalopathy, pulmonary encephalopathy, thyroid crisis, and severe hyponatremia. Since the patient in this case had a clear history of dog bites, rabies was considered first. Diagnosis and analysis can be made according to current symptoms and physical signs.

2. Diagnostic thinking

(1) Mental illness: Psychosis usually has a family history, and is preceded by major mental stimulation or long-term mental depression. Moreover, psychosis will not cause obvious fever and vomiting, and laboratory tests will not show an obvious elevation of hemogram. Combined with the course of the patient's illness, clinical symptoms, and laboratory tests, the disease can be ruled out.

(2) Tetanus: An early symptom of tetanus is trismus, followed by a "wry smile" and opisthotonos. Attempts to swallow can cause painful muscle spasms, in which the affected muscle groups maintain high tension during the spasmodic intervals, with few psychiatric symptoms. This patient never had muscle spasms, so tetanus could be ruled out.

(3) Poliomyelitis: Poliomyelitis is prevented by immunization, and the incidence is now very low. Paralytic poliomyelitis is easily confused with paralytic rabies. Paralytic poliomyelitis has a two-way fever onset with asymmetric flaccid paralysis of the bilateral limbs, and is often accompanied by paresthesia, with few psychiatric symptoms. This is different from the patient's clinical presentation in this case, and does not support the disease. Cerebrospinal fluid in poliomyelitis shows the phenomenon of cell protein separation, and its classification is mainly multinucleated granulocytes. Poliovirus can be isolated from the cerebrospinal fluid, pharynx, and feces. The presence of positive complement fixation antibodies and positive specific IgM antibodies can lead to a definitive diagnosis.

(4) Toxic bacillary dysentery: Toxic bacillary dysentery is commonly seen in children under the age of 10, and the body temperature can reach more than 40°C. In addition to the symptoms of encephalopathy, there are severe systemic toxemia and shock manifestations, and a large number of white blood cells can be found in the routine stool test. Sepsis can also present with systemic toxemia and shock manifestations. Careful gathering of medical history and physical examination should lead to the finding of the primary infectious foci. Toxic bacillary dysentery can be ruled out in this case.

(5) Parasitic infection: The brain-type malaria fever type is irregular. The disease begins with chills, fever, and sweating, and then develops into brain symptoms, and possibly splenomegaly and anemia. The patient in this case lacked these specific symptoms, so making a diagnosis was less likely. Specific serum antibodies and blood smears could be searched for plasmodium to assist in the diagnosis. If the patient has cerebral cysticercosis, cysticercosis images can be found by brain CT.

(6) Other non-infectious diseases: Patients with hepatic encephalopathy and pulmonary encephalopathy will have a history of chronic liver or lung disease. Thyroid crisis is common in females, and there will be significant abnormalities of thyroid function, which can be tested. Electrolytes were normal on admission, so hyponatremia can be ruled out for this patient.

(7) Meningitis or encephalitis caused by bacteria or viruses: Meningitis or encephalitis caused by bacteria or viruses have symptoms of intracranial hypertension, headache, projectile vomiting, bulbar conjunctival edema, meningeal irritation sign, and a large number of white cells in the cerebrospinal fluid of bacterial meningitis. None of the above features were present in this patient, and it can therefore be ruled out.

(8) Rabies: Rabies can either be manic or paralytic. Cases in China are mostly manic. Typical rabies cases are mostly of the manic type, presenting with rabies-specific symptoms such as hydrophobia, photophobia, and dysphagia, as well as manifestations of sympathetic hyperfunction such as irritability, excess salivation, spitting saliva, profuse sweating, accelerated heart rate, and increased blood pressure. The course of the illness lasts for three to six days in general. The paralytic type is rare. There is no excitatory stage or typical manifestation of hydrophobia. The course of the illness can be long, and the symptoms are mainly spinal cord changes accompanied by perioral spasms after stimulation, and muscle edema and hair erection after partial stimulation when the chest muscle is struck. This patient had a history of dog bites, but had no typical symptoms of hydrophobia or anemophobia. There was no sweating or salivation, but he showed spinal cord paralysis (urinary incontinence), muscle spasms, and bristling hair when stimulated. Paralytic rabies was highly suspected, but there was no confirmation from laboratory tests. Further viral neutralizing antibodies were needed to confirm the diagnosis.

3. Ward-round analysis on the first and second days after admission

On the first day after admission, the patient's abdomen was markedly distended, and the percussion note was tympanitic throughout the abdomen. Bowel sounds were significantly reduced and weakened. The plain abdominal film showed a large amount of gas, and some intestinal tubes were dilated, suggesting intestinal paralysis, with moderate fever. The patient's body temperature was 38.5°C. A CT scan of his head showed no abnormality, and his thyroid function was normal. On the second day after admission, he entered a shallow coma, with slow and shallow breathing, high fever, and a temperature of 39.7°C. No bacterial growth was found in multiple blood cultures. The titer of the anti-rabies neutralizing antibody was 4.1 U/ml, and the diagnosis of paralytic rabies was confirmed. After admission, the patient was given special care, fluid replacement, antipyresis, nutritional support, and antiviral treatment with ribavirin. The effect was not good.

V. Outcome

On the third day after admission, the patient went into a deep coma and finally died of respiratory and circulatory failure.

VI. Lessons learned

Paralytic rabies is relatively rare, and has no typical excitatory period or typical manifestations of hydrophobia. It is easily misdiagnosed due to a lack of specific changes. The diagnosis of this case was not confirmed at the start. Gathering epidemiological history was the key to a successful diagnosis.

(Hou Wei & Meng Qinghua)

Repeated joint swelling and pain for 21 years, rash for 20 years, and headache for 11 years

I. Medical history

Patient: Male, 24 years old, from Jinxi County in Jiangxi Province. He was hospitalized because of repeated joint swelling and pain for 21 years, a rash for 20 years, and headache for 11 years.

In 1987, the patient had left heel swelling and pain without any obvious causes, with slightly increased local skin temperature and no redness of the skin. He subsequently developed successive swelling and pain in his right heel, knees, elbows, and distal interphalangeal joints of both hands, without morning stiffness. After one week, the joint pain spontaneously resolved. Since then, the above symptoms have occurred intermittently, 6–7 times per year. In 1988, the patient presented with scattered red maculopapules on his extremities and trunk, about the size of a five-cent coin, with mild pruritus and without desquamation or pain. The rash resolved itself, and he did not see a doctor. In 1997, he experienced dull persistent pain in his forehead and occipital region without any obvious causes and no nausea or vomiting, accompanied by dizziness, a conscious decline in hearing and memory, and intermittent tinnitus. At the same time, bulbar conjunctival congestion of both eyes occurred frequently without convulsion and consciousness disorder. The patient did not note his body temperature before visiting the local hospital. At the local hospital, they found that his body temperature intermittently increased to 38.0°C. Routine blood tests showed that his white blood cells were $(13.4–14) \times 10^9$/L and platelets were $(453–467) \times 10^9$/L. Liver and kidney function was normal. An ESR of 48 mm/h and C-reactive protein of 7.11 mg/L were obtained. Anti-chain O antibodies were 369 IU/ml. He was considered as having chronic rheumatic arthritis, with headache to be investigated. The local hospital gave Levofloxacin by intravenous infusion, and his temperature returned to normal, but his headache and joint pain did not improve significantly. Since the onset of illness, the patient has been in a state of malaise and fatigue, saying few words, but without oral vulvar ulcer, Raynaud's phenomenon, a dry mouth, dry eyes, or light allergy, and no significant change in body weight.

The patient had previously been healthy, and denied any tuberculosis infection or contact with TB. He lived in the rural area of Jinxi County, and denied any history of contact with infected areas or pets. His cousin had a similar history of arthralgia and rash, and denied any allergies to food or drugs.

Thinking prompts: The patient was a young male who had a juvenile onset that was clinically characterized by multi-system involvement, manifested as multiple joint pain, a rash, and nervous system involvement. His joint pain was characterized by symmetrical swelling and pain in multiple joints without morning stiffness. The rash was made up of nodular erythema papules, and the nervous system manifestations were headache accompanied by hearing and memory impairment, and bulbar conjunctival congestion. Initial auxiliary examinations found increased white blood cells and platelets, increased ESR, and increased C-reactive protein. The patient had a clear manifestation of nervous system involvement. When asking about medical history, inquire about the nature, location, and degree of the headache, whether there is disordered consciousness, whether there is any manifestation of cranial hypertension such as projectile vomiting, and whether there are limb convulsions. In the physical examination, check whether there is any sign of meningeal irritation, central nervous system positioning signs such as cranial nerve involvement, muscle strength of the four limbs, and sensory disturbance. Check whether a lumbar puncture examination has been conducted. Cerebrospinal fluid pressure, routine, and biochemical test results are needed to help determine whether it is exudate or transudate. Ask if central nervous imaging such as CT or MRI has been performed.

The patient in this case presented with multi-system involvement, so infectious and autoimmune diseases should be considered in the initial differential diagnosis.

As for infectious diseases, when there is low fever, increased ESR, and fatigue, we should consider the possibility of tuberculosis infection. Reactive arthritis from tuberculosis infection can explain the joint pain. As for the fever, is it accompanied by night sweats and other symptoms of tuberculosis poisoning? Physical examination should investigate lymph node enlargement, lung signs, and hepatosplenomegaly. Other auxiliary examinations should be performed, such as chest imaging. The patient had joint pain, a rash, nervous system involvement, and suspicious low-grade fever, so the possibility of brucellosis and Lyme disease should also be considered for infectious diseases.

Brucellosis may present with osteoarthritis, fever, central nervous system involvement, so it should be ruled out if symptoms do not match. Epidemiological data should be collected. Lyme disease is characterized by migratory erythema, meningitis, myocarditis, and arthritis, and many patients have been to potential tick habitats such as woods and bushes, or have been bitten by ticks before the onset. When gathering medical history, ask for epidemiological data. Physical examination should note the characteristics of the rash and the presence of meningeal irritation. In addition, Lyme disease can feature cardiovascular system involvement. Physical examination should note any heart signs. When inquiring about medical history in cases of infectious disease, we should ask about the treatment and the patient's reaction, such as the use of antibiotics (type, dose, and treatment course) and their effects.

For autoimmune diseases, the possibility of juvenile idiopathic arthritis, also known as adult onset still disease (AOSD) in adults, should be considered, featuring a rash, joint pain, and fever, as well as increased inflammatory indicators such as white blood cells and ESR. This diagnosis should be considered according to the initial medical history of the patient, but a diagnosis of AOSD can only be made after ruling out other diseases, such as rheumatic fever. Patients with rheumatic fever usually begin suffering in childhood, with repeated joint swelling and pain, rashes, and nervous system involvement, accompanied by ESR and increased C-reactive protein. However, the typical rash of rheumatic fever is annular erythema, and the main manifestation of nervous system involvement is chorea. The characteristics of the rash and the presence of chorea should be noticed during physical examination. Juvenile ankylosing spondylitis should also be considered in autoimmune diseases. It may present as heel pain due to Achilles tendon attachment inflammation, and may be accompanied by joint pain, fever, and a rash. However, the patient in this case had no obvious waist symptoms, and unexplained central nervous system symptoms. For autoimmune diseases, ask about the treatment and reaction to it, such as whether glucocorticoids have been used, and record the dose and duration of treatment, and the therapeutic effect.

The patient in this case was a teenager at the time of onset. The possibility of lymphoma should be considered in terms of neoplastic diseases. Lymphoma may present with fever, rash, central nervous system involvement, enlarged lymph nodes, or hepatosplenomegaly. The characteristics of fever should be noticed in inquiries. Check whether examinations such as a bone marrow puncture have been conducted. Superficial lymph nodes and hepatosplenomegaly should be noted in the physical examination.

II. Physical examination on admission

The patient's body temperature fluctuated between 37.1°C and 38.3°C. His blood pressure was 105/65 mHg, and his heart rate was 80 times/min. He had a clear mind and speech, but his reactions were slightly dulled. On his bilateral upper limbs and bilateral thighs were scattered red maculopapules, which faded when pressed, with itching but no tenderness. There were 2–3 soybean-sized lymph nodes on the front of his neck on the left side, which were tough, movable, and free of tenderness. There was a 1 cm lymph node in left supratrochlear, and 1–2 soybean-sized lymph nodes in both inguinals, with the same characteristics as above. There was no icteric in the skin mucosa anywhere on his body; obvious congestion in the spherical conjunctiva; bilateral pupils were equal and round, and there was reaction to light. The eyes moved fully, and the nasolabial fold was symmetrical. No ulcers were seen in the oral mucosa. His tongue was in the middle, his neck was supple, and there was no feeling of resistance, no swelling of the thyroid, and no tenderness in the sternum. Percussion sounds were resonant in both lungs; clear respiratory sounds in both lungs, and no dry or moist rales were heard.

There was no elevation or tremor in the precordial region, and there was no enlargement of the cardiac boundary. The heart rhythm was even, and grade 2/6 blowing systolic murmur could be heard at the apex of the heart. The abdomen was flat and soft, without tenderness or rebound pain. The liver and spleen were not palpable below the costal margin, and no masses were palpated. The spine shape and range of motion were normal, with no tenderness. The limb joints were symmetrical without deformity or swelling. Limb muscle strength was level 5. His Achilles tendon reflexes were low, and his sensory coordination was normal. The straight chin-sternum distance was three transverse fingers. Kernig's sign and Babinski's sign were negative.

> **Thinking prompts:** For tuberculosis infection, routine blood, ESR, PPD test, protein electrophoresis, and tuberculosis antibodies should be checked. A chest CT should be taken to identify whether there is lung involvement and mediastinal lymph node enlargement. An abdominal CT can be taken to see whether there is liver damage from liver tuberculosis or abdominal lymph node enlargement. Antacid staining and tuberculosis culture can be performed on the cerebrospinal fluid. For brucellosis, the Brucella coagulation test should be performed. The patient in this case had central nervous system involvement including a headache, so he should undergo a spinal fluid puncture to check his cerebrospinal fluid pressure. Routine, biochemical, and pathogen examinations can help determine whether there is an infection of the central nervous system.
>
> In terms of autoimmune diseases, anti-nuclear antibodies, anti-double-stranded DNA, anti-solubility nuclear antigens, and rheumatoid factors were examined to check for autoimmune diseases. For juvenile ankylosing spondylitis, a CT of the sacroiliac joint can be taken.

III. Auxiliary examination

Routine blood: Leukocytes $(15.9-19.7) \times 10^9/L$, neutrophils 64.6%–87.3%, eosinophils $(0.22-0.36) \times 10^9/L$, hemoglobin 134–145 g/L, platelets $(402-536) \times 10^9/L$.

Routine urine and stool: No abnormality.

Examining parasite eggs in stool: Many times, negative.

Liver and kidney function: Alanine aminotransferase 9 U/L, total protein 91.5 g/L, albumin 43.5 g/L, lactate dehydrogenase 166 g/L, creatinine 89 μmol/L. ESR was 64 mm/h, C-reactive protein 9.83 mg/L. Complement: Normal.

Quantitative human blood immunoglobulin: IgG 15.5 g/L, IgA 3.67 g/L, IgM 1.70 g/L. IgE 2,018 IU/ml.

Protein electrophoresis: Albumin 46.1%, α_1 5.6%, α 211.6%, β 25.9%, γ 25.0%, A/G 0.8.

Immunoelectrophoresis: No abnormalities.

PPD test: Negative.

Tuberculosis antibodies: Negative.

Brucella coagulation test: Negative.

Anti-chain O antibody: 229 IU/L.

Mycoplasma antibodies, chlamydia antibodies, cold condensation test: All negative.

Blood calcitonin: Normal.

Toxoplasma gondii antibodies, rubella virus, herpes simplex virus antibodies, cytomegalovirus antibodies: Negative.

EBV antibodies: Negative.

Syphilis test: Negative.

Anti-nuclear antibodies, anti-double-stranded DNA, anti-soluble nuclear antigen, anti-neutrophil cytoplasmic antibodies, and anti-cardiolipin antibody: All negative.

Rheumatoid factor: Normal.

Anti-perinuclear antibodies, anti-keratin antibodies: Negative.

Enhanced chest CT: Clear lungs, no enlarged lymph nodes in hilar and mediastinum.

Enhanced abdominal CT: Multiple small lymph nodes seen behind the peritoneum.

Cardiac color ultrasound: No abnormality.

Bone marrow biopsy: Hyperplasia was active, the proportion and morphology of granulocytes and erythroid cells at all stages were normal, and the proportion of lymphocytes and monocytes was normal. The number of megakaryocytes and platelets was considerable.

CT of both hands, knees, feet, and sacroiliac joints: No abnormality found.

Brain MRI: Supratentorial brain sulci widened, ventricles enlarged, no abnormalities of venous sinus system and brain parenchyma were observed.

Multiple lumbar puncture examinations showed that the pressure of cerebrospinal fluid was more than 260 mmH$_2$O (reference value 80–180 mmH$_2$O). The cerebrospinal fluid was colorless and transparent. The number of cells was 0–18/mm^3, the number of leukocytes was 0–14/mm^3, protein was 49.4–70.9 mg/dl, glucose was 49–54 mg/dl, chloride was 119–127 mmol/L.

CSF bacterial smear, antacid stain, ink stain, bacterial culture, tuberculosis culture: All negative.

CSF porcine cysticercus antibody: Multiple times, negative.

IV. Initial diagnosis

The patient was a young male with a juvenile onset of illness. The clinical features were multi-system involvement, presenting as multiple joint pain, rash, fever, and nervous system involvement, among which the latter was prominent. The etiology of the disease was infectious or non-infectious.

1. The possibility of autoimmune diseases should be investigated when considering non-infectious diseases. Vasculitis may be characterized by joint pain, rash, fever, or central nervous system involvement, but multiple auto-antibodies in this patient were negative, and the features of his brain MRI did not support typical vasculitis. Ankylosing spondylitis can appear as inflammation of the Achilles tendon attachment point and heel pain. It can be accompanied by arthralgia, fever, and rash, but the CT of this patient's sacroiliac joint was normal, so it was ruled out. Other autoimmune diseases, such as AOSD, may be characterized

by fever, rash, joint pain, increased white blood cells, and increased hematopoiesis. However, AOSD is an exclusionary diagnosis, which means that other diseases should be ruled out before diagnosis, so it was ruled out. The possibility of lymphoma should be taken into account when considering tumor diseases. This patient's illness began at an early age, with fever and swollen lymph nodes. However, his condition had not deteriorated significantly for more than 20 years, which is inconsistent with the characteristics of tumor diseases. In addition, the patient had no liver and spleen enlargement, and the bone marrow smear and biopsy did not indicate lymphoma, so it was ruled out.

2. Infectious diseases

(1) Viral infection: Most viral diseases are acute, with a fever lasting 1–2 weeks. Some viruses, such as EB, can appear as a chronic process. The course of this patient's illness was more than 20 years, and it did not conform to the natural course of typical viral infections. In addition, the white cells in the peripheral blood infected by a virus do not increase in general, or mainly increase in lymphocytes, to which the patient's hemogram did not conform. Therefore, viral infection can be ruled out.

(2) Tuberculosis infection: The chronic course of TB infection can cause low fever, joint pain, swollen lymph nodes, and an increase in ESR. For patients with these symptoms, we should consider the possibility of tuberculosis infection. However, the patient in this case did not have the typical symptoms of tuberculosis infection, such as low fever in the afternoon and night sweats. The number of leukocytes in the cerebrospinal fluid was low; the biochemical chloride and glucose in the cerebrospinal fluid were normal; the protein was slightly increased; the course of the illness was too long, and there was no obvious abnormality in the central nervous system. These characteristics were not consistent with the manifestation of tuberculous meningitis (which is dominated by an increase of mononuclear cells). Moreover, a PPD test and multiple re-examinations of tuberculosis antibodies were negative, and no evidence supporting tuberculosis infection was found on the chest CT.

(3) Brucellosis: Osteoarthritis, fever, and central nervous system involvement may occur, which should be noted in diagnosis. Brucellosis patients have a clear history of contact with cattle and sheep, which this patient did not. Nor had he had contact with sick animals or corpses, and the Brucella Coagulation Test result was negative, so brucellosis can be ruled out.

(4) Common bacterial infection: The patient had increased white blood cells, so the possibility of bacterial infection should be considered. However, bacterial infection is usually characterized by an acute or subacute course. This patient had a long history of illness, and should have had a local infection. However, the number of leukocytes in his cerebrospinal fluid was low, and the fluid did not conform to the characteristics of bacterial infection, so it can be ruled out.

(5) Parasitic infection: The patient had a significant increase in IgE, so a parasitic infection could be a possibility. However, the patient had no elevation of eosinophils, and had not been to an area rife with parasites. Multiple examinations for parasite eggs were negative, so he could not be diagnosed. Cysticercus pigis can cause nervous system involvement in

parasite infection, and there can be signs and symptoms in certain parts of the body that are caused by neurological abnormalities. However, the patient's head imaging results did not show these issues, and the CSF antibodies for Cysticercus pigis were negative, so it can be ruled out.

(6) Lyme disease: Clinical manifestations are rash, meningitis, arthritis, and myocarditis. Prior to the onset the patient had entered a tick habitat and may have been bitten. The patient lived in a rural area with a lot of trees and grass. Although he did not think he had been bitten by a tick, the possibility cannot be ruled out. Moreover, his cousin lived in the same environment and had a similar rash, which could sway the diagnosis.

> **Thinking prompts:** Often, diagnosis focuses more on infectious diseases, among which common bacteria, viruses, and parasites are less likely. Therefore, we should focus on Lyme disease and TB infection. The pathogen of Lyme disease is tick-borne Borrelia burgdorferi. It is technically very difficult to isolate, so diagnosis mainly depends on the detection of high titer specific antibodies or increased double serum specific antibody titer in serum or cerebrospinal fluid. Syphilis and other known causes of false positives need to be ruled out. Serum and CSF antibodies for Lyme disease can be examined further. In addition, the patient had lymph node enlargement, so a lymph node biopsy should be performed to differentiate tuberculosis infection or lymphoma.

V. Further diagnosis and treatment

Lymph node biopsy: Reactive hyperplasia of lymph nodes (supratrochlear); neutrophils were seen in some lymphatic sinuses, and blood vessels were seen in the center of some lymphoid follicles; immunohistochemistry: CD3 (+), CD5 (+), CD20 (+), CD79α (+).

Cerebrospinal fluid check for Lyme disease: Negative.

The serum antibody IgG of Lyme disease was 1:32 by IFA; ELISA was used to detect antibodies of Lyme IgM (+), and Western blot was used to detect IgM 83 kD (one protein band) and IgG 83/41/17 kD (three protein bands).

Therefore, the diagnosis was clearly Lyme disease.

Due to a penicillin allergy, an intravenous infusion of ceftriaxone sodium was started on 11 January 2005 for two weeks, and then changed to doxycycline 100 mg three times a day. Mannitol was administered to reduce cranial pressure. Considering that craniocerebral hypertension was caused by chronic inflammation of the central nervous system, 40 mg prednisone was added once a day, with gradual reduction. The patient did not show any increase in body temperature. His rash subsided, and his joint pain and headache decreased.

Routine blood re-examination: Leukocytes 14.06×10^9/L, neutrophils 65.13%, platelets 409×10^9/L. ESR: 7 mm/h; C-reactive protein: 1.38 mg/dl. IgE 832.4 IU /ml. Cerebrospinal fluid pressure 310 mmH$_2$O, total cerebrospinal fluid cells 1/mm^3, protein 42.6 mg/dl, glucose 58 mg/dl. The patient continued to take doxycycline, as well as treatments for dehydration and reducing intracranial pressure. The CSF pressure was 225 mmH$_2$O and the protein was 58.8 mg/dl.

The patient continued to take doxycycline and prednisone after discharge. Doxycycline was taken for four weeks and then discontinued. Prednisone was gradually reduced, and stopped on 20 April. On 28 April, a red rash appeared again on his bilateral upper limbs, with the same nature. The patient occasionally had a low fever, sometimes reaching 37.5°C, and an aggravated headache.

Routine blood re-examination: Leukocytes 17.09 × 10^9/L, neutrophils 78.8%, platelets 607 × 10^9/L. ESR: 70 mm/h. C-reactive protein: 11.2 mg/dl. Cerebrospinal fluid pressure: 260 mmH$_2$O, clear and transparent cerebrospinal fluid; total number of cells 13/mm^3, leukocyte count 0/mm^3, protein 55.8 mg/dl, glucose 52 mg/dl. Review of the cerebrospinal fluid bacterial smear, antacid stain, ink stain, bacterial culture, tuberculosis culture, and Cysticercus pigis antibodies: All negative. Re-examination of the cerebrospinal fluid for Lyme disease antibodies (IFA method): IgG 1:16, blood Lyme disease antibodies (IFA method): IgM 1:16.

Ceftriaxone sodium infusions were continued for eight weeks, as well as prednisone 20 mg twice daily, starting to reduce to 5 mg per week after one month. The patient was also treated for dehydration and intracranial decompression. His bilateral upper limb rash subsided. His blood and cerebrospinal fluid were negative for Lyme disease antibodies; ESR 2 mm/h, C-reactive protein 0.45 mg/dl. However, the cerebrospinal fluid pressure was still 310 mmH$_2$O, accompanied by headache symptoms with the same nature. A ventriculoperitoneal shunt was performed on 3 August. After operation, the headache symptoms were obviously reduced. The CSF pressure was 130 mmH$_2$O–150 mmH$_2$O. There was no rash or joint pain, and the patient's temperature was normal. Glucocorticoids were gradually reduced, and antibiotics were stopped. Re-examination of routine blood and ESR: Normal. CSF pressure: 130 mmH$_2$O. In August, his blood and cerebrospinal fluid were once again negative for Lyme disease antibodies.

VI. Follow-up
Antibiotics were discontinued at discharge, and prednisone was reduced to 5 mg once daily. The patient's headache symptoms were relieved; his body temperature was normal, and there was no joint pain or rash. A re-examination of routine blood and ESR was normal. No major complaint was found six months after discharge, and his temperature was normal.

VII. Lessons learned
The pathogen of Lyme disease is the tick-borne Borrelia burgdorferi, the clinical manifestations of which are erythema chronicum migrans, meningitis, myocarditis, and arthritis. Patients have often been to tree-rich tick habitats, or have been bitten by ticks prior to becoming ill. According to clinical manifestations, Lyme disease has three phases:

Phase I – early infection: Several days to weeks after infection, with erythema chronicum migrans as the typical clinical manifestation, and systemic poisoning symptoms such as fever, chills, muscle pain, joint pain, and conjunctivitis;

Phase II – disseminated infection: Several weeks to several months after infection, with many nerve, heart, and eye symptoms (nervous system symptoms most prominent); can manifest as lymphocytic meningitis; cerebrospinal fluid indicates increased lymphocyte and protein; heart involvement can occur in different degrees of atrioventricular block;

Phase III – late infection: Mostly occurring months to several years after infection; can be prolonged into chronic arthritis, and can also cause chronic neurological lesions.

This patient had a clear involvement of the central nervous system, especially cranial hypertension. His cerebrospinal fluid pressure was found to be more than 300 mmH$_2$O many times. Cerebral ventricle edema and cistern enlargement were identified through a nuclear magnetic resonance examination, but the cerebrospinal fluid reflux was smooth, so communicating hydrocephalus was considered. After treatment with ceftriaxone sodium and doxycycline, the rash and joint symptoms improved, but the symptoms of high cranial pressure did not relieve. After anatomical variation of the venous sinus system was ruled out by imaging, arachnoiditis could be considered. The patient's cerebrospinal fluid protein was significantly increased. Therefore, the possibility of chronic high cranial pressure was considered due to the formation of skull base adhesions because of increased protein.

The diagnosis and treatment of this patient were complex, and several lessons were learned in the process.

Diagnostic skills and tips:

1. In patients suffering from problems with their skin, nervous system, and joints, as well as heart lesions and the possibility of tick exposure, Lyme disease should be considered. The diagnosis needs to be determined by specific Borrelia burgdorferi antibodies. This case was diagnosed by detecting these antibodies in the blood and cerebrospinal fluid.

2. For diseases involving multiple systems, the possibility of autoimmune diseases as well as other infections and diseases should be considered. Relevant examinations should be performed to rule out them one by one.

3. The patient in this case had meninges, and cranial pressure was increased. The cerebrospinal fluid displayed an increase in protein, accompanied by a small number of white blood cells. Meningitis caused by other pathogens needs to be identified, especially tuberculous meningitis, which is characterized by increased protein in the cerebrospinal fluid and increased cranial pressure.

4. Judging from the time of the onset of symptoms, the patient was suffering from an advanced infection without formal treatment, and had serious neurological complications such as cranial hypertension. Treatment can be carried out with penicillin, ceftriaxone sodium, or doxycycline. The course of treatment is usually 3–4 weeks for patients with central nerve damage. Some scholars have also suggested that the duration of antibiotic use should be extended for patients with advanced neurological complications from Lyme disease.

5. In patients with persistent increased intracranial pressure, do we need to continue

the use of antibiotics? The most likely cause of chronic cranial high pressure is the long-term elevation of protein in the cerebrospinal fluid and the formation of skull base adhesions. Antibiotics should not be used continuously for cranial hypertension, because the skull base adhesions have formed, and this pathological state cannot be changed. Whether antibiotic treatment is required should be judged in combination with indicators that suggest active infection such as leukocytes, ESR, and C-reactive protein. These indicators plus the presence of Borrelia antibodies in the cerebrospinal fluid can be used as indexes of active infection.

6. The patient's treatment was tortuous. After receiving ceftriaxone sodium and doxycycline, the ESR and C-reactive protein returned to normal, leukocytes and platelets decreased, and cerebrospinal fluid pressure and protein lowered, indicating that the infection was under control. However, similar symptoms returned after a relapse, including increased cranial pressure, increased white blood cells, platelets, ESR, and C-reactive protein, suggesting that active infection may have occurred again. The reasons may be as follows:

(1) The treatment was not complete: For patients with central nervous system complications, the initial treatment course may be short, and Borrelia can occur again after the withdrawal of antibiotics.
(2) Re-infection in the original living environment after discharge.

7. When treating the complications of intracranial hypertension, in addition to administering anti-infection medication, other measures should be taken to relieve communicating hydrocephalus. Reducing intracranial pressure by dehydration with Mannitol does not work; a ventriculoperitoneal shunt can be performed.

(Luo Ling & Li Taisheng)

Diarrhea for seven days, and loss of consciousness for seven hours

I. Medical history

Patient: Male, 48 years old, a prisoner at the Shenyang Public Security Detention and Education Institute. He was hospitalized between 2 and 7 September 2005 due to diarrhea for seven days and loss of consciousness for seven hours.

The patient suffered from diarrhea without inducement, and defecated large amounts of watery stool with mucus 4–5 times a day. He experienced abdominal pain accompanied by tenesmus, with nausea and vomiting several times, and a normal body temperature. He was treated with intravenous ofloxacin and oral furazolidone for three days, which reduced the diarrhea to once or twice daily, but his abdominal pain did not improve. On the seventh day after the onset, his consciousness gradually became unclear, and he went into a lethargic state, offering no response to questioning. There was no head pain or projectile vomiting, and no convulsions or restlessness after the onset.

The patient had previously been healthy. He had been detained at the Shenyang Public Security Detention and Education Institute for the past year. He had no obvious history of eating contaminated food, and denied any drug or food allergies. Similar cases had been reported recently. He had been drinking an average of 250 g/d for 20 years.

> **Thinking prompts:** The patient was treated with ofloxacin and furazolidone. The instances of diarrhea were significantly reduced, and his body temperature was always normal, indicating that the antibacterial treatment was effective. But why did his abdominal pain not improve? His infection poisoning symptoms were not heavy, and his body temperature had been normal, so why did he lose consciousness on the seventh day after the onset? Were these symptoms consistent with cerebral toxic bacillary dysentery? Further examination was required.

II. Physical examination on admission

T 36.5°C, BP 120/80 mmHg, P 78 times/min, R 18 times/min. Unconscious, shallow coma state, no restlessness, response to external stimuli, unable to answer questions, no stiff neck.

Both pupils were equally large and sensitive to light reflexes. No bulbar conjunctival edema. Skin elasticity, no dewatered appearance. No abnormal positive signs were found in the heart and lungs. A painful expression when the abdomen was pressed, rebound tenderness, mild muscle tension. Shifting dullness was suspiciously positive, and bowel sounds were normal. The limbs moved independently. Tendon reflexes were not hyperactive and pathological reflexes were negative.

> **Thinking prompts:** Why did this patient have signs of peritonitis and suspicious ascites? Severe acute bacillary dysentery (known as bacillary dysentery) can lead to complications such as peritonitis, shock, sepsis, myocarditis, and pneumonia, but was there any other reason? The analysis should be broad-minded: Since bacillary dysentery can be controlled with effective antimicrobial therapy, abdominal pain should also improve. However, abdominal pain persisted in this case, indicating that the cause also persisted.
>
> In order to determine abdominal condition, we must perform abdominal B-ultrasonography and abdominal X-ray plain film, and detect blood and urine amylase, to determine whether there are common acute abdominal illnesses such as suppurative cholangitis, pancreatitis, gastrointestinal perforation, appendicitis, or intestinal obstructions. In addition, it is necessary to perform an ascites assay to understand the nature of ascites (e.g., exudative, transudative, bloody, or chylous), which is important to determine the etiology of peritonitis. For coma, if the existing clinical data cannot explain it, a cranial CT scan and lumbar puncture of cerebrospinal fluid should be performed as early as possible to determine whether there are problems with the central nervous system, such as infection, stroke, or intracranial space-occupying lesions.

III. Auxiliary examination upon admission

Routine blood: WBC 13.0×10^9/L, N 77.0%.

Serum ion: Na^+ 124 mmol/L, K^+ 3.3 mmol/L, Cl^- 83.0 mmol/L, blood sugar 12.50 mmol/L.

Blood gas analysis: Suggesting metabolic alkalosis.

Routine stool examination (external hospital and internal results): 18–20 WBC/HP.

Abdominal X-ray plain film: No subphrenic free gas, slight flatulence in the intestinal canal, no fluid levels.

Abdominal B-ultrasound: Normal liver volume, smooth surface of liver, fine enhancement of echo in liver parenchyma, 43.40 cm² spleen area. The maximum dark liquid area of ascites was 6.65 cm, indicating fatty liver, large spleen area, and ascites.

Blood and urine amylase were normal.

Liver function: ALT 10 U/L, AST 21 U/L, total bilirubin 30.2 μmol/L, conjugated bilirubin 14.5 μmol/L, total protein 55.0 g/L, albumin 26.2 g/L, cholinesterase 1,842 U/L, γ-globulin 14.68%.

Immunoglobulin assay: IgG 16.1 g/L, IgM 2.9 g/L, IgA 9.2 g/L.

Hepatitis B and C virus serologic markers were negative. Osmotic pressure of blood ketone bodies and plasma was normal.

Blood ammonia: 65 mmol/L.

Routine ascites: Total number of cells 380/mm^3, Lobulated nucleus cells 60%, Rivalta test negative. Ascites biochemical examination: Total protein 10.0 g/L, glucose 12.87 mmol/L.

No abnormality was found on the plain CT scan of the head.

Cerebrospinal fluid assay: Clear and transparent appearance, pressure 150 mmH$_2$O, cell number 0/mm^3, glucose 10.03 mmol/L, protein 0.16 g/L. The gram stain, ink stain, and antacid stain of the cerebrospinal fluid smear were all negative.

IV. Treatment

1. Preliminary diagnosis

The onset of the illness occurred when summer changed to autumn, and there were similar cases in the surrounding areas. Diarrhea occurred, with the patient defecating large amounts of watery stool with mucus 4–5 times a day, with abdominal pain accompanied by tenesmus. Routine blood and stool examination showed significantly increased white blood cells, although there were no stool culture results. The patient was still diagnosed with bacillary dysentery. He had not regained consciousness after seven days.

In cases of severe central nervous system symptoms, toxic bacillary dysentery (cerebral) must be considered, but the patient had a lot of symptoms that did not support such a diagnosis. Cerebral toxic bacillary dysentery occurs more in children, and the onset is rapid. The central nervous symptoms often occur within 24 hours, and the temperature and general state of infection and poisoning symptoms are very serious. In this case, the progress of the course of disease was relatively slow, without fever. The loss of consciousness occurred only one week after the onset, and there was no progressive aggravation. Other vital signs such as respiration, heart rate, and blood pressure were very stable, so differential diagnosis was required. Also, the patient had low potassium and low chlorine metabolic alkalosis. Was this related to his disordered awareness? Further analysis was required.

> Thinking prompts: Diarrhea and loss of consciousness were the two major symptoms. Were they caused by the same cause, or two diseases? Can bacillary dysentery be diagnosed? If dysentery could be diagnosed, was it common or toxic? What other diseases should be investigated?

2. Diagnostic thinking

(1) Differential diagnosis of bacillary dysentery

Because there are many diseases that cause bloody purulent stool, its presence was not necessarily caused by infection from the Shigella pathogen. Diseases that cause bloody purulent stool can generally be divided into two categories: Infectious diseases in the gut or outside the gut, and non-infectious diseases in the gut. Infectious diseases include bacillary dysentery, bacterial gastrointestinal food poisoning (e.g., Salmonella, Proteus, Escherichia coli, and Staphylococcus aureus), amoebic dysentery, intestinal infection caused by other pathogenic bacteria (e.g., enteroinvasive scherichia coli, Campylobacter jejuni, Plesiomonas, and Aeromonas), and acute necrotizing hemorrhagic enteritis. A small amount of bloody purulent stool can also occur in individual cases of septicemia or peritonitis. Among the non-infectious diseases are colon cancer, chronic non-specific ulcerative colitis, intestinal polyps, and ischemic enteritis. These diseases must be carefully identified before bacillary dysentery is diagnosed.

Diagnostic criteria for bacillary dysentery: The disease can be diagnosed if symptoms align with one of the first three items and one of the second two items below: ① A clear history of contact with bacillary dysentery patients within a week of the onset; ② There was tenesmus; ③ Obvious tenderness in the lower left abdomen; ④ In microscopic stool examination of ten high power microscopic fields, the average number of white blood cells in each field was more than 10, or more than five white blood cells can be examined by microscopy two consecutive times; ⑤ Fecal culture positive for dysentery bacillus.

This case meets items ①–④ , so bacillary dysentery can be diagnosed.

(2) Identification of cerebral toxic dysentery

Characteristics: ① Cerebral (brain edema or respiratory failure) toxic bacillary dysentery occurs in children aged 2–7 years; shock type is more common in adults. ② Cases are urgent, the incubation period is short, the progress is fast; often the disease deteriorates rapidly within 24–48 hours. ③ The disease is dangerous, mostly with sudden high or ultra-high fever (42°C), with symptoms such as repeated convulsions and unconsciousness. ④ In many cases, diarrhea symptoms appear later than poisoning symptoms, and are light, therefore easily ignored.

Thinking prompts: The pathogenesis of this case was very different from that of toxic bacillary dysentery. The patient did not have a constant fever, the symptoms of infection poisoning were not obvious, and the progress of the illness was slow. The neurological symptoms appeared on the seventh day after the onset, and cerebral toxic bacillary dysentery was not supported.

So why did the patient experience neurological symptoms? There are many clinical diseases that cause coma, such as febrile convulsions, Japanese encephalitis, viral encephalitis, epidemic cerebrospinal meningitis, cerebral malaria, intracranial space occupation (tumors, abscesses), and diseases that can cause symptoms of the central nervous system. Since the body temperature in this case had been normal, febrile convulsions, Japanese encephalitis, and epidemic cerebrospinal meningitis can be ruled out. Cases of encephalitis caused by other viral infections without fever symptoms have also been found clinically, but the cerebrospinal fluid biochemistry and cranial CT scan of the patient were normal, excluding other viral infections, and also excluding intracranial space-occupying lesions. In addition, check for metabolic encephalopathy (such as diabetic ketoacidosis, hypoglycemia, uremia, hypernatremia, and hyponatremia), brain lesions (such as cerebrovascular accidents, and intracranial tumors and infections) and toxic encephalopathy (such as poisoning from alcohol, drugs, and heavy metals).

The patient in this case was found to have high blood sugar on admission, and had no previous history of diabetes. The infection could induce ketosis and hypertonic coma in diabetic patients, but his blood sugar, ketone body, and osmolality did not meet the criteria for diabetic ketosis and hypertonic coma. Low potassium and low chlorine metabolic alkalosis cause neuromuscular excitatory symptoms such as agitation, excitement, delirium, mouth-lip numbness, hand-foot twitching, and tendon hyper-reflexes, which were inconsistent with this case.

Because the patient had a history of heavy drinking for 20 years, a B-ultrasound examination of the abdomen indicates chronic liver injury and a large spleen area, which can lead to a diagnosis of alcoholic liver disease. The pathological change of alcoholic cirrhosis is characterized by the small and evenly distributed regenerated nodules formed by the hepatic pseudolobules, at the size of 0.2–0.5 cm. The nodules do not contain the portal area and central vein. The surrounding fibrous bundles are narrow and neat, and the uneven appearance of the liver surface is not obvious. It is difficult to identify a non-smooth liver surface by B-ultrasonography, which is very different from the serrated appearance of the common liver surface after hepatitis cirrhosis.

In addition, the patient's serum IgA was significantly increased, so alcoholic cirrhosis cannot be ruled out in this case.

Infection is the main cause of hepatic encephalopathy in severe liver disease. Hypokalemic hypochlorous alkalosis can promote the absorption of ammonia from the intestinal tract. The patient had hyperammonemia, so the possibility of hepatic encephalopathy cannot be ruled out.

(3) Cause of ascites

Transudative or exudative ascites should be distinguished. In this case, the plasma albumin was very low and there was a basis for the formation of transudative ascites, which was related to the loss of albumin in diarrhea and the reduction of intake. However, the intestinal lesions of bacillary dysentery are mainly in the colon, with the sigmoid colon and rectum lesions most prominent. The acute phase is diffuse fibrin exudative inflammation. Therefore, it cannot affect intestinal protein uptake. The half-life of albumin was 21 days, and the patient was able to eat normally every day despite poor appetite. Without other causes of protein reduction, it was difficult to explain the reduction of albumin to 26.2 g/L in this case. The result of the routine urine examination was normal, and hemoglobin was normal in the routine blood tests. Hypoproteinemia caused by loss of protein from the urine or malnutrition anemia can be ruled out. At the same time, the patient had an inverted alb/glb ratio, so a reduction in albumin synthesis due to liver disease must be considered.

The patient's ascites were exudative, with abdominal tenderness, rebound tenderness, and mild muscular tension. According to the results of the abdominal B-ultrasonography, abdominal X-ray plain film, and blood and urine amylase detection, common acute abdominal disease was basically excluded, meaning that spontaneous bacterial peritonitis (SBP) was highly likely. SBP occurs more in patients with cirrhosis, severe hepatitis, and nephrotic syndrome due to the translocation of intestinal bacteria (on the basis of damage to the intestinal mucosal barrier, intestinal bacteria pass through the intestinal epithelial cells into parenteral tissue). Dysentery produces ulcers that are mostly superficial, rarely penetrating the muscular layer of the mucosa and causing perforation leading to peritonitis. Shigella septicemia may cause primary peritonitis, but most cases occur in children and those with low immune function. The clinical symptoms in this case were mild. There was no fever, and the patient was treated with effective antimicrobial agents early on, so Shigella septicemia was very unlikely.

This case had the basis of liver disease, low albumin in ascites, and vulnerability to SBP. In such cases, antibiotics must be selected in combination with common SBP bacteria before bacterial culture and drug sensitivity results are available. The common SBP bacteria are Escherichia coli, Klebsiella pneumoniae, and Streptococcus pneumoniae, and enterococci; anaerobic bacteria are rare. Although the quinolone antibiotics used before admission were effective for the above common bacteria, the curative effect was worse than that of third-generation cephalosporin (common cefoperazone, ceftriaxone sodium, ceftazidime, and cefotaxime). It was completely correct to apply cefoperazone to anti-infection after admission. If possible, it is better to combine third-generation cephalosporins with quinolones and supplement albumen properly, as it helps to prevent hepatorenal syndrome.

3. Ward-round analysis on the fourth day after admission

After admission, cefoperazone was given to resist infection, supplemented with sodium chloride and potassium chloride to control blood sugar. The electrolyte disturbance of low sodium, low chlorine, and low potassium was quickly corrected. The patient's blood sugar also decreased to normal, and blood gas was not rechecked. After 8.5 hours of admission, the patient regained consciousness, but still experienced abdominal pain and distension. His body temperature was consistently normal. On the third day of hospitalization, he discharged unformed yellow stool once. Samples were taken, and were normal. Blood ammonia re-examination: 21 mmol/L and blood routine returned to normal.

Acute bacillary dysentery usually resolves in about a week. The patient's hepatitis virus serum marker was negative. Because alcoholic cirrhosis could not be ruled out, further examination should have been conducted, including gastroscopy, a CT scan of liver, and liver biopsy if necessary to determine whether there is cirrhosis. Unfortunately, the patient refused further examination. His rapid regaining of consciousness may be related to a decrease in ammonia absorption after the correction of alkalosis with low potassium and low chlorine.

4. Condition at discharge (the sixth day after admission)

The patient's consciousness was clear. His abdominal pain and distention were reduced, and his body temperature was normal. There was a slight yellow staining of the sclera. There was still tenderness, rebound tenderness, and mild muscle tension in the abdomen. Shifting dullness positive. Routine stool examination was normal and stool culture was negative. He was transferred to the Security Detention medical clinic to continue anti-inflammatory treatment.

V. Follow-up

The patient was reviewed one month after discharge. He had a normal body temperature, slight yellow staining of the sclera, flat abdomen, and no tenderness or suspicious shifting dullness. The results of laboratory examination were as follows: ALT 12 U/L, AST 28 U/L, total bilirubin 30.1 μmol/L, conjugated bilirubin 14.4 μmol/L, total protein 67.0 g/L, albumin 32.4 g/L. Abdominal B-ultrasonography: Enhanced and thickened hepatic parenchyma echo, large spleen area, and small amount of ascites.

VI. Lessons learned

The diagnosis of bacillary dysentery in this case was easy, but it was difficult to classify. However, if the clinical characteristics of toxic bacillary dysentery were mastered and a differential diagnosis of cerebral toxic bacillary dysentery was made (especially through detailed inquiry into personal history, such as long-term heavy drinking), the complications of such combined diseases as alcoholic liver disease (e.g., hepatic encephalopathy) should be taken into account. The causes of hepatic encephalopathy should be attributed to intestinal infection (bacillary dysentery) and electrolyte disturbance. It is also worth noting that patients with liver disease must avoid intestinal infection, otherwise it is easy to develop spontaneous bacterial peritonitis.

Bacillary dysentery is an intestinal infectious disease caused by Shigella. It is a common disease in summer and autumn in China and elsewhere. For many years, Shigella flexneri (group B) was the main epidemic flora in most regions of China. In recent years, Shigella dysentery group A has been widespread in a few areas. Clinically critical cases have increased. The prognosis of bacillary dysentery is affected by many factors. Early detection, accurate diagnosis, and correct treatment are the keys to reducing mortality.

(Liu Pei)

Repeated convulsions for 21 hours, and diarrhea for 15 hours

I. Medical history

Patient: Male, four months old. He was hospitalized between 19 June and 3 July 2008 with repeated convulsions for 21 hours and diarrhea for 15 hours.

The patient was suffering from convulsive seizures without any obvious cause. During the convulsions, both eyes rolled upwards, and his limbs were tetanic, lasting for about a minute. The patient's condition was relieved by pressing the philtrum and sedation, but the convulsive seizures recurred, but there was no obvious disturbance of consciousness. Diarrhea occurred six hours later (15 hours before admission), with five incidents of bloody mucous purulent stool in small amounts. There was no fever, no vomiting, and no crying before defecation.

The patient was born by Cesarean section in the city of Jinan on 15 February 2008, and returned to Faku County in Shenyang one month ago. He was partly breastfed and partly formula fed. His intelligence was normal, and he had learned to roll over. There was a clear recent history of eating contaminated food (watermelon slices had been placed in the refrigerator on returning home, and squeezed into a juice with gauze before eating).

II. Physical examination and related auxiliary examinations

1. Physical examination on admission

T 37.0°C, BP 80/30 mHg; breathing was steady when not convulsing, clear consciousness. Head circumference normal; fontanelle not closed, with no bulge or depression. Normal complexion, no stiff neck. There was no edema in the bulbar conjunctiva, and both pupils were equally large and sensitive to light. No dehydrated appearance. No abnormal positive signs were found in the heart or lungs. The liver was palpable 1 cm below the right part of the costal margin. His abdomen was soft, and bowel sounds were active. His limbs could move independently. Normal muscle strength and muscle tension. There was no hyperreflexia of the tendon, and bilateral Babinski's signs were positive.

2. Auxiliary examination

Routine blood: WBC 18.0×10^9 /L, N 64.6%.

Serum Ion: Na^+ 135 mmol/L, K^+ 3.6 mmol/L, CL^- 93.0 mmol/L, Ca^{2+} 2.40 mmol/L. Blood sugar 6.5 mmol/L.

Routine stool: WBC 40–50/HP, RBC 20–30/HP.

CT scan of the head showed no abnormality.

B-ultrasound: Plenty of pneumatosis in the abdominal intestinal canal.

3. Further examination after admission

Blood gas was normal. The results of repeated routine blood tests and routine stool tests were the same as before. Stool cultures were negative. Cerebrospinal fluid pressure, routine tests, and biochemistry were normal, and cerebrospinal fluid smear Gram staining, ink staining, and acid-fast staining were negative.

III. Diagnosis

The pediatric patient developed the illness in the summer, and had a clear recent history of eating contaminated food. The onset was sudden, with repeated convulsions as the initial symptom, followed by the discharge of a small amount of typical bloody purulent stool with mucus. A routine blood test and stool examination showed that white blood cells were significantly increased. Although there was no stool culture result, cerebral toxic bacillary dysentery was considered first, as it is common in children. However, this patient had symptoms that did not support such a diagnosis. Although the onset was rapid, there was no fever or acute inflammatory response syndrome, suggesting that the infection and poisoning were not serious. Besides, the child's consciousness was clear when not convulsing, with stable respiration, no vomiting, no refusal of milk, no bulging fontanelle, and no obvious clinical manifestation of cerebral edema. The neurological symptoms of cerebral toxic bacillary dysentery are the result of diffuse cerebral edema caused by toxemia, metabolic disorders, and hypoxia. Was the cause of frequent convulsions in this patient cerebral edema or cerebral parenchymal lesions? An MRI examination of the head and lumbar puncture cerebrospinal fluid test were necessary to confirm the presence of intracranial organic lesions and central nervous system infection.

> **Thinking prompts:** In this case, are the diarrhea and unclear consciousness caused by the same illness, or are there two? Can bacillary dysentery be diagnosed? If dysentery can be diagnosed, is it common or toxic? What other diseases should be considered?

1. The differential diagnosis of bacillary dysentery

Detailed in Case 29.

Diagnostic criteria for bacillary dysentery: The illness can be diagnosed if symptoms align with one of the first three items and one of the second two items below: ① Clear history of contact with bacillary dysentery patients within one week before the onset; ② Tenesmus;

③ Obvious tenderness in the lower left abdomen; ④ Microscopic stool examination of ten high-power microscopic fields, in which the average number of white blood cells in each field is more than 10; or, more than five white blood cells can be examined by microscopy two consecutive times; ⑤ Fecal culture is positive for dysentery bacillus.

This case meets the criteria of items ②, ③, and ④, so bacillary dysentery can be diagnosed.

2. Identification of cerebral toxic dysentery
Detailed in Case 29.

> **Thinking prompts:** Hyperpyrexia, severe cerebral edema, cerebral hypoxia, respiratory tract obstruction, and cerebral parenchyma lesions can all cause convulsions. Frequent convulsions should be distinguished from febrile convulsions, seizures (e.g., infantile spasm), cerebral cysticercosis, low calcium, encephalitis B, other forms of viral encephalitis, epidemic cerebrospinal meningitis, cerebral malaria, intracranial space occupation (tumors, abscesses), and other diseases that may cause symptoms of the central nervous system. However, this patient's body temperature was normal. There was no projectile vomiting and no central respiratory failure. Hyperpyrexia convulsions and central nervous system infection (such as encephalitis B and epidemic cerebrospinal meningitis) can be ruled out. Although some forms of viral encephalitis may not be febrile, the cerebrospinal fluid and head CT of the pediatric patient were normal, so it was not supported. Intracranial space occupying lesions and developmental deformities can also be ruled out. So, since the patient's convulsions were not brain edema, nor were there substantial brain lesions, nor was the low calcium, what exactly was the cause of his illness?

IV. Ward-round analysis on the seventh day after admission
After admission, cefoperazone was given to fight infection, as well as mannitol, scopolamine, and diazepam for symptomatic treatment. The patient's diarrhea improved significantly, but the convulsions were still frequent, and their duration was longer than before – up to ten minutes. Low fever occurred, with a body temperature of around 37.6°C. The patient defecated a total of three times, with bloody, mucopurulent stool (showing abnormal results on a routine stool examination) and two bouts of mucopurulent yellow stool (showing normal results on a routine stool examination).

After a consultation, the Department of Pediatric Neurology completed an EEG examination, which showed that both sides of the frontal and temporal parts of the fulminant spike wave were slow, indicating abnormal brain rhythm. A cranial MRI showed bilateral frontal and temporal extracerebral space widening, no brain atrophy, nodular focus, low density shadow, brain softening focus, and cerebral hemorrhage focus. Considering that common dysentery could be diagnosed, cerebral toxic bacillary dysentery could be ruled out, but symptomatic infantile spasm was not excluded.

Infantile spasm is a type of epilepsy that occurs in infants, usually at 4–6 months of age, and can either be symptomatic and cryptogenic, often complicated with dysnoesia. Cryptogenic infantile spasm may be related to genetic metabolic factors, and neurological examination and neuroimaging may not be abnormal. Symptomatic infantile spasm can be caused by hypoxic-ischemic encephalopathy, nodular sclerosis, and brain development malformation. Neurological examination and neuroimaging can reveal abnormal findings. The widening of the extracerebral space in infants can either be physiological or pathological widening. Because the child in this case had frequent epileptic seizures and local abnormalities on the EEG, pathological widening should be considered. Because there was no enlargement of the head circumference nor a bulging fontanelle, the possibility of frontal and temporal lobe brain dysplasia was considered. This combination of bacillary dysentery can be the cause of epileptic seizures. Because the results of two routine stool examinations had been normal, the patient was transferred to pediatric neurology for treatment.

V. Condition at discharge (fourteenth day after admission)

The patient had no fever and no diarrhea, and the results of routine examinations were normal. After combined treatment with valproate and nitrazepam, the number of seizures began to decrease, and he was discharged to continue treatment at home.

VI. Follow-up

After one month, the patient was defecating normally. The number of epileptic seizures had been significantly reduced, no psychomotor retardation had been found, and medication was continued.

VII. Lessons learned

The diagnosis of bacillary dysentery was easy to make in this case. The cause of convulsions should be differentiated from cerebral toxic dysentery, which manifests as high fever and severe infection poisoning symptoms. Convulsions are based on a consciousness disorder, and brain edema is obvious. The patient in case had only frequent convulsions, and was just 4–6 months old at the onset. The possibility of infantile spasm should be considered. In addition to cranial imaging, performing a timely EEG is very important. An MRI is far superior to a CT scan for cranial neurological examination.

(Liu Pei)

Abdominal pain and diarrhea
for nine hours, decreased blood pressure,
and low urine output for one hour

I. Medical history

Patient: Male, 47 years old. He was hospitalized between 01:50 and 09:45 on 24 July 2005 because of abdominal pain, diarrhea for nine hours, decreased blood pressure, and low urine output for one hour.

The patient had a sudden onset of chills without any inducements. His body temperature was not detected, and he had diarrhea ten times with a large amount of watery yellow mucous stool (about 1,000 mL in total). He had persistent abdominal colic with tenesmus, but no nausea or vomiting. He had received temporary fluid replacement and anti-infection treatment at another hospital. After eight hours (one hour before admission), his blood pressure dropped to 70/40 mmHg, and he was producing little urine.

The patient lived in a suburb of the city of Shenyang, and had occasional diarrhea. There was no clear history of eating contaminated food, nor recent contact with similar patients.

II. Physical examination and related examinations

1. Physical examination on admission

T 35.8°C, P 170 times/min, tachypnea 36 times/min, BP 50/40 mmHg. Poor skin elasticity, moderately dehydrated, and cold limbs, with ecchymosis at the injection site. Conscious, dispirited, and with a pained expression. No stiff neck. No edema in the bulbar conjunctiva. No positive signs were seen in either of his lungs. His abdomen was soft, and there was tenderness in the lower left portion. Bowel sounds were slightly active. All four limbs could move independently. There was tendon reflex without hyperfunction.

2. Auxiliary examination on admission

Routine blood: WBC 16.7×10^9/L, N 89.8%, Hb 160 g/L.

Routine stool: WBC 30–50/HP.

3. Emergency examination after admission

PT 75.8s, Fibrinogen 13 g/L, PLT 35×10^9/L. Cr 246 μmol/L. Blood gas suggests metabolic acidosis criteria. PaO_2 67 mmHg, $PaCO_2$ 28 mmHg. ECG: Sinus tachycardia. The results of routine blood re-examination and routine stool re-examination were the same as before.

III. Diagnosis and treatment
1. Initial diagnosis and treatment

The patient was a young male with a summer onset and no clear recent history of eating unhygienic food. The onset of his illness was rapid, with chills, abdominal pain, and diarrhea as the initial symptoms. His stool was yellow, mucous, and watery in large amounts, with abdominal pain and tenesmus. Eight hours after the onset, his blood pressure dropped to 70/40 mHg. He was producing less urine, and there was ecchymosis at the injection site. The total number of leukocytes and the proportion of neutrophils in a routine blood examination were significantly increased. The leukocytes and erythrocytes in a routine stool examination were significantly increased. The prothrombin time was significantly prolonged, fibrinogen and platelets were significantly decreased, and the serum creatinine was increased. Because of the acute onset, toxic shock and DIC occurred within 24 hours. Dysentery was indicated in a routine examination. Although blood culture and stool culture results have not been obtained, shock-type toxic bacillary dysentery should be considered first. At that point, T < 36.0°C, H > 160 times/min, R > 32 times/min, WBC > 12.0×10^9/L were consistent with systemic inflammatory response syndrome. Coagulation function and renal function were involved, and there was multiple organ failure.

On admission, the patient had no fever. Although he was treated quickly with the correct acidosis, expansion, anisodamine, heparin, and cefotaxime to fight infection, his blood pressure had not recovered. He passed watery yellow stool once. Test results: 30–50 WBC/HP, 5–10 RBC/HP. After admission, he did not produce urine, and fell into a coma with a large amount of ecchymosis on his skin. He died of circulatory failure eight hours after admission.

> **Thinking prompts:** Diarrhea and shock were two of this patient's major symptoms, and should pertain to the same disease. The diagnosis of bacillary dysentery should be clear. The cause of shock needs to be identified.

2. Diagnostic thinking

(1) Identification of shock: The common forms are cardiogenic shock, hemorrhagic and fluid-loss shock, anaphylactic shock, and toxic shock syndrome. Although the factor of fluid loss existed in this case, it was obviously inconsistent with the intractable shock of this patient, because it takes a certain amount of fluid loss to cause shock, and fluid replacement therapy was easy to correct. Therefore, in combination with the results of the routine stool test, the diagnosis of toxic shock was clear. Toxic shock caused by infection occurs frequently in fulminant epidemic cerebrospinal

meningitis, pneumonia, suppurative cholangitis, intraperitoneal infection, bacillary dysentery, and various types of food poisoning. Bacillary dysentery has the fastest onset.

(2) Identification of bacillary dysentery: Diseases that cause dysentery-like stool are generally either infectious enteral or parenteral diseases or non-infectious intestinal diseases. Infectious diseases include bacillary dysentery, bacterial gastrointestinal food poisoning, amoebic dysentery, and intestinal infections caused by other pathogenic bacteria such as Escherichia coli and Campylobacter jejuni. Among the non-infectious diseases are colon cancer, chronic non-specific ulcerative colitis, intestinal polyps, and ischemic enteritis. These diseases must be carefully identified before bacillary dysentery is diagnosed.

Diagnostic criteria for bacillary dysentery: The disease can be diagnosed if the symptoms align with one of the first three items and one of the second items mentioned below: ① Clear history of contact with bacillary dysentery patients within one week before the onset; ② Tenesmus; ③ Obvious tenderness in the left lower abdomen; ④ Microscopic stool examination of ten high-power microscopic fields, with the average number of white blood cells in each field being more than 10; or, more than five white blood cells can be examined by microscopy two consecutive times; ⑤ Stool culture positive for dysentery bacillus.

This case meets the criteria of items ②, ③, and ④, so bacillary dysentery can be diagnosed.

(3) The identification of this case is shock-type toxic bacillary dysentery or Shigella septicemia. Shigella septicemia mostly occurs in children, mainly manifesting as high fever, abdominal pain, diarrhea, nausea, and vomiting. Stool is mucous watery, bloody, or mucous bloody. Most patients suffer from severe dehydration; few have no diarrhea. They suffer drowsiness, coma, and convulsions; rashes may also occur, as well as liver and spleen enlargement. Severe cases have hemolytic anemia, septic shock, hemolytic uremic syndrome, renal failure, and DIC.

Clinical features of this case: ① Middle-aged male with a history of diarrhea; ② Clinical symptoms of infection and poisoning and gastrointestinal symptoms are very serious, especially frequent diarrhea, a large amount of watery mucous stool, continuous abdominal colic, and tenesmus. The disease progresses rapidly, with septic shock as the main manifestation, followed by multiple organ failure, especially early-onset DIC; ③ Septic shock was difficult to correct, leading to death within 24 hours of the onset.

The clinical manifestation of this case is highly consistent with the manifestation of sepsis. However, there are two points to note: ① Why did the patient have no clinical manifestation of persistent high fever? ② Why did the patient rapidly develop multiple organ failure without the typical clinical course of sepsis?

The fever caused by infection is mainly a result of pathogens, toxins, and pathogen metabolites stimulating inflammatory cells to produce inflammatory cytokines to act on the fever center. After infection with dysentery bacilli in this case, there was one clinical manifestation of hypothermia. However, due to the serious condition and rapid progress of the disease, the patient quickly developed shock, T < 36°C. The progression of sepsis was slower than that of toxic bacillary dysentery. It is mainly due to the pathogen entering the body, as it must pass through a short bacteremia period before developing into sepsis. The immune function of the human body and the virulence and quantity of bacteria determine the speed of onset. Toxic bacillary dysentery is caused by a strong allergic reaction to the endotoxin released by Shigella, resulting in an increase of many kinds of vasoactive substances such as catecholamine in the blood, leading to small vasospasms in the whole body. Therefore, the clinical manifestation of the disease is rapid and dangerous. Therefore, the diagnosis of shock-type toxic bacillary dysentery in this case is correct. It should be noted that bacterial blood culture results are the only indicator of confirmed Shigella sepsis.

(4) Diagnosis of DIC: The patient's prothrombin time (PT) was significantly prolonged; fibrinogen and platelets were significantly decreased, and skin ecchymosis appeared and gradually increased. Although there were no results of fibrin degradation products (FDP) and D-dimer, the diagnosis of DIC was unquestionable. The cause is the exposure of collagen to vascular endothelium caused by infection poisoning and shock, which initiates the endogenous coagulation pathway.

Stool culture results after the patient's death: Shigella dysenteriae grew; blood culture bacteria did not grow.

IV. Lessons learned

In this case, it is easy to make a diagnosis of shock-type toxic bacillary dysentery. Adults mainly suffer from shock-type, with the disease progressing rapidly, and death occurring within 24 hours. It was a very typical case. The occurrence of toxic bacillary dysentery is related to the sensitivity of the human body to endotoxins, in addition to the strength of the bacterial virulence. Early diagnosis and treatment are the keys to improving prognosis. Early application of anisodamine may reduce mortality.

(Liu Pei)

Fever for four days, and consciousness disorder for one day

I. Medical history

Patient: Male, 16 years old, hospitalized on 21 April 2008 for fever for four days and consciousness disorder for one day.

The patient developed a fever without any obvious causes on 17 April 2008, accompanied by aversion to cold and chills, severe headache, vomiting once, non-projectile. The vomitus was stomach contents. After taking medicine for a cold, it was relieved, but symptoms persisted, and there was aggravation. On 19 April 2008, the patient complained of a stiff neck, and found a non-itchy red rash mostly on his lower limbs but also on his buttocks. He went to his local village clinic for an infusion treatment (details unknown), but his condition did not improve. On 21 April, he began to suffer with disordered consciousness and apathy. He went to the county hospital and was diagnosed with meningitis. He was then transferred to our hospital and admitted to our department by the outpatient department with an infection of the central nervous system. Since the onset of the disease, the patient has had no abdominal pain or diarrhea, no cough or expectoration, and no urinary frequency, urgency, or pain. He had poor mental health, appetite, and sleep, but normal defecation. There was nothing notable in his medical, family, or personal histories.

> **Thinking prompts:** The onset of illness was acute and the course was less than a week. Fever was the first symptom, accompanied by infection poisoning symptoms such as aversion to cold. Infectious fever should be considered first. Fever is a common clinical manifestation of infectious diseases, and lacks specificity. In addition to fever, the patient presented with a severe headache, vomiting (probably a manifestation of increased intracranial pressure), apathy, and disturbance of consciousness suggestive of intracranial infection. A rash is another common clinical manifestation of infectious diseases. When it appears, the patient should be asked in detail about its morphology, color, growth, and decline, and whether there is a relationship between the rash and fever, as this has implications for diagnosis and identification. For example, a rash appears within 24 hours with chicken pox fever, and on the second

day with scarlet fever. As well as thinking about pathogens, attention should be paid to collecting epidemiological data for infectious diseases, and inquiring whether there are other cases in the surrounding area, as well as whether there is any history of a contaminated diet. This is because epidemic cerebrospinal meningitis and toxic bacillary dysentery (which can also cause damage to the central nervous system) are transmitted through the respiratory tract, and there are likely to be multiple similar patients around. The latter is spread from feces to mouth, often in patients with a history of unclean eating. During physical examinations, special attention should be paid to vital signs, consciousness, the presence of meningeal irritation signs, pathological reflection, the distribution and nature of the rash, and whether there is hepatosplenomegaly.

Further medical history: There were no similar patients around, and no history of eating a contaminated diet.

II. Physical examination

T 39.4°C, P 96 times/min, R 18 times/min, BP 100/50 mmHg. Normal nourishment, moderately developed, clear mind, appearance of acute illness, active demeanor, lack of cooperation with physical examination. Skin and sclera were not icteric, scattered bleeding points seen on the lower limbs and buttocks, with some fusion into ecchymosis, red or purplish red, clear boundary; the color does not fade with pressure. There was no enlargement of the superficial lymph nodes anywhere in the body; normal head shape; both pupils were equally round. Slight congestion of the pharynx, with stiff-neck trachea in the middle; no varicose jugular vein, no abnormality of the heart and lungs, abdominal rigidity, could not be palpated; obvious tenderness, dissatisfaction with liver and spleen palpation, normal bowel sounds. No edema in either of the lower limbs. Muscular tension normal, habitual knee reflex present, Klinefelter's sign positive, Babinski's sign negative.

> Thinking prompts: The physical examination revealed that the rash was hemorrhagic, and the patient had significant meningeal irritation. Therefore, the likelihood of septicemia (whether gram-negative bacteria – normal blood pressure, no signs of peripheral circulatory failure) or gram-positive bacteria (non-congestive rash, with significant meningeal irritation) in this patient is less likely. In viral infectious diseases, the manifestation of simple hemorrhagic rash is less. The distribution characteristics of hemorrhagic rash in viral hemorrhagic fevers such as epidemic hemorrhagic fever are not consistent with the rash distribution on this patient. An infection of the central nervous system caused by a virus is mainly manifested by brain parenchyma damage, sometimes with signs of membrane stimulation. However, this patient tested negative for muscle strength, muscle tension, and

pathological reflex, so the likelihood of a virus was low. According to the time of the onset (April), the symptoms of acute fever with headache and vomiting, a rash on the lower limbs and buttocks, ecchymosis, stiff neck, positive Kirschner's sign, and other positive meningeal irritation signs support the diagnosis of epidemic cerebrospinal meningitis. Further laboratory tests are required to confirm the diagnosis.

III. Laboratory examination on admission

Routine blood: WBC 12.9 × 10⁹/L, N 85%, L 15%, RBC 4.18 × 10¹²/L, Hb 116 g/L, PLT 76 × 10⁹/L.
    Urine, routine stool: Normal.
    Liver function: A/G 35.4/27 g/L, TB/CB 38.6/15.6 μmol /L, ALT/AST 12.8/18.4 U/L.
    Chest X-ray, liver, gall bladder, and spleen ultrasound examination: Normal.

IV. Diagnosis

1. Initial diagnosis

The patient developed acute rapid-onset high fever with infection poisoning symptoms such as a headache and an aversion to cold. The patient had positive meningeal irritation signs, hemorrhagic spots and ecchymosis on the skin of the lower limbs, peripheral hemogram, and elevation of white blood cells and neutrophils. An infection of the central nervous system could be diagnosed clinically, with a high possibility of epidemic cerebrospinal meningitis.

> **Thinking prompts:** The patient suffered acute rapid-onset fever, with the course of the illness lasting for less than one week, accompanied by infection poisoning symptoms such as aversion to cold and headache. Fever caused by infectious diseases is mainly considered in clinical practice. Fever is common in all infectious diseases, and it is often the first symptom. In the early (prodromal) stage of an infectious disease, the main manifestations are fever and symptoms of systemic infective poisoning, plus a lack of characteristic manifestations of the disease. Therefore, it is often difficult to find the exact cause of fever and the clinical diagnosis of the disease in the early stage. It is necessary to observe the progress of the disease and the appearance of some characteristic manifestations closely, and combine the necessary laboratory tests, especially the three routine examinations (blood, urine, and stool) to carry out the preliminary clinical analysis and diagnosis in the early stage. For example, in this case, the first symptom was fever, and the initial characteristic manifestation was lacking. The illness was considered as a cold, and symptomatic treatment was ineffective. On the second and third days after the onset of the illness, the patient's headache and vomiting worsened, and a hemorrhagic rash appeared. On the fourth day, a consciousness disorder appeared along with the typical symptoms of infection of the central nervous system. A routine blood examination showed that the white

cells and neutrophils were significantly increased, suggesting bacterial infection. In addition, the patient had a hemorrhagic rash (one of the manifestations of sepsis), and its onset was in April. Although no similar patients were identified in the surrounding areas, the clinical manifestations were sufficient to suggest a purulent bacterial infection of the central nervous system, with epidemic cerebrospinal meningitis being the most likely. Other infectious diseases that cause fever should be ruled out when the primary diagnosis is considered.

2. Diagnostic thinking

(1) Viral infectious diseases: Acute fever, symptoms of infective poisoning, and short course; the possibility of viral infection should be considered. A routine blood test showed that the increase in the total white blood cells and neutrophils did not support viral infectious diseases. However, in the early stage of some viral infectious diseases, the total white blood cells and even neutrophils can be increased. These diseases include epidemic encephalitis B, epidemic hemorrhagic fever, rabies, and infectious mononucleosis.

1) Epidemic encephalitis B: There is obvious seasonality of incidence in this area (temperate zone), and the epidemic is related to the local mosquito density. The general onset season is from July to September. The season in this case did not match. Here, the clinical manifestations were not convulsions, changes in muscle strength and tension, and changes in consciousness, but rather headache, vomiting, and signs of meningeal irritation, with non-prominent brain parenchyma damage, which did not conform to the clinical characteristics and progression of epidemic encephalitis B. Therefore, this diagnosis can be ruled out. Examination of the cerebrospinal fluid can help to identify the disease.

2) Epidemic hemorrhagic fever: A common viral infectious disease in this area, with no obvious seasonality. November to January and April to June are the peak times of onset. Therefore, this case could be epidemic hemorrhagic fever since the onset was in April, but the patient lacks clinical features such as congestion extravasation (red eyes, red face, redness of the skin on the anterior chest, eyeball conjunctival edema). Although there were hemorrhagic spots, they did not conform to the rash distribution in epidemic hemorrhagic fever, which is usually found in the oral maxillary mucosa and axillary skin. Also, laboratory tests do not support a diagnosis of epidemic hemorrhagic fever. White blood cells can increase, but there is mainly an increase in lymphocytes, as well as the presence of abnormal lymphocytes. Another change in the blood is a decline in platelets, which was not observed in this case. A positive and progressive increase in urinary protein is the early laboratory basis for a diagnosis of epidemic hemorrhagic fever, which this case also lacked, so it can be ruled out.

3) Rabies: Although WBC can be increased, our patient lacks epidemiological data and the main clinical features of rabies, such as hydrophobia and wind phobia. It can therefore be ruled out.

4) Infectious mononucleosis: Patients in the early stage may have similar clinical manifestations to the patient in this case, but the rash should be pleomorphic and congestive,

and there should be no meningeal irritation. The main change in the routine blood test is the increase of lymphocytes, particularly abnormal ones. Therefore, infectious mononucleosis can also be ruled out.

(2) Spirochete infection: The main acute spirochete infection prevalent in the region in question is leptospirosis, which mainly occurs in the autumn harvest season in rural areas. Obviously, there is no supporting epidemiological evidence in this case. In addition to fever and other symptoms of infective poisoning, leptospirosis in the early stage can be marked by fatigue, body pain, significant muscle pain, conjunctival and facial congestion, and lymph node enlargement. This case, however, lacks these clinical features, so leptospirosis can be ruled out. Spirochete infections in this area also include Lyme disease, which is a natural epidemic disease transmitted through tick bites. Patients generally work in fields, or have sat or lain in grass. In the early clinical stage, there are skin manifestations such as migratory erythema and features such as lymph node enlargement, which are all absent in this case. Spirochete infection can therefore be ruled out.

(3) Mycoplasma and chlamydia infection: Mycoplasma and chlamydia often have a slow onset; acute onset of high fever is rare. It is commonly found with infections of the respiratory tract and urinary and reproductive systems, with few symptoms of central nervous system infection. Hemorrhagic rash is rare in such infections. Therefore, from the clinical features of this case, mycoplasma and chlamydia infections can be ruled out.

(4) Parasitic infection: An infection of the central nervous system caused by a parasite is usually a chronic process. Although acute schistosomiasis can lead to the manifestations of acute meningoencephalitis, the symptoms of infective poisoning are generally mild, with no skin hemorrhage or ecchymosis, and obvious eosinophilia in routine blood examination: ① In addition to the clinical manifestations, epidemiological data is required for a diagnosis of acute schistosomiasis, i.e., the patient had contact with contaminated water (equivalent to the incubation period of acute schistosomiasis) about two months before the onset. This patient lacks this data, so acute schistosomiasis is highly unlikely. ② Cerebral malaria may be manifested as high fever and headache, with varying degrees of unconsciousness and convulsions. Cerebral malaria is often caused by an infection of Plasmodium falciparum. There were no cases of this in the patient's locality. Plasmodium vivax can cause cerebral malaria, but it is unlikely to occur during the non-epidemic season. ③ Primary amoebic meningoencephalitis is very rare in China. It has not been reported in our patient's locality, and the epidemic season does not match. Our patient had not gone swimming in the week before the onset of illness. The lack of epidemiological support means that primary amoebic meningoencephalitis can be largely ruled out.

(5) Rickettsia infection: The rickettsia infections that can occur in the patient's region are typhus (both epidemic and endemic), scrub typhus, and cat scratch disease: ① Typhus may cause symptoms of high fever, headache, and even more obvious infections of the central nervous system, but the white blood cells are often not increased in routine blood examinations. Typhus is largely under control due to improved sanitation, and is therefore unlikely. ② The

incidence of scrub typhus (tsutsugamushi disease) has been increasing recently in our region, but is more common in summer and autumn and is related to outdoor activities. Obviously, this patient lacked the support of epidemiological data, and there were many unsupported clinical characteristics. For example, he did not have eschars or ulcers on the parts bitten by chigger mites (head and neck, both axilla and four limbs), enlarged lymph nodes, or a rash on the corresponding parts. He had an acute onset, and the symptoms of infective poisoning were manifested as systemic soreness, severe headache, appetite deficiency, and nausea. There were few manifestations of consciousness disorders and meningitis. Peripheral white blood cells were generally not high, so scrub typhus was not considered. ③ Similarly, because there is no support from epidemiological data (frequent contact with or being scratched by cats and dogs), there is a lack of clinical features of cat scratch disease, i.e., a local scratch and corresponding lymph node enlargement. Moreover, cat scratch disease generally starts slowly, with low and moderate fever, mild systemic symptoms, and rapid recovery, which can be self-limited. Therefore, it can be ruled out.

(6) Fungal meningitis: The fungus that causes meningitis is cryptococcus neoformans. Other fungi, such as Candida albicans and Aspergillus, can cause infections of the central nervous system: ① Fungal infection is common in areas with poor sanitation, and also in people with low immunity. In this case – a 16-year-old immunocompetent adolescent – meningitis caused by Candida albicans and Aspergillus was almost impossible. ② Cryptococcus neoformans meningitis is a common fungal infection of the central nervous system. There would be obvious headache and vomiting, but the consciousness disorder generally does not develop quickly, and there would be no hemorrhagic rash or ecchymosis. Examination of the cerebrospinal fluid helps to identify bacterial meningitis from cryptococcal meningitis. Based on this patient's clinical features, cryptococcus neoformans meningitis is unlikely.

(7) Bacterial infections of the non-central nervous system: Bacterial infections are considered when there is leukocytosis in the peripheral blood. Besides fever, headache, and vomiting, our patient had no symptoms of infection of the respiratory tract, digestive tract, and genito-urinary tract. The possibility of septicemia should be considered when there are signs of infection but no evidence of a localized infection. Septicemia manifesting as an increase in the total white blood cells should first be considered as gram-positive bacterial septicemia. Both staphylococcus and streptococcus in gram-positive bacteria can produce rash toxins, which can cause congestion and hemorrhagic rash. Therefore, a rash caused by these bacterial infections should show pleomorphism rather than a single hemorrhagic spot and ecchymosis. Severe infections can cause toxic encephalopathy, which can manifest as severe headache, vomiting, and even disordered consciousness. It is also possible that migratory lesions may cause infections of the central nervous system, such as brain abscesses; examination of the cerebrospinal fluid helps in differential diagnosis. A mild increase in peripheral hemogram does not completely rule out Gram-negative bacterial infection. However, infections with Gram-negative bacteria rarely cause hemorrhagic rash and ecchymosis unless it is meningococcal.

(8) Bacterial meningitis, especially epidemic cerebrospinal meningitis: Both bacterial meningitis and epidemic cerebrospinal meningitis present as purulent meningitis. Epidemic cerebrospinal meningitis refers to pyogenic meningitis caused by Neisseria meningitidis, also known as pyogenic meningitis caused by meningococci. Therefore, a differential diagnosis is difficult to make in terms of clinical manifestations and purulent changes in the cerebrospinal fluid. A diagnosis is made mainly by culturing cerebrospinal fluid to identify the causative organism and to obtain a definitive diagnosis of the pathogen. However, a source of bacterial infection other than Neisseria meningitidis can develop from a nearby lesion, or can be caused by blood-derived transmission; hemorrhagic rash and ecchymosis are rarely seen during the development of the disease.

Neisseria meningitidis usually infects the respiratory tract, causing purulent meningitis-related changes through the bloodstream by a process of bacteremia. In this process, a hemorrhagic rash and ecchymosis are often caused by a bacterial embolism of the microvessels. Therefore, if hemorrhagic rash and ecchymosis are found during the development of the illness, they can often be important signs for the clinical diagnosis of epidemic cerebrospinal meningitis. In this case, there was acute onset of fever, severe headache and vomiting with hemorrhagic rash and ecchymosis, positive signs of meningeal irritation, increased peripheral blood white cells, and increased neutrophils. The onset of the disease coincided with the epidemic season in the local area. Therefore, the basis for the clinical diagnosis of epidemic cerebrospinal meningitis in this case is adequate.

V. Diagnosis and treatment after admission

Because purulent meningitis was considered as a diagnosis on admission, and because the possibility of epidemic cerebrospinal meningitis was high, bacteriological examinations were performed immediately after admission, including blood culture, ecchymosis tissue fluid smear and culture, and Gram staining for Neisseria meningitidis. Examination of the cerebrospinal fluid is very important for diagnosis. Upon confirmation that the patient's vital signs were stable, a lumbar puncture was performed immediately. Cerebrospinal fluid was taken for routine, biochemical, and smear bacteriological examination, and sent for bacterial culture.

1. Examination results after admission

(1) Intracranial pressure measured by lumbar puncture was 230 mmH$_2$O; opalescent cerebrospinal fluid outflow.
(2) Cerebrospinal fluid inspection results (21 April):

Cerebrospinal fluid routine test: Pandy's test positive, the total number of cells was 12,000 × 10^6/L, the number of white cells was 3,250 × 10^6/L, the number of multinucleated cells was 90%, and the number of mononuclear cells was 10%.

Cerebrospinal fluid biochemistry: Protein 2.12 g/L (0.20–0.45 g/L), glucose 0.02 mmol/L (2.5–4.5 mmol/L), and chloride 114.3 mmol/L (120–130 mmol/L) (Note: Normal values are shown in parentheses).

Etiological examination: ① Cerebrospinal fluid smear, Gram-negative diplococcus was observed in the cytoplasm of white blood cells stained by Gram-negative; acid-fast staining was negative, and ink staining was negative. ② TB antibody IgG and IgM tests were negative. ③ Results of bacterial culture: No bacterial growth.

(3) Blood culture: Including ordinary culture and anaerobic culture: No bacterial growth.
(4) Bacteriological examination of ecchymosis tissue fluid: Gram staining was performed on the smear, and Gram-negative diplococcus was occasionally observed; both normal culture and anaerobic culture of bacteria: No bacterial growth.

2. Treatment after admission, and outcome

After obtaining bacteriological specimens after admission, a large dose of penicillin was administered immediately in four intravenous instillations of penicillin sodium at 12.8 million U/d. Mannitol and Glycerin fructose were administered to decrease the intracranial pressure. Symptomatic treatment, such as physical cooling, was given. After 24 hours of treatment, the patient felt that his symptoms had significantly improved, and his body temperature had decreased significantly. The cerebrospinal fluid was re-examined on 24 April, and routine examination results showed that it had a clear appearance; Pandy's test was weakly positive. The total number of cells was 430×10^6/L, and the number of white cells was 200×10^6/L.

Biochemical test results of cerebrospinal fluid: Protein 0.36 g/L, glucose 2.38 mmol/L, and chloride 120.2 mmol/L. Gram stain, acid-fast stain, and ink stain of the cerebrospinal fluid smear were negative. The cerebrospinal fluid was re-examined on 28 April, and the routine examination results showed that it had a clear appearance; Pandy's test was weakly positive; the total number of cells was 20×10^6/L and the number of white cells was 10×10^6/L.

Cerebrospinal fluid biochemistry: Trace protein 0.23 g/L, glucose 2.8 mmol/L, and chloride 123 mmol/L.

The symptoms disappeared after nine days of treatment, and the patient was discharged after recovery.

VI. Lessons learned

In this case, the clinical manifestations were typical. Acute sudden-onset fever accompanied by severe headache, vomiting, and positive signs of meningeal irritation indicated an infection of the central nervous system. Along with peripheral blood leukocytosis and an increased percentage of neutrophils, it appeared that the infection was mostly bacterial. Therefore, the possibility of acute suppurative meningitis caused by bacteria was high. At the same time, it was found that the patient had scattered hemorrhagic spots, with some having fused into ecchymosis, further confirming that epidemic cerebrospinal meningitis caused by Neisseria meningitidis was the most likely diagnosis. Routine and biochemical cerebrospinal fluid examinations after admission showed changes typical of purulent meningitis, supporting the diagnosis of epidemic cerebrospinal meningitis. So far, the clinical diagnosis of epidemic cerebrospinal meningitis had been established. At the same time, Gram-negative diplococcus was found in the patient's cerebrospinal fluid and ecchymosis tissue fluid, establishing a pathogenic diagnosis of epidemic cerebrospinal meningitis even though the bacterial culture failed to reveal the pathogenic bacteria. This reminds us that for the etiological examination of epidemic cerebrospinal meningitis, the positive rate of a culture may be low due to the autolysis of the pathogen itself. Prompt examination of Gram staining of smears from infected specimens may improve the pathogen detection rate. In addition, an antigen or antibody of Neisseria meningitidis in the cerebrospinal fluid may be detected by an immunological detection method. Otherwise, a PCR technique may be used to detect Neisseria meningitidis DNA in cerebrospinal fluid for etiological examination, to improve the diagnosis rate of this disease.

Penicillin is the first choice for the treatment of epidemic cerebrospinal meningitis. The therapeutic effect in this case is very obvious. After effective treatment, the most common type of epidemic cerebrospinal meningitis has a high cure rate and no sequelae. Therefore, cerebrospinal fluid re-examination does not need to be performed when a significant clinical effect is achieved by treatment. The cerebrospinal fluid examination results for this patient after treatment also reflect the improvement and rules of detection indexes after treatment. With bacterial meningitis, there is a proliferation of bacteria, and a rise in glucose in the cerebrospinal fluid. Therefore, glucose in the cerebrospinal fluid decreases most significantly when treatment is effective. Bacterial reproduction is controlled, the consumption of glucose is reduced, and glucose levels in the cerebrospinal fluid recover quickly. Thus, the recovery of glucose in the cerebrospinal fluid represents the control of bacterial reproduction, and is the earliest biochemical indicator of an improvement in purulent meningitis. Therefore, observing the change of glucose content in cerebrospinal fluid is beneficial for evaluating the progression and curative effect of purulent meningitis.

(Tan Deming)

Continuous fever, headache, and muscle soreness for two weeks; deafness for two days

I. Medical history

Patient: Female, 15 years old, a student from Wenshui County in Shanxi Province, onset in May. She was hospitalized between 9 and 22 May 2005 with a fever, headache, muscle soreness for two weeks, and deafness for two days.

The patient felt cold, and had chills without any obvious inducements two weeks ago. Her temperature subsequently increased to 39°C–40°C, with persistent non-decline, accompanied by obvious headache, generalized muscle soreness and lumbearlier abdominal pain, nausea, and vomiting. After seeing a doctor at her local county hospital, and taking dexamethasone 10 mg/d for three days, her body temperature dropped briefly. At the same time, standard antibiotics (penicillin, azithromycin, cefoperazone, macrolide, and ribavirin) were given successively or in combination, but had no effect, and she developed deafness in the past two days. Since the onset of illness, the patient had not suffered from coughing, expectoration, sore throat, frequent micturition, urgent urination, painful urination, diarrhea, tinnitus, or purulence in the external auditory canal. Her spirit and appetite were poor, but her sleep was good, and defecation was basically normal.

The patient had previously been healthy. She denied any history of headaches, dizziness, nausea, vomiting, and otitis media, and was not allergic to any drugs or food. She had always lived in the countryside, and maintained high standards of cleanliness. There were mice inside and outside of her house, and she had no history of eating leftovers. She did not keep any animals. She denied any history of contact with contaminated water. There was no history of hereditary diseases or infectious diseases in her family, and there was no similar history of diseases in the surrounding population.

II. Physical examination on admission

Body temperature 40°C. The patient was in a generally fair condition, with moderate nutrition but very poor hearing. She appeared feverish, but was clear-minded, and cooperated with the physical examination. Facial flushing, scattered dark red maculopapules on chest and back. No masses or subcutaneous nodules anywhere on her body; no pathological enlargement of the superficial lymph nodes nor conjunctival congestion; no yellow stains on the sclera, and no ulcers or white secretions observed in the oral cavity. The external auditory canal was unobstructed, and no secretion was seen. Both lungs had thick respiratory sounds; no dry or moist rales were heard, and no abnormal signs were seen in the heart. The abdomen was flat and soft, and there was tenderness around the navel without rebound pain. The liver was not palpable below the costal margin, and percussion pain in the liver area was significant. The spleen was palpable about 2 cm under the rib, and it was substantial and without tenderness. The ascites sign was negative, and percussion pain in the kidney area was significant. Neurological tests showed no positive signs.

III. Auxiliary examination on admission

Routine blood: White blood cells 8.1×10^9/L, neutrophils 62%, lymphocytes 38%, platelets 138×10^9/L, hemoglobin 130 g/L, and red blood cells 4.89×10^{12}/L.

Urinalysis: Urine protein (+), red blood cells (+).

Liver function: ALT 108 U/L, AST 86 U/L, and other indicators were normal.

C-reactive protein 120 g/L, ESR67 mm/h, and both PPD tests were negative.

Multiple blood cultures (the blood was collected when the patient was cold and trembling, or when her body temperature was 38.5°C), bone marrow cultures, ANA, ENA polypeptide zymogram, ANCA, RF, immunoglobulin, anti-HIV, and tuberculosis antibodies were all negative.

No abnormality was found in the chest radiograph and bone marrow smear.

B-scan ultrasound of abdomen: Diffuse changes in the liver, trace amount of ascites, and no abnormality elsewhere.

Brucellosis agglutination test, Widal test, Weil-Felix test, and a fluorescent antibody test for hemorrhagic fever were negative.

Electrical audiometry: Indicating nervous deafness.

IV. Diagnosis and treatment
1. Initial diagnosis

The patient was a female adolescent with a body temperature of more than 38°C for more than two weeks. She had many severe symptoms of toxemia, and her condition was complex. A definitive diagnosis had not been made, and she was hospitalized with a fever of unknown origin (FUO). The patient had damage to multiple organs and systems, so we should be alert to connective tissue disease and hematological system diseases. However, infectious diseases cannot be ruled out.

> Thinking prompts: The causes of FUO are either infectious diseases or non-infectious diseases. All pathogenic microorganisms, protozoa, and helminth infections in infectious diseases can cause fever. Non-infectious diseases that can cause fever are usually tumors and connective tissue diseases. What kind of fever did this patient have? Further analysis should be undertaken.

2. Diagnostic thinking

(1) Tumors: The patient was 15 years old, and solid tumors are rare in this age group. At the same time, no space-occupying lesion was found in chest radiography and B-ultrasonography of the abdomen, and no positive sign was found on neurological examination. The patient had a fever for two weeks, and her liver and lymph nodes could not be palpated or swollen. Her spleen was slightly swollen. No abnormality was found in peripheral blood and bone marrow images. There was no bleeding tendency or progressive anemia. Hematological diseases were not considered. In conclusion, tumors can be ruled out.

(2) Connective tissue disease: The patient had a fever for two weeks, but no joint pain. She experienced whole-body muscle soreness and ESR of 67 mm/h, but no muscle weakness. In addition to fever, lupus erythematosus is often accompanied by manifestations of damage to the skin and other organs and systems, which this patient did not have. At the same time, laboratory tests showed that ANA, ENA polypeptide enzyme spectrum, ANCA, RF, and immunoglobulin were negative, and C-reactive protein was 120 g/L. Taking 10 mg/d dexamethasone for three days at the start of the disease was ineffective, so connective tissue disease can be ruled out.

(3) Bacterial infectious diseases: The patient had a fever for two weeks, with a temperature of 39°C–40°C, accompanied by chills and obvious symptoms of toxemia such as a headache, systemic muscle soreness, and deafness. Bacterial infection cannot be completely excluded. Infectious diseases featuring long-term fever include typhoid fever, brucellosis, and tuberculosis. The patient was treated with penicillin, azithromycin, and cefoperazone successively at her local county hospital, all of which failed. The above antibiotics have good curative effects on most bacteria (including Salmonella and Brucella), and the patient grew up in rural areas where antibiotics were not frequently used, so drug resistance is less likely. It cannot be ruled out that administering dexamethasone in the early stage of the disease affected the curative effect, but repeated blood and bone marrow cultures were negative. The patient had a persistent high fever all day without night sweats and weight loss. Two PPD tests and a tuberculosis antibody test were negative. No signs of tuberculosis were found in chest radiography and a B-scan ultrasound of the abdomen. Bacterial diseases, including tuberculosis infection, were therefore not considered.

(4) Spirochete infection: Spirochete infection has good sensitivity to most antibiotics such as penicillin and cefoperazone. In this case, standardized drug use for two weeks by the patient outside the hospital was ineffective, so spirochete infection can be ruled out.

(5) Chlamydia, mycoplasma, and parasitic infections: Chlamydia and mycoplasma infections are more common in the respiratory tract and genito-urinary tract, and antibiotics such as macrolides have good curative effects. Such antibiotic therapy failed in this patient, so chlamydia and mycoplasma infections can be ruled out. Parasitic infections can be protozoan and helminth infections, generally with an epidemiological history of mosquito bites, animal scratches, or contact with contaminated water, and usually with a change of the mononuclear phagocyte system, possibly accompanied by a significant increase in eosinophils. The patient had no such manifestations, so parasitic infection was not considered.

(6) Fungal infections: Fungal infections should be considered due to the longer duration

of the patient's combination of antimicrobials. However, for double fungal infection, the body temperature is often around 38°C, and oral Candida albicans infection is common. The patient had a persistent high fever, a headache, and generalized muscle soreness. There were no white oral secretions and no diarrhea, and the chest X-ray was normal, so fungal infection can be ruled out.

(7) Viral infectious diseases: There were mice inside and outside of the patient's home. She suffered from fever, headache, lumbearlier facial flushing, conjunctival congestion, positive waist percussion pain, urine protein (+) and urine red blood cells (+). A B-scan ultrasound of the abdomen showed diffuse changes in the liver with trace ascites, similar to hemorrhagic fever with renal syndrome. However, in patients with hemorrhagic fever accompanied by renal syndrome, rashes are mostly distributed on the neck, chest, and axilla. They are often scratch-like hemorrhagic rashes, and platelets in the peripheral blood decrease significantly in the early stage. The patient in this case did not conform to the characteristics of hemorrhagic fever with renal syndrome. The duration of fever for other viral infectious diseases is generally not more than 7–10 days. Herpes viruses (such as Epstein-Barr viral infection) can cause a fever lasting for up to a month, often accompanied by enlargement of the liver, spleen, and lymph nodes. Abnormal lymphocytes can be seen in the peripheral blood. However, early treatment with ribavirin was ineffective and anti-HIV negative in this case. This, combined with the patient's medical history, viral infectious diseases were not considered.

(8) Epidemic typhus: Epidemic typhus, also known as louse-borne or classic typhus, is an acute infectious disease caused by Rickettsia prowazekii and transmitted by human lice as a vector. Rickettsia enters the body of a louse when it bites an infected human and is excreted in lice feces after multiplication. Lice excrete feces when they bite people. When a person scratches the bite, rickettsia from the louse feces enters the skin. Because lice prefer to live in an environment of about 29°C, epidemic typhus occurs mostly in winter and spring in cold regions, as well as in people with poor personal hygiene. After entering the human body, Rickettsia prowazekii multiplies in the small blood vessels and capillary endothelial cells, causing vascular lesions and spreading to the adjacent endothelial cells, producing small infection foci. It can also spread with blood flow to distant endothelial cells of the arterioles and venules.

Epidemic typhus is caused by vascular lesions directly caused by pathogens and pathogen-induced allergic reactions. Small vessel vasculitis is its most basic lesion. The main clinical manifestations are as follows: ① Fever: The onset is usually rapid, and the body temperature quickly increases to above 39°C within 1-2 days, accompanied by systemic toxemia symptoms such as chills, fatigue, severe headaches, and congestion in the face and conjunctiva. ② Rashes: An important sign. More than 90% of cases develop a rash on the fourth to fifth day of the illness, initially on the chest and back, then spreading all over the body within 1–2 days. There is usually no rash on the face. It begins as a bright red, congestive maculopapule that fades under pressure and then becomes dark red or turns into petechiae. Rashes are often isolated, with no fusion. After one week, the rash disappears, but the petechiae can last for two weeks. There is often pigmentation or desquamation, but no eschars. ③ Central nervous system symptoms: These are more obvious, and appear early, characterized by severe headaches accompanied by dizziness, tinnitus, and hearing loss. It can also cause slow reactions or panic, delirium, occasional meningeal irritation signs, hand and tongue tremors, incontinence, and coma. ④ Hepatosplenomegaly: About 90% of patients develop splenomegaly, and a few patients have mild hepatomegaly. ⑤ Cardiovascular system symptoms: Pulse rate may be increased, accompanied with myocarditis; there may be low and blunt heart sounds, arrhythmia, galloping rhythm, hypotension, and circulatory failure. ⑥ Others: Respiratory tract and digestive tract symptoms as well as acute renal failure may occur. Since small vessel vasculitis is the most basic lesion of epidemic typhus, abdominal pain, liver damage, and ascites may occur in some patients due to the exudation of abdominal blood vessels.

Laboratory tests: Routine white blood cell counts in blood and urine are usually within the normal range; neutrophils are often increased, eosinophils are significantly reduced or have disappeared, and platelets are often decreased. Urine protein is often positive. The Weil-Felix test (Proteus bacteria OX_{19} agglutination test) is positive in the first week after the onset of the illness, and reaches a peak in the second to third week, lasting for several weeks to three months. The titer ≥ 1:160 or the increase of duplicate serum more than four times in the course of the illness is of diagnostic value. Treatment with tetracycline and doxycycline can be effective.

The patient's medical history was analyzed, and there were cases of epidemic typhus locally. In conclusion, the patient was diagnosed with epidemic typhus, to be treated with doxycycline after further re-examination of the Weil-Felix test.

3. Ward-round analysis of the fourth day after admission

Considering that the patient had obvious gastrointestinal symptoms, and that quinolone antibiotics were also effective for Rickettsia, after admission, levofloxacin injections were given –0.2 g per time, twice a day by intravenous infusion, as well as liver protection, symptomatic treatment, and support treatment. The patient's body temperature decreased slightly to around 38°C–39°C; the subjective symptoms decreased slightly, but there was no significant recovery in hearing. Consider that quinolone antibiotics are less sensitive to Rickettsia than tetracycline and doxycycline, and that Rickettsia might be resistant to quinolones. On the fourth day after admission, the patient was switched to doxycycline – 0.2 g each time, administered orally once a day. The following week, re-examination of the Weil-Felix serum reaction, fluorescent hemorrhagic fever antibody, liver function, ESR, and other indicators were planned.

4. Ward-round analysis on the ninth day after admission

The day after the patient began a course of 0.2 g doxycycline administered orally once a day, her body temperature significantly decreased, and she completely recovered three days later (i.e., the seventh day after admission). Her mental condition and appetite were better, and she felt that her symptoms had disappeared and her hearing had significantly recovered.

Re-examination of liver function: ALT 53 U/L, AST 42 U/L, C-reactive protein

15 g/L, ESR 23 mm/h, blood and urine analysis were in the normal range, and an abdominal B-ultrasound showed diffuse changes in the liver and negative ascites.

Weil-Felix test: OX_{19} 1:640 was positive, while the Brucella agglutination test, Widal test, and fluorescent hemorrhagic fever antibodies were negative (re-examination on the eighth day after admission).

Epidemic typhus was diagnosed. Doxycycline was continued at 0.2 g/time, once a day for 4–5 days, while liver protection and symptomatic treatment were given.

V. Condition at discharge (thirteenth day after admission)

The patient's body temperature remained normal without any discomfort. Her spirit, appetite, and sleep were good, and her rash disappeared. Routine blood and urine tests were normal. Liver function, ESR, and C-reactive protein were completely normal. The patient recovered and was discharged.

VI. Follow-up

Follow-ups at the first month, the third month, and the sixth month after discharge showed that the patient's body temperature was normal and she did not feel any discomfort. She went to school as usual, and underwent re-examination. The routine blood test, urine test, liver function, ESR, and B-ultrasound of her abdomen were all normal.

VII. Lessons learned

The patient's body temperature exceeded 38°C for more than two weeks, with many symptoms, including severe toxemia. Her condition was complex. In the early stage, hormone therapy was administered without the application of effective antibiotics, further complicating the situation. She could not produce antibodies, and epidemiological data did not support the diagnosis. In addition, the patient developed some rare manifestations of epidemic typhus, such as ascites, deafness, severe toxemia symptoms, and ineffective antibiotic treatment, which made clinical diagnosis difficult. However, a diagnosis was made after gathering detailed medical history, performing thorough physical examinations, analyzing her condition, and following up based on any suspicious symptoms or signs that appeared, as well as laboratory tests, and necessary re-examinations. When antibacterial drug treatment is ineffective, we must investigate whether there is resistance, whether the antibacterial spectrum is wide enough, whether the coverage is wide enough, and whether there are any specific pathogenic bacterial infections. Do not rule out infectious diseases. In recent years, living standards and sanitary conditions in China have improved. Particularly in the rural areas, the incidence of epidemic typhus has been significantly reduced. As a result, clinicians' understanding of the disease has been weakened, which is an important reason why it cannot be diagnosed easily in the early stage.

(Zhao Longfeng)

Fever and headache for ten days, and slow responses for three days

I. Medical history

Patient: Male, 67 years old, from Taiyuan in Shanxi Province. He was hospitalized between 2 and 11 August 2004 with fever and headache for ten days, and slow responses for three days.

The patient complained of fatigue due to overwork ten days earlier followed by a headache, distress to both lower limbs, and chills. His body temperature measured 38.5°C, and he had a mild cough. He thought he had caught a cold, and took oral anti-virus granules at home for two days, which were not effective. On the third day after the onset, he was treated at a municipal staff hospital. His peripheral blood leukocytes were 3.7×10^9/L, neutrophils 70%, lymphocytes 29%, eosinophils and 0. No abnormality was found in a routine urine test. Liver function was normal. The Widal serum reaction was H 1:320, O 1:160. The Weil-Felix test was OX_{19} 1:40, OX_k 1:80. He was diagnosed with typhoid fever and received hospital treatment.

After admission, the patient was given a ceftriaxone sodium powder infusion of 4.0 g/d by intravenous drip, and four days of symptomatic and supportive treatment. His body temperature did not decrease significantly, and his headache persisted. He had an apathetic expression and slow reactions, as well as occasional tinnitus. A 0.2 g/time levofloxacin injection was added twice daily, by intravenous drip for three days. The patient's body temperature was still about 38°C, and his other symptoms were not relieved. For further diagnosis and treatment, he was transferred to our department. According to his medical history, since the onset of illness, the patient had a mild cough, no expectoration, no sore throat, and no frequent, urgent, or painful urine; no abdominal pain, diarrhea, nausea, vomiting, joint pain, or rash. Poor mental health, appetite, and sleep; dry stool, and normal urination.

The patient had previously been healthy. He denied any medical history of hypertension, diabetes, or infectious diseases, and claimed to have no allergies to drugs and food, nor any addiction to tobacco and alcohol. He had been living in Taiyuan, and had visited relatives in Handan in Hebei Province one month before his illness, staying there for two weeks. He had not seen any mice inside or outside of his home, nor did he keep animals. He denied any history of contact with contaminated water, hereditary diseases, or infectious diseases in his family, or similar diseases among the people around him recently.

II. Physical examination upon admission

His temperature was 37.5°C, and he was in a fair condition with good nutrition and hearing. His consciousness was clear, his position was free, and he cooperated with the physical examination, although he moved slowly. No papules, no palpable masses, and no subcutaneous nodules were observed anywhere on his body, and no pathological swelling was palpated in the superficial lymph nodes. There was no congestion in the conjunctiva, no icteric sclera, and no ulcers or white secretions were observed in the oral cavity. Both lungs had thick respiratory sounds, but no rhonchi or moist rales were heard, and no abnormal signs were seen in the heart. The abdomen was flat and soft, and there was no tenderness or rebound pain anywhere. The liver and spleen could not be palpated below the costal margin. There was no sign of ascites, and no percussion pain in the kidney area. Pathological reflections such as Klinefelter's sign and Brudzinski's sign were negative, and no positive signs were found in other examinations.

III. Auxiliary examinations on admission

Routine blood: Leukocytes 4.3×10^9/L, neutrophils 72%, lymphocytes 24%, eosinophil count 0.02×10^9/L, platelets 208×10^9/L, hemoglobin 130 g/L, and erythrocytes 4.76×10^{12}/L.

Urinalysis and liver function were normal; stool occult blood was negative.

C-reactive protein 28 g/L, erythrocyte sedimentation rate 57 mm/h, negative PPD test.

Multiple blood cultures, bone marrow cultures, and stool cultures were negative.

ANA, ENA, ANCA, RF, immunoglobulin, anti-HIV, and tuberculosis antibodies were all negative.

No abnormality was found in chest radiography, bone marrow smear, head CT, or abdominal B-ultrasound.

Widal test H 1:80, O 1:40, Weil-Felix test OX_{19} 1:320, OX_k 1:80.

IV. Diagnosis and treatment

1. Initial diagnosis

On the basis of epidemiology, comprehensive consideration, the main clinical manifestations of the patient, and laboratory tests, the preliminary diagnosis was a fever of unknown origin and endemic typhus. However, fever due to a tumor, connective tissue disease, or typhoid fever should not be ruled out.

2. Diagnostic thinking

The patient was a senior citizen, and had a low-grade fever for more than ten days. The onset was in the summer, and antimicrobial therapy had a poor effect. Tumor fever and connective tissue disease had to be ruled out. A detailed analysis of his symptoms, signs, and laboratory tests was performed, taking the following into account:

(1) Connective tissue disease: Connective tissue disease causes fever in the elderly, which is characterized by non-specific vasculitides, such as giant cell arteritis and rheumatic polymyalgia. However, this patient had no corresponding clinical features, and laboratory tests showed negative

ANA, ENA, ANCA, RF, and immunoglobulin. Therefore, autoimmune diseases can be ruled out.

(2) Tumors: No space-occupying lesion was found in the chest radiograph, abdominal B-ultrasound, or head CT, and the stool occult blood was negative. Besides a loss of appetite, there were no digestive or urinary tract symptoms. The routine urine test was normal, so space-occupying lesions were not considered. The patient was febrile for ten days. The liver, spleen, and lymph nodes could not be palpated or swollen. Peripheral blood and bone marrow images were normal. There was no bleeding and no progressive anemia. Hematological diseases were not considered. In conclusion, tumors can be ruled out.

(3) Viral infection: The patient's fatigue, headache, soreness of both lower limbs, and chills were mainly due to overwork. His body temperature was measured at 38.5°C, and he thought he had a cold. Oral antiviral granules had no effect after two days of treatment, but the patient had no catarrhal symptoms such as a sore throat, nasal congestion, and runny nose. The duration of fever in viral infectious diseases generally does not exceed 7–10 days. In light of the patient's medical history, viral infection can be ruled out.

(4) Typhoid fever: The diagnostic bases for typhoid fever are as follows: ① Epidemiological history: No previous history of typhoid fever, onset in summer and autumn, recent history of contact with typhoid fever, mostly affecting children and young adults. ② Clinical manifestations: Continuous fever for more than a week, accompanied by systemic poisoning symptoms, indifferent expression, appetite deficiency, and abdominal distension; gastrointestinal symptoms of abdominal pain, diarrhea, or constipation; signs of relative bradycardia, rose rash, and hepatosplenomegaly. If complicated with intestinal perforation or bleeding, it is more helpful for diagnosis. ③ Laboratory tests: The number of white blood cells in peripheral blood has decreased, the proportion of lymphocytes has increased, and the eosinophils have either decreased or disappeared. The Widal test is only of reference value for the diagnosis of typhoid fever, and should be dynamically observed. A diagnosis can be made if the serum antibody titers increase more than fourfold in two copies at intervals of a week. Positive blood and bone marrow cultures are important for a definitive diagnosis.

The patient fell ill in August, with general fatigue, headaches, drowsiness in both lower limbs, chills, indifferent expression, and slow reactions. He sometimes had tinnitus, with a mild decrease in peripheral blood leukocytes, an eosinophil count of zero, and only one increase in the Widal serum reaction, which led to a diagnosis of typhoid fever. However, this was not consistent with the diagnostic basis of typhoid fever by comprehensive analysis. Multiple blood, bone marrow, and stool cultures were negative. Although there was a slight decrease in the peripheral white blood cells of $3.7 \times 10^9/L$ and the eosinophil count was zero, it was not specific to typhoid fever. In the early stages of illness, the patient's Widal serum reaction was H 1:320, O 1:160, and re-examination after one week was H 1:80, O 1:40. Meanwhile, the titers of H and O antibodies decreased. The increase of H antibodies in the early stages of the illness may have been an anamnestic reaction, but the O antibodies should not be affected. The increase may be due to a laboratory error. Comprehensive analysis can rule out this illness.

(5) Other pathogenic microbial and parasitic infections: See Case 33 for details.

(6) Endemic typhus: Endemic typhus, also known as flea-borne or murine typhus, is caused by Rickettsia mooseri, also known as Rickettsia Typhi, and is an acute infectious disease spread by rat fleas. The house rat is the main source of infection, and Rickettsia mooseri is transmitted from rat to rat through fleas. Rats do not die immediately after infection, while fleas infect humans by biting them only after the death of the rats. Endemic typhus has a high incidence in China's Hebei and Henan provinces, and is endemic there, especially in late summer and autumn. The incubation period is 1–2 weeks, and the clinical manifestations are similar to that of epidemic typhus. However, the disease is milder, and its course is short. Clinical manifestations include fever, headaches, rash, hepatosplenomegaly, and rarely nervous system symptoms. It can be complicated with pneumonia, hepatitis, pericarditis, adult respiratory distress syndrome, multiple organ failure, acute renal failure, and DIC. The total number and classification of leukocytes are mostly normal, and a few patients develop thrombocytopenia early in the course of the disease. The Weil-Felix test is positive, but the antibody titer is low. Doxycycline is more effective than tetracycline.

Comprehensive analysis of the patient's medical history: ① He fell ill in August, having previously spent time in Handan in Hebei Province, which was an endemic area for endemic typhus. ② The main clinical manifestations included fever, headaches, general fatigue, soreness in both lower limbs, coughing, and indifferent expression; ③ Weil-Felix test OX_{19} 1:40, OX_K 1:80. After one week, re-examination showed that OX_{19} 1:320, OX_K 1:80. In conclusion, the epidemiological data showed that the patient had no history of flea bites. However, Spain recently reported that only 3.8% of the 104 patients with endemic macula injury admitted being bitten by fleas. Therefore, we cannot overstress this patient's history of flea bites. Clinical manifestations: The patient had no rash, but not 100% of cases report it; laboratory tests showed an eight-fold increase in the OX_{19} antibody titer. Therefore, the patient's diagnosis was compatible with endemic typhus.

3. Ward-round analysis on the third day after admission

After the patient was admitted to our hospital, he was given doxycycline 0.2 g/time, once a day orally, as well as symptomatic treatment. After treatment, his body temperature decreased rapidly, and his headache was significantly alleviated. After the rest of the symptoms disappeared, his spirit and appetite improved. He was asked to continue taking doxycycline and to undergo consolidation treatment for 4–5 days after his body temperature returned to normal.

4. Ward-round analysis on the eighth day after admission

On the fourth day after the patient's body temperature returned to normal, there was no discomfort, and his spirit, appetite, and sleep were good. After re-examination, C-reactive protein < 6 mg/L, ESR 13 mm/h, routine liver function, blood, and urine were all in the normal range. Widal test: H 1:80, O 1:40, Weil-Felix test: OX_{19} 1:640, OX_k 1:80.

V. Condition at discharge (the ninth day after admission)

The patient's body temperature remained normal, and he was not suffering any discomfort. His spirit, appetite, and sleep were good. He was urinating and defecating normally. No positive signs were found on physical examination. The laboratory tests were all in the normal range. The patient was discharged from hospital with a diagnosis of endemic typhus.

VI. Follow-up

The patient's body temperature was normal one month, three months, and six months after discharge, and he was not suffering any discomfort. Routine blood and urine tests, liver function, erythrocyte sedimentation rate, and B-ultrasound of the abdomen were all normal after re-examination.

VII. Lessons learned

The patient fell ill in August, with fever, headaches, general fatigue, soreness of both lower limbs, coughing, indifferent expression, slow reactions, occasional tinnitus, mild decline in peripheral blood leukocytes, an eosinophil count of zero, and only one increase in the Widal serum reaction, which led to a diagnosis of typhoid fever. The main causes of previous misdiagnosis were as follows: ① Basic primary clinicians and non-infectious disease physicians were not familiar with typhus and typhoid. The incidence of typhus was low in recent years, so they were not alert enough to the disease. ② The main lesions of typhus are systemic small vessel vasculitis and perivascular inflammation, as well as toxemia and allergy caused by rickettsial toxin. The lesions can affect all systems of the body, causing complex and diverse clinical manifestations, and there has been an increase in atypical cases in recent years. ③ Clinicians' diagnosis is excessively dependent on laboratory results, and their understanding of the clinical significance of the Widal test and Weil-Felix test is not adequate. ④ Some epidemiological data was not noticed. One month before falling ill, the patient visited relatives in Handan in Hebei Province, where he stayed for two weeks. The area was endemic to typhus.

In conclusion, as long as detailed medical history is gathered, physical examination is conducted, and the patient's condition is analyzed carefully, a correct diagnosis can generally be made based on epidemiological data, clinical manifestations and laboratory tests, necessary re-examination, and comprehensive consideration.

(Zhao Longfeng)

Recurrent chills and fever for two weeks, accompanied by a rash for five days

I. Medical history

Patient: Male, 62 years old, hospitalized because of recurrent chills and fever for two weeks, accompanied by a rash for five days.

The patient developed chills and persistent fever after overwork two weeks earlier with a temperature of up to 39°C. There was no coughing or expectoration, no chest distress and chest pain, no abdominal pain and diarrhea, no frequent, urgent, or painful in urination, and no arthralgia. After treatment with acetaminophen (Tylenol) and amoxicillin, his body temperature decreased. However, his fever reappeared five days earlier with his body temperature reaching 38.5°C, accompanied by multiple rashes all over his body, no obvious chest distress or palpitations, no coughing or expectoration, no dyspnea, and no joint pain.

The patient had previously been healthy, and denied any history of tuberculosis or hepatitis B. He also denied any food or drug allergies.

> **Thinking prompts:** This case was characterized by acute fever, and the patient's body temperature decreased and then increased. The cause of the fever was first considered to be infectious. We asked whether he had been to an epidemic area, and whether any febrile diseases were prevalent there. However, the patient's fever returned, possibly caused by double infection or drug fever. Therefore, when gathering medical history, we should focus on asking about the accompanying symptoms of fever, the type of fever, whether there is coughing and expectoration, the sequence of the rash, and the use of drugs. Clinically, medications that cause drug fever are sulfa drugs, antibacterial drugs, iodine agent, arsenic agent, salicylic acid, phenytoin sodium, and barbital. When gathering medical history, we should also focus on whether there is a history of taking the above drugs, as well as plant-based medication, and Traditional Chinese Medicine and healthcare products. In addition, we should observe the characteristics of the rash, and whether it is related to fever. For example, the rash caused by adult-onset Still's disease is characterized by fever, and disappears when the fever goes down. 87%–90% of patients' skin can be

covered with red or pink papules, which fuse into sheets. Typical rashes are target-shaped or measles-like, mostly distributed on the anterior chest, trunk, and limbs, but rarely on the face. The rash is transient, and leaves no trace after resolution.

II. Physical examination and auxiliary examination on admission
1. Physical examination:
Body temperature 38.8°C, blood pressure 140/60 mmHg. There were red maculopapules on the skin of the whole body, especially the chest, abdomen, and back; no swelling of the superficial lymph nodes, pharyngeal reddening, and no swelling of tonsils; a heart rate of 100 beats/minute, no heart murmur through auscultation, clear respiratory sounds from both lungs, no dry or moist rales; flat and soft abdomen, no tenderness, no palpable liver and spleen below the costal margin, and negative shifting dullness.

2. Auxiliary examination:
Routine blood: Leucocytes 10×10^9/L, neutrophils 45.1%, eosinophils 10%, hemoglobin 110 g/L, and platelet 100×10^9/L.

CRP 10 mg/L was found, and the NAP score in the peripheral blood was 30 points, with a positive rate of 20%.

No abnormalities in ESR, rheumatoid factor test set, biochemistry, blood culture, ANA, and ANCA examination.

The chest radiograph was normal, and the results of the B-ultrasound of the liver, gallbladder, spleen, pancreas, and urinary system were normal.

III. Diagnosis and treatment
1. Ward-round analysis on admission:
Supplementary medical history: The patient developed a fever accompanied by catarrhal symptoms in the upper respiratory tract. Members of his family had a history of successive fever. They were in a stable condition and had no rash. Before the rash appeared, he took acetaminophen and amoxicillin.

2. Diagnosis on admission:
① Influenza; ② Drug reaction/fever.

> Thinking prompts: The patient had a short-term fever, so infectious fever should be considered first. He also had catarrhal symptoms of the upper respiratory tract, as did his family members or close contact, so influenza should be considered first. The patient had a second fever with a rash, and had previously taken acetaminophen and amoxicillin. Therefore, a drug reaction should be considered.
>
> The typical clinical manifestations of influenza include sudden onset of high fever, severe systemic symptoms, and mild respiratory symptoms, manifested as

an aversion to cold, fever, headaches, fatigue, and generalized soreness and pain. The body temperature can reach 39°C–40°C, which generally lasts for 2–3 days and then gradually decreases. The systemic symptoms gradually improve, but the upper respiratory tract symptoms, such as nasal obstruction, nasal discharge, sore throat, and dry cough, can be more significant. The secretions discharged from the airways can last for 6–8 weeks before complete recovery. A few patients may have epistaxis and mild gastrointestinal symptoms such as appetite deficiency, nausea, constipation, or diarrhea. The diagnosis of influenza depends on the detection of the influenza virus in the culture of the respiratory secretions.

Drug fever refers to a fever caused by drugs themselves. In clinical settings, it is often confused with fever caused by diseases, and is not easy to identify. In particular, some patients have fever before taking medication, which persists after medication, so it is necessary to identify whether the fever is caused by disease or the medication. It is very important to distinguish between the two. If the fever is caused by drugs, the patient should stop taking the medication immediately. Conversely, if the fever is caused by the disease itself, the medication should be continued. Therefore, we should be vigilant about drug fever, and make a timely differential diagnosis. In order to facilitate this, the following points should be noted: ① It is necessary to understand which drugs can cause drug fever. Clinically, the medications that cause drug fever are sulfa drugs, antibacterial drugs, iodine agent, arsenic agent, salicylic acid, phenytoin sodium, and barbital. ② It is necessary to know when drug fever can occur after taking medication. In general, drug fever occurs 8–9 days after the second dose, but it can also occur after the first dose. ③ Drug fever is the human body's allergic reaction to medication. It can be accompanied by rashes, lymph node enlargement, angioneurotic edema, and increased eosinophils in the peripheral blood. However, sometimes fever is the only symptom. ④ If the decreased fever reoccurs or increases during medication, consider the possibility of drug fever. ⑤ If the fever decreases after the original medication is stopped or other drugs are used, the diagnosis of drug fever can be made.

3. Diagnosis

(1) Common cold: Common colds usually start slowly, with mild symptoms and no obvious poisoning symptoms. The patient in this case had a distinct cluster of symptoms, of which fever was particularly severe. Virologic testing is helpful for identification.

(2) Epidemic meningoencephalitis (epidemic cerebrospinal meningitis): The early symptoms of epidemic cerebrospinal meningitis are often similar to influenza, but epidemic cerebrospinal meningitis has a clear seasonality, and is more common in children. Severe headaches, meningeal irritation, petechiae, and herpes labialis in the early stage can distinguish it from influenza. Cerebrospinal fluid examination can confirm the diagnosis. It can be ruled out in this case.

(3) Legionnaires' disease: Legionnaires' disease is more common in summer and autumn, with clinical manifestations of severe pneumonia, increased white blood cell count, and liver and kidney complications. However, mild cases are similar to influenza. Antibiotics such as erythromycin, rifampin, and gentamicin are effective against it, and etiological examination can help confirm the diagnosis. It can be ruled out in this case.

(4) Mycoplasma pneumonia: Mycoplasma pneumonia is similar to the X-ray manifestations of primary viral pneumonia, but the former is milder, and the cold agglutination test and MG streptococcus agglutination test can be positive. It can be ruled out in this case.

(5) Adult-onset Still's disease: Adult-onset Still's disease can manifest as fever, sore throat, rashes, joint muscle pain, enlarged lymph nodes, hepatosplenomegaly, abnormal liver function, and increased white blood cells and neutrophils. Antibiotic therapy is ineffective. Adrenocortical hormone is effective, but there is no specific diagnostic index. Diagnosis depends on the exclusion of the above-mentioned diseases. It can be ruled out in this case.

4. Treatment

Based on the patient's medical history, physical examination, and auxiliary examinations, there is an insufficient basis for infection at present. After admission, the patient was only given anti-allergic treatment with cetirizine, intravenous injection of 5 mg dexamethasone needle, and local topical application of calamine lotion. The fever and rash subsided on the second day. After three days of medication, the patient's body temperature was completely normal, and the rash had completely disappeared. After two days of observation after discontinuation of the medication, his condition remained normal, and he was discharged. On discharge, routine blood tests showed white blood cells 6.8×10^9/L, neutrophils 68.3%, eosinophils 0.5%, hemoglobin 117 g/L, platelets 120×10^9/L, and ESR 5 mg/L.

IV. Lessons learned

If patients with influenza have no complications, their white blood cell counts will usually be normal. However, the duration of fever and catarrhal symptoms will be longer than that of the common cold. Symptomatic support is the main treatment. Antibacterial drugs can be used to treat patients who are infected with bacteria, but antibiotic allergies may occur.

(Yan Dong & Huang Jianrong)

Fever, swelling, and pain in the left cheek for three days, and abdominal pain for one day

I. Medical history

Patient: Male, 34 years old, worker. He was hospitalized between 14 and 22 December 2004 for fever, swelling, and pain in his left cheek for three days, and abdominal pain for one day.

The patient developed fever, swelling, and pain in his left cheek without any obvious inducements three days ago. He suspected that he had gingivitis, but did not get better after taking self-prescribed anti-inflammatory drugs. The swelling and pain worsened, accompanied by headache, chills, and fever. His highest temperature was 40°C, but there was no nausea or vomiting. He went to his local hospital, where a preliminary diagnosis of either epidemic parotitis or gingivitis was made.

After two days of treatment with ribavirin, the pain in his left cheek was alleviated, but his fever and headache were not improved. He developed severe middle and upper abdominal pain one day earlier without shoulder or radiating back pain. He experienced nausea, and vomited stomach contents, but there was no diarrhea, abdominal distension, hematemesis, or melena.

At the outpatient department of our hospital, we found that his blood amylase was 908 U/L, urine amylase was 8,991 U/L, and blood routine was normal. The patient was admitted with acute epidemic parotitis complicated with acute pancreatitis. Since the onset of illness, he had been in generally good spirits, with no rashes, joint pain, coughing, or expectoration.

A parotitis epidemic had broken out in the patient's local area, and his daughter had caught it three weeks earlier. He denied any medical history of cholecystitis, cholelithiasis, tuberculosis, or hepatitis. He had been smoking 3–4 cigarettes a day for 15 years, and drinking a small amount of alcohol.

> **Thinking prompts:** The patient's diagnosis was considered as parotitis at the local hospital. The pathogen of this illness is the parotitis virus. In addition to entering the parotid gland and nearby tissues, it can also invade other glandular tissues such as the testes, ovaries, pancreas, and thymus. Even non-glandular tissues such as the myocardium, liver, brain, and meninges can be affected. There will be corresponding complications when the above tissues are invaded. Therefore, when gathering

medical history, physicians should focus on the following points:

1. Whether there are meningitis manifestations such as headache, nausea and vomiting, and nuchal rigidity. This is because epidemic parotitis can cause meningitis, meningoencephalitis, and encephalitis, and the symptoms of this complication can occur within six days before or two weeks after parotid gland swelling. Therefore, it is important to consider the presence of complications during inquiries, and to conduct cerebrospinal fluid examination when necessary.

2. Whether there is testicular swelling or pain, because 14% to 35% of male patients post-puberty experience high fever, chills, and obvious tenderness when parotid gland enlargement begins to subside after about one week, causing orchitis.

3. If a patient presents with abdominal pain, we should pay special attention to its location, nature, rhythm, and accompanied symptoms, with or without inducing factors, because about 5% of adults with parotitis can develop pancreatitis 3–4 days or one week after parotid swelling. However, alcohol-related or biliary pancreatitis needs to be ruled out. During inquiries, ask for details about any history of overeating before the onset of illness, and whether there was a history of heavy drinking, gallstones, melena after meals, hematemesis, and digestive tract ulcers.

4. Cardiac involvement should be noted in any inquiry or physical examination, because cases of parotitis can be complicated with myocarditis, which is more common in a course of five to ten days, and can occur at the same time as or after the recovery of parotid gland swelling. Therefore, changes in cardiac sounds, heart rhythm, cardiomegaly, systolic murmur, and ECG should be noted.

5. The source of parotitis infection is current patients and recessive infected patients. Patients with parotitis are infectious from three days before the onset to nine days after swelling of the parotid gland. It is transmitted through the respiratory tract by droplets, and the population is generally susceptible. Therefore, during inquiries, it is necessary to confirm whether the patient has been to an affected area or has had contact with similar patients, as this is important in determining the diagnosis.

6. During physical examination, confirm whether the local swelling of the parotid glands is obvious, whether it is bilateral or unilateral, whether there is a feeling of fluctuation, and whether pus flows out of the parotid duct during extrusion (different from suppurative parotitis: The local swelling and tenderness of the latter is obvious; most of it is unilateral, there is a feeling of fluctuation, and pus flows out of the parotid duct during extrusion); careful examination should also be carried out, so that the swelling of lymph nodes in the neck or in front of the ear is not mistaken for parotid gland swelling (the swollen lymph nodes are not centered on the earlobe, and tenderness is obvious). We must also check for neck resistance. During abdominal physical examination, be alert to any tenderness or rebound pain, positive Murphy's sign, palpable enlarged pancreas, redness and tenderness of the testes, and cardiac signs.

II. Physical examination and auxiliary examination on admission

Physical examination on admission: Body temperature 38.4°C. General physical conditions were good. The neck was supple, no yellow stain or rash on the skin or mucosa. The superficial lymph nodes were not enlarged. The left parotid gland was enlarged by 2 cm × 2 cm; no redness, with medium hardness. There was mild tenderness, but no pus overflow from the parotid duct. There was mild congestion in the pharynx, but no swelling in tonsils. There were clear respiratory sounds in both lungs. There were no abnormalities in the cardiac examination. The abdomen was flat and soft, and there was mild tenderness in the left middle and upper abdomen. Murphy's sign was negative. The liver and spleen could not be palpated below the costal margin. No enlarged pancreas was palpable. There were no special testicular abnormalities, and no edema in either of the lower limbs. No neurological pathological signs were educed.

Auxiliary examination on admission: Blood amylase was 908 U/L, urine amylase was 8,991 U/L, and the blood routine test was normal.

> **Thinking prompts:** On the basis of the patient's complete history and physical examination, further cerebrospinal fluid examination and head CT are needed to rule out parotitis combined with encephalitis and meningitis. Examination of lipase, abdominal B-ultrasound, or a CT scan can identify the biliary system and pancreatic lesions. Myocardial enzymes, chest radiography, ECG, ultrasonic cardiogram to exclude cardiac lesions. Ask the Department of Stomatology for consultation to exclude gingivitis. Liver and kidney function, blood glucose, and electrolyte examination can rule out liver and kidney diseases.

III. Diagnosis and treatment

1. Initial diagnosis: Parotitis.

> **Thinking prompts:** The 34-year-old male patient developed fever, swelling, and pain in his parotid gland. Routing blood tests were normal. He had increased blood and urine amylase, and a history of exposure to parotitis three weeks earlier, which established the clinical diagnosis of parotitis. However, the patient had abdominal pain and headache, and further examination was required to ascertain whether there were complications such as acute pancreatitis or meningitis.
>
> The pathogen of epidemic parotitis is the parotitis virus, which belongs to the paramyxovirus family and is a secondary virus that invades a variety of organs. Therefore, parotitis is considered as a systematic disease involving multiple organs, meaning that the clinical manifestations are varied. Adult parotitis combined with pancreatitis is not uncommon. In addition to swelling and pain in the parotid gland, the main manifestations include headaches, abdominal pain, nausea and vomiting, acute pancreatitis, and meningitis. Other complications should be considered, and they should be carefully distinguished from other acute abdominal issues.

2. Treatment after admission: Symptomatic support treatment such as respiratory tract isolation, temporary fasting, antiviral medication, enzyme inhibition, acid inhibition, and anti-inflammatories, plus the application of diethylstilbestrol to prevent orchitis.

3. Ward-round analysis on the third day after admission

Further examination results after admission: Cerebrospinal fluid examination was normal; CT scan of the head was normal; abdominal B-scan ultrasonography of the liver, gallbladder, and spleen were normal, but the pancreas was slightly enlarged. Myocardial enzymes, chest radiograph, ECG, and ultrasonic cardiogram were all normal. Liver and kidney function and electrolytes were normal. Fasting blood glucose 7.2 mmol/L. Stomatology consultation ruled out gingivitis.

(1) Diseases that can be ruled out: ① Biliary tract disease: The patient had a fever, middle and upper abdominal pain, nausea, and vomiting stomach contents, and there was no radiating pain in the shoulder and back. The patient denied any medical history of cholecystitis and cholelithiasis, and there was no history of overeating and heavy drinking before the onset of illness. Murphy's sign was negative, and B-ultrasound examination of the abdomen did not indicate any biliary abnormalities. ② Gastrointestinal diseases: The patient denied any history of gastrointestinal ulcers, and there was no hematemesis or melena. ③ Meningitis and encephalitis: The patient had a fever, headache, nausea, and vomiting, but on physical examination there was no neck stiffness. CSF was normal, and the head CT was unremarkable.

(2) The possibility of complications with pancreatitis should be considered if the parotid gland duct is partially blocked and the discharge of saliva is blocked due to epidemic parotitis. The amylase in saliva enters the blood circulation through the lymphatic system, resulting in an increase of blood amylase and its exclusion from urine. Therefore, 90% of patients with acute pancreatitis have mild to moderate increases in blood and urine amylase. However, when serous enzyme glands of the pancreas and small intestine are involved, the amylase in blood and urine can also be significantly increased. In acute pancreatitis, 5% of adult patients have pancreatic involvement, which usually occurs in the first, third, or fourth week of parotid gland swelling. The main manifestations are severe pain and tenderness in the middle and upper abdomen. The enlarged pancreas can sometimes be palpable. If the serum lipase increases more than two times, and the amylase in blood and urine is more than three times higher than the maximum limit, this can suggest pancreatitis. The patient in this case had a typical clinical history of parotid gland enlargement, upper and middle abdominal pain, tenderness, and gastrointestinal symptoms. Amylase in the blood and urine was more than three times higher than the maximum limit at the time of admission, and mild enlargement of pancreas was detected by B-ultrasonography of the abdomen after admission, all suggesting that concurrent acute pancreatitis should be considered. However, pancreatitis caused by gallbladder issues, alcohol, and hyperlipidemia should be ruled out. According to the patient's medical history, physical signs, B-ultrasonography of his abdomen, and denial of overeating and heavy drinking before the onset, pancreatitis can be ruled out.

4. The original treatment was continued, and the changes in the disease were observed. The patient's body temperature returned to normal three days after admission, and after one week, his abdominal pain subsided and his blood and urine amylase returned to normal. He was hospitalized for nine days and discharged in a stable condition.

5. Final diagnosis: Parotitis complicated with pancreatitis.

IV. Lessons learned

Parotitis is a common respiratory infectious disease caused by the parotitis virus in children and adolescents, of which the prominent manifestations are non-suppurative swelling and pain in the parotid gland. The virus can also invade various glandular tissues as well as the nervous system, liver, kidneys, heart, and joints, often causing complications such as meningoencephalitis, orchitis, pancreatitis, mastitis, and oophoritis. It is an RNA virus, and can come on all year round, with spring and winter the most likely seasons. Lasting immunity can be acquired after a single infection, and secondary infections are rare.

A diagnosis of epidemic parotitis can be made according to the local situation and the characteristics of parotid gland enlargement. Serological examination can be conducted. Positive parotitis virus IgM antibodies indicate present infection, and the most prominent clinical manifestations are non-suppurative salivary gland swelling and tenderness. Unilateral or bilateral parotid glands are involved in most cases. The symptoms of parotitis in young adults are more severe than those in children, and systemic infection other than salivary glands can often occur. Further blood lipase examination should be conducted for the diagnosis of pancreatitis complications, for a stronger diagnostic basis. In addition to antiviral and symptomatic treatments for parotitis, diethylstilbestrol should be used early on to prevent orchitis in adult male patients.

(Sheng Jifang)

Parotid gland enlargement with fever for four days, headache for three days, and vomiting once

I. Medical history

Patient: Male, 38 years old, hospitalized for parotid gland enlargement with fever for four days, headache for three days, and vomiting once.

Four days earlier, the patient became aware of bilateral parotid gland enlargement and mild tenderness without any obvious inducements. That night, he developed a fever, and found his temperature to be around 38.0°C. At that time, he had no headache, dizziness, nausea, or vomiting, and no sore throat and runny nose, coughing and expectoration, or diplopia. He went to his local hospital and was suspected of having epidemic parotitis. No special treatment was given. Three days earlier, he had a mild and persistent headache, which was focused on his bilateral temporal and occipital regions. He was hospitalized locally. His routine blood tests showed WBC 13.7×10^9/L, N 65.7%, Hb 134 g/L, and PLT 144×10^9/L. After anti-inflammatory and symptomatic treatment, his body temperature decreased and his headache subsided slightly. A day earlier, he developed a fever again, with the highest body temperature of 38.5°C. His headache worsened and became pulsating, accompanied by projectile vomiting of the stomach contents. He was admitted to our hospital for parotitis and viral meningitis by the outpatient department. The patient arrived with clear consciousness, moderate spirits, moderate appetite, slightly poor sleep, no abnormality in urination or defecation, and no significant change in weight. He had tested positive for hepatitis B HBsAg, HBeAb, and HBcAb for about 20 years, and had normal liver function. No antiviral treatment was given.

Thinking prompts: The patient was a middle-aged man who was not at the age of susceptibility to epidemic parotitis. He had a sudden onset, and had no previous history of parotitis. The main symptoms in the early stage were bilateral parotid gland enlargement and fever. A hemogram suggested that the total number of white cells was slightly increased. According to this basic medical history, viral parotitis, auricular lymphadenitis, and suppurative parotitis were considered. The most common form of viral parotitis is epidemic parotitis: ① Parotitis can be caused by the parotitis virus, parainfluenza virus types 1 and 3, influenza A virus, coxsackievirus type A, herpes simplex virus, lymphochoroidal meningitis virus, and cytomegalovirus. It can only be identified by etiological examination. ② The enlarged part of preauricular lymphadenitis is limited to the auricular area, and it is nucleate, with a relatively hard texture, clear edges, and obvious tenderness. Superficial examples can move, and tissue inflammation can be found in relevant areas. Symptoms include a sore throat and an increase in the total number of white cells and the proportion of neutrophils. ③ Pyogenic parotitis mainly occurs on one side, with obvious local swelling and tenderness, and fluctuation in the late stage. Pus flows out of the opening of the parotid duct during extrusion, causing an increase in the total number of leukocytes and the proportion of neutrophils in the hemogram. The body temperature is generally higher.

The patient in this case had bilateral parotid gland enlargement, and his body temperature was consistently low-grade feverish. His condition was generally good, and no obvious signs of bacterial infection were seen. He was diagnosed with epidemic parotitis at another hospital – a self-limited disease for which there is no specific therapy. After symptomatic treatment, his condition improved for a time, and then parotid gland enlargement and recurrent fever symptoms appeared. He suffered a headache with projectile vomiting, but there were no other complaints of the nervous system. Considering that the central nervous system had already been involved, the possibility of concurrent meningitis was high. Parotitis is a systemic infection. Sterile meningitis, meningoencephalitis, and encephalitis are the most common complications, along with polyneuritis, orchitis, pancreatitis, and myocarditis. In the current clinical consideration of parotitis combined with meningitis, attention should be paid to the involvement of other organs. During the gathering of medical history, note the presence of related complaints from patients, such as palpitations, chest tightness, abdominal pain, testicular pain, and the manifestation of parenchymal brain damage. During physical examination, attention should be paid to enlargement of the parotid gland, parotid duct, local superficial lymph nodes, pharynx, eyes, testes, and other local signs, as well as signs of meningeal irritation, limb muscle strength, pathological signs, and skin sensations. Corresponding laboratory tests should be performed to identify and rule out related diseases.

II. Physical and auxiliary examination

1. Physical examination on admission

T 37.9°C, R 20 times/min, P 86 times/min, BP 102/66 mmHg. The patient was conscious and in moderate spirits, and could answer questions normally. There was no rash, no yellow staining of the sclera, and no palpable obvious enlargement of the superficial lymph nodes. There were palpable nodular masses under both earlobes, about 2–3 cm on the left side and 4–5 cm on the right side. They had clear boundaries and a relatively soft texture. There was no obvious shiny skin or redness in the local auricular area appearance. No pus discharge was seen from the opening of the oral parotid duct. There were no notable results of the physical examination of the heart, lungs, and abdomen, but the patient had mild neck resistance. Kernig's sign, Brudzinski's sign, and pathological signs were negative. The muscle strength of the four limbs was normal, and no abnormal signs were found in the superficial and deep reflex examinations. Testicular examination revealed no abnormalities.

2. Auxiliary examination

(1) Local hospital examination:

Routine blood: WBC 13.7×10^9/L, N 65.7%, Hb 134 g/L, PLT 144×10^9/L. No obvious abnormality found in biochemistry and ESR.

(2) Examination after transferring to our hospital:

Routine blood: WBC 10.8×10^9/L, N 62.7%

Lumbar puncture: Clear cerebrospinal fluid, pressure of 230 mmH$_2$O, Pandy's test positive, red blood cells 25/μl, white blood cells 435/μl, lymphocytes 53%, mesothelial cells 30%, endothelial cells 17%, chlorine 114 mmol/L, sugar 3.5 mmol/L, and protein 6.16 g/L.

ESR, CRP, PT, tuberculosis antibodies, amylase, routine urine and stool test, and biochemistry were normal.

Hepatitis B HBsAg, HBeAb, and HBcAb test positive, HBV-DNA below test value.

No obvious abnormality was found in either the plain or enhanced MRI scans of the head. ECGs normal.

> **Thinking prompts:** A lumbar puncture examination after the patient was transferred to our hospital showed that the protein content of his cerebrospinal fluid was significantly increased and the white blood cell count was high. Therefore, the possibility of suppurative meningitis and tuberculous meningitis can be ruled out. However, the ESR, tuberculosis antibodies, and CRP tests were all normal. In addition, the patient had an acute onset, with no obvious chills and high fever, no obvious toxemia symptoms caused by tuberculosis or bacterial infection, and clear cerebrospinal fluid. Therefore, viral diseases were not ruled out.

III. Diagnosis, treatment, and follow-up

The patient was admitted to hospital for a diagnosis of parotitis complicated with meningitis. An electroencephalogram and cranial MRI were performed to exclude parenchymal brain lesions.

Five milligrams of dexamethasone were given intravenously to reduce cerebral edema and mannitol dehydration. Cytidine choline (nicorandil) was given to promote recovery of the nerve cell function, supplemented with pantoprazole gastritis capsules. During treatment, the patient's parotid enlargement, pain, fever, and headache were significantly reduced, and there was no more vomiting.

Eight days after treatment, the lumbar puncture was re-examined: The cerebrospinal fluid was clear, the pressure was 160 mmH$_2$O, Pandy's test was negative, red blood cells 1/μl, white blood cells 3/μl, lymphocytes 53%, mesothelial cells 30%, endothelial cells 17%, chlorine 117 mmol/L, sugar 4.2 mmol/L, and protein 0.61 g/L. Dexamethasone was reduced to 3 mg, followed by hormone reduction to 8 mg once daily methylprednisolone (Medrol) orally four days later. The patient was discharged after 14 days in hospital.

After one week's follow-up at the outpatient department, the patient recovered well and was no longer suffering from headaches and parotid gland enlargement. Hormone treatment was stopped. The treatment process proves that the etiological diagnosis was correct.

IV. Lessons learned

1. When the patient was admitted to hospital, the protein content in the cerebrospinal fluid from his first lumbar puncture had obviously increased, accompanied by a decrease in chlorine content. Tuberculous meningitis needed to be ruled out. He had no symptoms of tuberculosis poisoning, and laboratory tests did not support a diagnosis of tuberculosis. After symptomatic treatment and administration of dexamethasone, symptoms were obviously improved; the parotid gland enlargement receded, and the results of lumbar puncture re-examination were also obviously improved. In the absence of anti-tuberculosis treatment, recovery also excluded the existence of tuberculous meningitis.

2. The patient was hepatitis B HBsAg, HBeAb, and HBcAb test positive, and HBV-DNA negative. The hormone dose should not be too high and the course of treatment should not be too long, in order to avoid the replication of the hepatitis B virus, which causes hepatitis. In this case, dexamethasone was administered intravenously for 12 days, changing to 8 mg Medrol, and then reducing in dosage to zero. HBV-DNA was still below the test value at outpatient follow-up monitoring. Prednisone 30 mg/d for 5–7 days is generally considered as a treatment for parotitis combined with meningitis.

3. Symptomatic parotid gland enlargement: The patient tested positive for 20 years for hepatitis B HBsAg, HBeAb, and HBcAb. Frequent abnormalities to liver function can cause bilateral symmetrical parotid gland enlargement, with no swelling and pain, soft texture, or pathological manifestations of fatty degeneration. Generally, however, there are no other symptoms.

4. Parotitis is generally more serious in adults. This patient presented with mild parotid gland enlargement, obvious cranial hypertension symptoms, and signs of meningeal irritation, but no other organ complications. The prognosis was good after short-term hormone treatment.

(Sheng Jifang)

Recurrent fever for over ten days, and vomiting and diarrhea for four days

I. Medical history

Patient: Female, ten months old, from Guangzhou. She was hospitalized between 17 and 25 May 2008 due to recurrent fever for more than ten days, and vomiting and diarrhea for four days.

She developed a fever (up to 38°C) on 7 May 2008 without any obvious causes, with no chills or aversion to cold, no cough or expectoration, no vomiting or diarrhea, and no convulsions. The next day, she went to a children's hospital for routine blood tests, which showed that WBC was 13.9×10^9/L, L 30.3%, N 52.4%, Hb 97 g/L, and PLT 266×10^9/L; some red blood cells were annular and low in pigment. Ibuprofen suspension was given orally, and cefazolin sodium pentahydrate and cefuroxime sodium were given intravenously. The patient's condition did not significantly improve, and she still had a recurrent fever. On 14 May, she presented with vomiting and diarrhea, which was yellow watery stool with visible fecal residue. A routine blood test at the children's hospital showed WBC 8.0×10^9/L, L 33.3%, N 21.5%, Hb 98 g/L, PLT 497×10^9/L. A routine stool examination revealed fat globules (+), white blood cells (+), and red blood cells (−). Rehydration and other treatment were given but there was no improvement.

The patient was referred to our hospital for oral administration of dioctahedral smectite, intramuscular injection of metoclopramide, and intravenous administration of ribavirin and cefmenoxime hydrochloride. There was no significant improvement. Her temperature was 38.8°C on 17 May, and she was admitted to hospital. Since the onset of illness, the patient had been in poor spirits with a low appetite. She had diarrhea more than ten times the day before, then low urine volume and no significant weight loss when she was admitted.

The patient was born and raised in the same place, and was the first baby who was born full-term with eutocia, and no history of labor injury or suffocation. Her growth and development were normal. She had previously been healthy, with no history of infectious diseases such as hepatitis or tuberculosis. She had never undergone surgery, trauma, or blood transfusion, and had no history of food poisoning or drug allergies. She had received her scheduled vaccinations.

> **Thinking prompts:** In-depth and detailed inquiry can help clarify the development process of an illness, and can also provide clues for diagnosis and further examination. Gathering detailed history and careful physical examination are still the most important and basic means for diagnosis, and they are also basic skills that clinicians must be familiar with. First of all, we should ask about the chief complaint. For example, the most important symptoms in this case were fever, vomiting, and diarrhea. Inquiry should start from these aspects. For fever symptoms, we should note the causes of fever, whether the onset is acute or slow, the degree of fever, the daily temperature difference, accompanying symptoms, the duration and interval of the fever, and its reduction. As the patient in this case had a fever for ten days, we should also note auxiliary examination, diagnosis, and treatment outside the hospital, and we should ask about medication and its effects in detail. When asking about vomiting and diarrhea, we should attempt to understand the character, frequency, and quantity of the vomitus and stool, and whether there is mucus, pus, blood, and tenesmus. In addition, the accompanying symptoms should not be ignored, and the patient's mental status, skin dehydration, and urine volume should be noted. Special attention should be paid to the collection of epidemiological data for infectious diseases, such as whether the patient has been to an epidemic area, had contact with similar patients, and eaten any unclean food, as well as the onset season and age of the patient. Growth and development, vaccination status, and breastfeeding status should also be understood in order to comprehensively evaluate the current physical condition of the patient and assess the development and changes of the illness.

II. Physical examination

The patient's temperature was 38.6°C, with 35 breaths per minute. Her pulse was 130 times per minute, and she weighed 6 kg. She displayed normal development, general nourishment, poor spirits, and a lack of cooperation with the physical examination. The skin on her whole body was dry, and no icteric or bleeding points were seen. There was no palpable swelling of the superficial lymph nodes throughout the body, no cyanosis of the lips, no eruption or ulcers of the oral mucosa, no swelling of the bilateral tonsils, no obvious pharyngeal congestion, and no secretion. There was no limitation in neck movement, and her thorax was symmetrical. There was no limitation in movement and no three-concave inspiratory sign. Bilateral respiratory movements were symmetrical, bilateral respiratory sounds were clear, no obvious dry or moist rales were heard, and there was no abnormal pulsation and bulge in the precordial region. No tremors or friction; her heart rate was 130 beats per minute, and no pathological murmurs were heard in any valve auscultation area. The abdominal wall was soft, with no distension, no varicose veins, no gastrointestinal type and peristaltic wave, no cry when pressing the abdomen, no palpable liver and spleen, and active borborygmus. No deformity of the spine and limbs.

Thinking prompts: Physical examinations should be comprehensive and focused. Only after a thorough and meticulous physical examination combined with detailed history gathering can a clinician make a preliminary diagnosis. Focused and comprehensive physical examination should be carried out with emphasis on the relevant signs of the chief complaint. For example, fever, vomiting, and diarrhea were the most important signs in this case. Vital signs such as consciousness, blood pressure, pulse, respiration, oxygen saturation, and urine volume should be accurately grasped to understand dehydration and determine whether there is hypovolemic shock or renal failure. The color of lips should be noted for cyanosis. Manifestations of shock should be confirmed by checking the terminal temperature of the four limbs. Because of vomiting and diarrhea, be wary of acute pulmonary edema in the process of fluid replacement therapy – a critical condition caused by cardiac insufficiency. Attention should be paid to patients with heart failure symptoms (cold limbs, cyanosis, fast heart rate, weak heart sounds, liver enlargement; ECG showing T-wave and ST-segment changes and low voltage). At the same time, observe the patient's general conditions such as nutritional status and physical development. Because infants are easily dehydrated, attention should be paid to a pediatric patient's appearance, skin mucosal elasticity, invagination of the eye socket, and lacrimation while crying.

After the medical history inquiry and physical examination are complete, there should be a preliminary understanding of the patient's condition based on clinical symptoms and signs. Clinicians should select relevant examinations according to their preliminary judgment of the disease for clarification. As the WBC of the peripheral hemogram for this patient was not high, and no specific results were found in stool examination at the children's hospital, the diagnosis of infectious diarrhea with a high possibility of viral enteritis was initially considered. In addition to completing the three routine examinations on admission, the stool examination was particularly important, particularly stool culture and antigen and antibody tests for some common viral enteritis pathogens. A routine blood test, liver function test, renal function test, electrolyte test, and blood gas analysis should be conducted to find out whether the patient suffers from an electrolyte disorder, metabolic acidosis, or renal insufficiency. In addition, corresponding examinations should be conducted according to relevant complications: Chest radiography and B-ultrasound should be performed. Auxiliary examinations are the most important indicators for diagnostics and evaluation. Improper examinations may delay diagnosis and aggravate the economic burden on the patient.

III. Diagnosis

1. Initial diagnosis

According to the patient's age, onset season, fever, vomiting, and diarrhea, and the auxiliary examination results from the external hospital, the stool examination at the children's hospital the same day showed fat globules (+), white blood cells (+); white blood cells on the peripheral hemogram were not high. Infectious diarrhea with a high possibility of viral enteritis was considered after admission.

2. Differential diagnosis

> **Thinking prompts:** The patient developed a fever on 7 May, and was kept on anti-infection treatment at a children's hospital from 8 May. She presented with diarrhea on 14 May. The possibility of diarrhea caused by a flora imbalance was considered, combined with factors such as her age.

(1) This must be distinguished from infectious diarrhea caused by bacteria such as Shigella dysenteriae and Escherichia coli. Possibilities:

1) Bacillary dysentery: Occurring mainly in summer and autumn, with the main clinical manifestations of abdominal pain, diarrhea, tenesmus, and bloody purulent stool. It can be accompanied by fever and systemic toxemic symptoms, and severe cases may include septic shock and/or toxic encephalopathy.

2) Enteropathogenic E coli diarrhea: The most common form of E coli diarrhea, especially in infants. It is epidemic or sporadic. The carrier rate in the healthy population is about 1.2%–4%. Most have enteritis-like manifestations, and the feces are yellowish and watery or with a little mucus. Abdominal pain may be present, but not severe. Infants may suffer fever, vomiting, and abdominal distension.

3) Yersinia enterocolitica infection: Common in some cold countries and regions or in cold seasons because Yersinia grows easily at low temperatures. Also known as refrigerator disease. Outbreaks in recent years have been rare and mainly sporadic. Gastroenteritis is prominent in infants and children, and enteritis is the main manifestation in adults. Its onset is acute, with fever, abdominal pain, and diarrhea as the main manifestations. The duration of the fever is two to three days, and the diarrhea lasts one to two days. In severe cases, the illness lasts for one to two weeks. The feces are mostly watery and contain mucus, and there may be bloody purulent stool. Abdominal pain is common, and it can be confined to the right lower abdomen, accompanied by muscle tension and rebound pain. It is easily misdiagnosed as appendicitis, especially in young children. It can cause a variety of parenteral illnesses, such as erythema nodosum and arthritis.

4) Proteus infection: Proteus is a common opportunistic pathogen of hospital infection, especially in those who use broad-spectrum antibiotics with decreased resistance. It can cause a variety of infections under certain conditions, such as suppurative infection, urinary tract infection, gastroenteritis, acute gastritis, and endocarditis. The main manifestations are fever, nausea, vomiting, abdominal pain, and diarrhea. Abdominal pain is located in the upper abdomen and around the navel. The diarrhea is mild, occurring several times a day, or 20–30 times when severe.

5) Antibiotic-associated diarrhea: Mostly caused by Clostridium difficile, and known as Clostridium difficile associated diarrhea (CDAD), or pseudomembranous enteritis. Its incidence has been increasing in recent years, making it the main cause of hospital-infectious diarrhea. Most cases present with mild to moderate watery diarrhea, fever, abdominal distension, and spasmodic pain in the lower or whole abdomen. In severe cases, mucous stool is also observed; bloody stool is rare. Severe complications include dehydration, hypoproteinemia, electrolyte disturbance, enteroparalysis, and intestinal perforation. The mortality rate is 2%–5%. The only cause related to death is delayed diagnosis.

6) AIDS-related diarrhea: 30%–80% of AIDS patients have diarrhea during the course of illness. The main pathogens of bacterial diarrhea are Shigella, Salmonella, Campylobacter jejuni, Mycobacterium avium, C. difficile, and invasive E. coli. Diarrhea is often the first symptom and cause of death in AIDS patients with fever, general malaise, nausea, vomiting, anorexia, and weight loss. Acute diarrhea usually lasts no longer than two weeks, and chronic diarrhea can last for weeks or months.

(2) It should be distinguished from adenovirus and viral Norwalk enteritis.

1) Adenovirus gastroenteritis: Widely distributed in all parts of the world, especially in children, second only to rotavirus enteritis. It is more common in under-fives, and is generally sporadic, with an incubation period of about ten days. The main symptom is diarrhea, consisting of watery or loose stool of uncertain volume. Pediatric patients defecate 8–9 times at most every day, and the course of the illness is generally 4–8 days. The duration of diarrhea caused by adenoviruses varies, and diarrhea caused by enteroadenovirus gastroenteritis lasts the longest. Most patients vomit for 1–2 days, and a few have fever. Patients with non-intestinal adenovirus diarrhea are more prone to fever. About 20% of patients with adenovirus gastroenteritis have respiratory symptoms. The virus is excreted in the feces for about one week.

2) Norwalk virus and Norwalk virus enteritis: Norwalk virus was isolated from patients' feces in October 1968 when gastroenteritis broke out in a primary school in Norwalk, Ohio, USA. Patients and healthy carriers of the virus are the sources of infection, and outbreaks can occur in crowded places. The incubation period of this disease is 24–48 hours, and the onset is acute or gradual. Acute abdominal pain and nausea come first, then vomiting and diarrhea, or diarrhea alone. Some patients have low fever, headaches, and myalgia. They pass moderate watery stool with a little mucus 4–8 times a day. The course of the illness is about 2–3 days.

3. Final diagnosis

Stool cultures and associated common enterovirus antigen tests were routinely performed after admission to clarify the etiological diagnosis. The results showed no bacteria in stool cultures, suggesting rotavirus antigen (+), adenovirus antigen (−) and Norwalk virus antigen (−). Therefore, rotavirus enteritis was finally diagnosed.

IV. Treatment

The treatment of viral enteritis is mainly symptomatic and supportive therapy along with the prevention and treatment of complications. According to the patient's medical history, physical examination, and chest radiography, it was determined that she had fever, dehydration, and malnutrition. Immediately after admission, she was given symptomatic and supportive treatment, including fluid replacement to supplement blood volume, electrolyte disorder correction, and acidosis correction and nutrition. The prevention and treatment of complications were strengthened. For example, ribavirin antiviral therapy was applied. Due to the patient's cough, azithromycin was given to fight infection, and aerosol symptomatic and supportive treatment led to an improvement in her condition.

The patient's HBDH (hydroxybutyrate dehydrogenase) level of 269 U/L was re-examined after admission. A routine blood test showed that her lymphocytes were 5.39×10^9/L, her hemoglobin was 96 g/L, and her creatinine was 27 μmol/L. Rehydration was given to correct dehydration and electrolyte disorders. Ribavirin was given for antiviral treatment, and diarrhea was alleviated. The patient had a cough during hospitalization, so azithromycin was given to fight infection, as well as symptomatic nebulization, and supportive treatment, and her condition improved.

After seven days of symptomatic treatment, her body temperature was normal, and there was no abdominal pain or diarrhea. No abnormality was found in routine stool re-examination, and she was discharged on recovery.

V. Lessons learned

1. Diagnosis: Infectious diarrhea can have many causes, particularly viruses and bacteria. Therefore, etiological diagnosis is particularly important. If it is infectious diarrhea caused by bacteria, corresponding sensitive antibiotics must be used for pathogenic treatment. In cases of viral infectious diarrhea, antibiotics are not required. Therefore, it is very important to make an active and rapid etiological diagnosis of diarrhea with unknown causes.

2. Treatment: For diarrhea of undetermined etiology, dehydration, blood volume supplement, acidosis correction, and water and electrolyte balance should be quickly and effectively corrected, supplemented by active supportive therapies such as plasma, albumin, gamma globulin, and red blood cells. If combined medical history and auxiliary examination cannot exclude bacterial infectious diarrhea, three generations of cephalosporins (such as ceftriaxone sodium) can be given as anti-infection treatment (note that infants and patients cannot take quinolone antibiotics, as they affect bone development). In the process of active fluid replacement, emphasis should be placed on preventing heart failure and pulmonary edema. Infantile diarrhea is characterized by rapid changes. Clinical attention should be paid to it, and comprehensive and effective treatment measures should be taken as soon as possible to prevent severe complications such as dehydration, acidosis, electrolyte disorders, renal insufficiency, and pulmonary edema due to heart failure.

3. Prevention: For patients with diarrhea, note digestive tract isolation and offer active treatment. Carry out close observations on nearby contacts and suspected patients. Look at food, water, and personal health, make sure that feces are properly dealt with. Encourage hand washing, maintaining high standards for aquatic products, keeping good personal hygiene habits, and avoiding raw, cold, or bad food. The rotavirus vaccine has been approved for clinical use. Breastfeeding should be promoted because of the presence of specific rotavirus IgA in breastmilk, and because breastfed infants rarely or never suffer from rotavirus enteritis.

(Hou Jinlin & Jiang Ronglong)

Fever for one week, and a rash for two days

I. Medical history

Patient: Female, seven months old, from Guangzhou. She was hospitalized between 17 July and 15 August due to a fever for one week and a rash for two days.

The patient developed an irregular-type fever without any obvious inducements. Her body temperature fluctuated in the range of 38°C–39°C, and was most obvious at night. The effect of taking antipyretic outside the hospital was not obvious. The patient developed a reddish rash after intravenous infusion of medication (details not specified), which first appeared in her neck and then spread to the face, trunk, and limbs. She had been treated many times in our outpatient department, with unsatisfactory effects. A chest radiograph showed bilateral lung bronchopneumonia. She was in poor spirits and had a low appetite as well as a mild dehydrated appearance.

The patient had previously been healthy (according to her relative), with no history of allergies to any drugs or food. She had no history of contact with contaminated water or similar patients.

> **Thinking prompts:** The two most important symptoms in this case are fever and rash, so inquiries should start from these aspects. For the fever symptoms, we should note the inducements of fever, onset priorities, degree, daily temperature difference, duration and interval, and conditions of reduction. Because the patient had experienced fever for one week, attention should also be paid to treatment outside of the hospital. Ask what medication was used for the fever, and what the therapeutic effect was. When asking about the rash, attention should be paid to its location and sequence, size, number, color, and shape, as well as the subsidence. Concomitant symptoms should not be ignored. Investigate whether the patient had a cough, expectoration, sore throat, nausea, vomiting, abdominal pain, diarrhea, or chills before the onset of fever. For infectious diseases, special attention should be paid to the collection of epidemiological data: Whether the patient had been to the epidemic area or been in contact with similar patients, the onset season and age of the patient, the growth and development of the patient, and her vaccination and breastfeeding, to comprehensively evaluate her current physical condition and assess developments and changes to the disease.

II. Physical examination and auxiliary examination on admission

Physical examination: The patient's body temperature was 39.3°C, and she had dysplasia, poor spirits, drowsiness, a hoarse cry, appearance of mild dehydration, facial measles, conjunctive membrane congestion of the eyes, many secretions, and no cyanosis on her lips. Pharyngeal reddening, congestion (++), bilateral tonsils I° swelling, and typical oral mucosal spots were observed. A large number of papules scattered with dark red stains were visible on the skin, with some fused into flakes. The rash was visible on the palms of her hands and feet, and the skin between the rash was normal. Respiratory sounds in both lungs were slightly rough, and there were no dry or moist rales. Her heart rate was 148 beats/min, with a regular rhythm, and there was no murmur in either valve area. Her abdomen was soft, and her liver was palpable 1.5 cm below her costal margin, with sharp edges and a soft texture. The spleen was not palpable below her costal margin, and her bowel sounds were normal. There was no edema in either of her lower limbs.

> **Thinking prompts:** Physical examination should be comprehensive, focusing on the signs related to the chief complaint. For example, the rash is the most serious sign in this case, so the skin and mucosa of the whole body should be taken as the focus of physical examination, and attention should be paid to the site of the rash (color, size, presence of fusion), the condition of the skin around the rash, the subsidence, and whether there is pigmentation, desquamation, or oral mucosal plaque after subsidence, which are the most important signs for the diagnosis of measles. Careful examination should be conducted for organs that may be involved. For conjunctivitis, check for the presence of congestion and edema of the ocular surface membrane. For laryngitis, note any throat congestion, edema, hoarseness, or presence of a dry irritant cough. For pneumonia, investigate whether the patient has shortness of breath, nasal flaps, cyanosis of the lips, bilateral lung auscultation, dyspnea, and the three-concave respiratory sign.
>
> Myocarditis and cardiac insufficiency often occur in children with pneumonia, resulting in critical illness. Therefore, attention should be paid to whether the patient has symptoms of heart failure: Cold limbs, cyanosis, a high heart rate, weak heart sounds, and an enlarged liver. An ECG showed T-wave and ST-segment changes and low voltage. Although our patient had liver enlargement at the time of admission, it was a normal sign considering her age and clinical manifestations. At the same time, observe the patient's general conditions such as nutritional status and physical development. Because infants are easily dehydrated, note their appearance, mucosal skin elasticity, eye socket invagination, and lacrimation while crying. Only with a detailed medical history and a complete and focused physical examination can a preliminary diagnosis be made, along with an assessment of the severity and prognosis of the illness.

After gathering a complete medical history and physical examination, we have a preliminary understanding of the patient's condition based on clinical manifestations and signs. The attending physician should select some relevant examinations based on the preliminary judgment of the disease for clarification. For example, considering severe measles in this case, in addition to completing the three routine examinations on admission, we should start with the measles-related examinations: Sending samples for a measles antibody test, conducting a secretion smear test to examine the specificity of multinucleated giant cells, and checking liver function, kidney function, and electrolytes to understand the patient's general situation. We should also carry out corresponding examinations according to related complications: A chest radiography for pneumonia, and myocardial enzyme spectrum, troponin, and myoglobin for myocarditis. Auxiliary examination is the most important indicator for confirming the diagnosis and evaluating the condition. Improper examination may delay the diagnosis and lead to an incorrect judgment of the condition. Its importance is self-evident.

Auxiliary examination on admission: A chest radiograph showed bronchopneumonia in both lungs.

III. Diagnosis and treatment after admission

1. Initial diagnosis: According to the patient's age, season of onset, fever, and rash characteristics, she was diagnosed with severe measles on admission, accompanied by pneumonia, laryngitis, conjunctivitis, and mild dehydration.

(1) Measles in the eruption stage should be distinguished from other eruptive diseases: ① Drug eruption: The patient had a one-week history of fever and a recent history of medication. Her rash occurred after an intravenous drug infusion, so the possibility of drug eruption cannot be ruled out. However, drug eruption has various forms, which are characterized by the fact that the rash does not develop and gradually disappears after discontinuation of the drug. ② Exanthema subitum: Occurring in infants with sudden high fever, but generally characterized by a scattered, rose-colored rash when the fever subsides, which is not consistent with the characteristics of the rash in this case. ③ Scarlet fever: Fever accompanied by a sore throat for 1–2 days, with a scarlet pin-head rash all over the body and flushing of the skin around it. This is not in accordance with the rash in this case. Laboratory tests showed that the number of white cells had increased, and the majority of them were neutrophils, which was different from a viral infection. Scarlet fever can be identified by pharyngeal swab culture.

(2) Classification of measles: Mild measles has a short course and mild symptoms with a good prognosis, while severe measles has a long course and severe symptoms with many complications. It is life-threatening, and has a poor prognosis. Judging a patient's condition according to their clinical characteristics and medical history is important for evaluating the prognosis. The patient

in this case was not breastfed, and had low immunity, malnutrition, bronchopneumonia, high fever, severe poisoning symptoms, and intensive rash fusion. There is a possibility of a diagnosis of severe measles, which may have a poor prognosis.

(3) Treatment and prevention of related complications: The most common complication of measles is bronchopneumonia, which accounts for 95%–98% of patient mortality. While the measles virus itself can cause giant-cell pneumonia, secondary pneumonia can occur in all stages of the disease, especially in the eruptive stage, where it is commonly found as Staphylococcus aureus, pneumococcus, and adenovirus. Complicated with pneumonia, the systemic symptoms worsen, and the body temperature continuously increases with shortness of breath, flaring of the alae nasi, cyanosis, and medium to small moist rales in the lungs. It can be complicated with empyema, pyopneumothorax, myocarditis, heart failure, and circulatory failure. Severe pneumonia is the main cause of death for measles, followed by myocarditis and cardiac insufficiency. Severe measles should be considered when the condition is serious. Myocardial function can be affected due to severe fever and poisoning symptoms, especially in malnourished patients and those with pneumonia. The prevention, diagnosis, and treatment of other common complications of measles, such as diarrhea and laryngitis, also need to be noted.

2. Initial treatment plan: No specific antiviral drug has yet been found for the measles virus, so treatment focuses on improving nursing care, symptomatic treatment, and the prevention and treatment of complications. According to medical history, physical examination, and chest radiography, it can be determined that the patient in this case currently had fever, bronchopneumonia, dehydration, and malnutrition. After admission, she was immediately given fluid replacement, electrolyte disturbance correction, antipyresis, nutrition, and other symptomatic support. The prevention and treatment of complications were improved, including anti-infection with ceftriaxone, myocardial nutrition, diarrhea arrest, sore throat elimination, and nursing care. Comprehensive treatment is the key, and the treatment plan should be adjusted according to the development and changes of the disease.

3. Progression

(1) Ward-round on the third day after admission: Routine blood test: WBC 9.75×10^9/L, N 59.7%, Hb 112 g/L and PLT 402×10^9/L. Serum potassium, sodium, chlorine, calcium, phosphorus, magnesium normal, normal renal function; Moderate to high fever, old rash all over her body, fused into flakes, heart rate of 180 beats/min, respiratory rate of more than 40 breaths/min, rough respiratory sounds in both lungs, no rales were heard, poor peripheral circulation of all four limbs, and oxygen saturation of 98%–100%. The abdomen was soft, and the liver was palpable 1.5 cm below the costal margin, with sharp edges and soft texture.

Considering the confirmation of a diagnosis of severe measles, with complications such as pneumonia, laryngitis, conjunctivitis, and dehydration, the patient's condition did not significantly improve after three days of treatment. Her heart rate and accelerated breathing were considered to be related to high fever. Anti-infection treatment with ceftriaxone sodium was ineffective.

When the patient's mother came to our hospital, she told us that her daughter was allergic to cephalosporin (details unclear), so we switched to azithromycin to fight infection treatment, and dexamethasone was given for temperature reduction and anti-allergic treatment. Low-flow oxygen inhalation was used to relieve dyspnea, and fluid replacement and nutritional support were strengthened to maintain the balance of water and electrolytes. Symptomatic treatments such as ganciclovir and ofloxacin (telithromycin) eye drops and temperature reduction were conducted, and we improved the nursing care to prevent further aggravation of the disease.

(2) Ward-round on the sixth day after admission: Electrolyte potassium was 2.6 mmol/L, sodium and chlorine were normal, and the peripheral blood WBC was 9.65×10^9/L, N 41.6%, and PLT was 21×10^9/L. The patient still had a moderate or high fever; could not eat, urine volume was reduced, tachypnea, no obvious cyanosis, and the liver was obviously larger than before admission (navel level below the rib); the texture was medium to hard, and there was no new rash. The respiratory sounds of both lungs were rough, and no rales were heard. The monitoring of ECG oxygen saturation showed that the heart rate was 180–190 beats/min, and the oxygen saturation was about 50%. The patient's illness worsened further, with manifestations of heart failure.

Furosemide was given for diuresis, Lanatoside C to protect the heart, and diazepam and phenobarbital for sedation. The low-flow oxygen supply was changed to mask oxygen supply to restore the blood's oxygen saturation. It was also necessary to maintain the balance of discrepancy, correct the electrolyte disorder, monitor renal function and electrolytes daily, keep the infusion speed under 15 ml/h, and prevent heart failure. After the above treatment, the patient's condition was still not controlled. In the afternoon, hypoxemia occurred again with blood oxygen saturation of 80%–90%, and antifebrile treatments such as Lanatoside C to protect the heart, diuretic furosemide, phenobarbital for sedation, dexamethasone, and antipyretic treatments such as compound aminobarbital were given again. Urgent blood gas examination showed type II respiratory failure. The patient was put on ventilator-assisted breathing with an oxygen concentration of 100%, but her oxygen saturation fluctuated at 50%–60%, and both pupils became unequal. Considering the formation of hypoxic encephalopathy and cerebral hernia, she was given 20% mannitol for dehydration and furosemide for diuresis (alternating). Due to the presence of hypovolemia, treatments such as rehydration and correction of electrolyte disorders were given, the blood oxygen saturation gradually increased to 77%. Phentolamine was given to improve microcirculation, doxofylline was given to relieve spasms, Lanatoside C was given to protect the heart, and furosemide was given for diuresis. The patient was also given sodium fusidate, meropenem combined with ribavirin to fight infection, 100 mg methylprednisolone (once/12 hours, used continuously for three days, and gradually reduced after three days), immunoglobulin to enhance immunity, and an alkali supplement to correct acidosis. Indwelling gastric tube, sputum aspiration, and intensive care were given, and the patient's blood oxygen saturation increased to more than 90%. Both pupils were equal, and symptoms such as respiratory failure, heart failure, and cerebral edema were improved. Finally, her condition was under control.

Thinking prompts: The patient suffered from respiratory failure, heart failure, hypoxic encephalopathy, and various complications, and was in a critical condition with a high mortality rate. Basic treatment is the key at this stage, and symptomatic support is the top priority. First, vital signs should be stabilized, the water and electrolyte balance maintained, acid-base imbalance prevented, and energy supply ensured. Anti-infection should be strengthened on the basis of the above treatment to prevent other complications such as renal insufficiency.

(3) Ward-round on the tenth day after admission: Her vital signs were stable. Her blood oxygen saturation was maintained above 90%; oxygen concentration was 60%, and heart rate was 120–140 beats/min. Her blood pressure was 92–100/49–68 mHg. Both pupils were about 3 mm – equal, round, and sensitive to light. However, she still had a high fever, restlessness, and intermittent stimulating cough. The routine blood test showed that WBC was 14.13×10^9/L, N 67.9%, Hb 100 g/L, and PLT 462×10^9/L. Renal function, myocardial enzyme spectrum, and electrolytes were basically normal, and blood gas analysis indicated slight metabolic acidosis (pH 7.343).

After four days of symptomatic support and anti-infection treatment after being ventilated, the patient's condition eventually stabilized. However, the hemogram was higher than before, and the infection was aggravated further. Therefore, the dosage of methylprednisolone was reduced to 50 mg, symptomatic support and anti-infection treatment were continued, and nursing care was improved, together with atomization, sputum aspiration, and oral care, to prevent further aggravation of the infection. The patient's condition was still serious, and she was still not out of danger.

(4) Ward-round on the fourteenth day after admission: After eight days of ventilator-assisted respiratory therapy, the patient was in a stable state with an oxygen concentration of 35%, maintaining blood oxygen saturation of more than 90%, peak inspiratory pressure of 22 cmH$_2$O, an inspiratory to expiratory ratio of 1:2, heart rate of fewer than 150 times/min continuously, blood pressure fluctuation of 87–97/47–57 mHg, and stable vital signs. She was removed from the ventilator, and calcium gluconate was given before extubation to reduce laryngeal edema for the switch to mask oxygen. Her blood oxygen saturation was maintained at 98%–100%. The patient continued to receive atomized inhalation of dexamethasone, budesonide, and terbutaline, as well as an intravenous drip of ambroxol to eliminate phlegm and relieve tracheal spasms. She was also given phentolamine for microcirculation, anti-infection, fluid replacement, and energy support. The methylprednisolone was reduced to 25 mg/d, and meropenem was discontinued after 12 days of treatment.

The patient's condition improved gradually, and she recovered slowly. Re-examination of the chest radiography showed that the pneumonia was gradually improving, and her body temperature was normal. The flakes of skin had completely fallen off, and her food intake was good. Due to laryngeal edema, she occasionally coughed when drinking water, and her voice was still hoarse. She was in a generally good condition with spontaneous breathing. Treatment measures such as anti-infection medication, fluid replacement, and nutritional support were stopped.

4. Follow-up: As the prognosis and rehabilitation process required a long recovery period, it was recommended that the patient should be transferred to a rehabilitation department for further treatment.

IV. Lessons learned

Ensure good communication with patients and their families. Gather detailed medical history, and make an early assessment of the development and changes of the disease after physical examination. Recognize the severity of the illness, and explain the condition to the patients and their families to keep them informed and prevent doctor-patient conflict caused by the patient's lack of understanding when their condition changes.

There are many complications of severe measles (in this case including pneumonia, respiratory failure, cardiac insufficiency, hypoxic encephalopathy, brain hernia, laryngitis, and conjunctivitis). The symptoms were severe and the condition changed rapidly. Therefore, in clinical practice, comprehensive and effective treatment measures should be taken as early as possible to prevent serious complications such as respiratory failure, heart failure, and brain hernia.

Severe measles with complications has a high mortality rate and poor prognosis. However, with the improvement of medical conditions, the mortality rate can be reduced with treatment. For infants and young children, even if hypoxic ischemic encephalopathy occurs, the prognosis can also be restored to a relatively ideal state. Therefore, active treatment should be conducted for such patients, to reduce the mortality rate.

(Hou Jinlin & Zhu Youfu)

A recurring perineal rash for six years, with systemic dissemination for one month

I. Medical history

Patient: Female, 24 years old, from Guangan in Sichuan Province. She was admitted to the infectious disease department at 09:00 on 13 April 2006 due to a recurring perineal rash for six years, with systemic dissemination for one month. She died at 23:30 on 13 April 2006.

The patient developed perineal and perianal papules accompanied by local pruritus without any obvious inducements when working in Guangdong in 2000. The rash presented as sporadic papules protruding above the skin surface. After receiving medical treatment (details unclear) at a local hospital, the rash improved, but remained around the anus. One month earlier, the patient's perineal rash increased again, with obvious itching. A similar rash appeared on her head, face, four limbs, and trunk. The rash protruded above the skin surface, and was uniform – about the size of a mung bean. At the same time, anorexia, nausea, and vomiting occurred, and the vomitus was stomach contents. For further diagnosis and treatment, she came to our hospital with a rash yet to be investigated, and suspected AIDS, and was admitted to our department. Since the onset of her illness, she had been in poor spirits, with occasional stomachache, but no abnormal urination or defecation. She had lost 5 kg in a month. She had been a sex worker in Guangdong since 1998.

II. Physical examination and auxiliary examination on admission

1. Physical examination on admission

Body temperature 36.4°C, pulse 86/min, breathing 20 beats/min, blood pressure 100/60 mmHg. She had normal development, clear consciousness, poor spirits; she was carried to the ward on a doctor's back; fluent speech, active demeanor, cooperative with physical examination, no yellow staining on the skin anywhere on her body' no liver palm or spider angioma. Mung bean-sized papules were scattered on her head, face, neck, limbs, and trunk, with uniform size. The surface of her skin was covered with scabs due to scratching, and there was no congestion or tenderness. There was no deformity or blackening; uniform distribution of the five facial features of the head. There was no edema or drooping of the eyelids. Her eyelid conjunctiva was pale. The sclera had no yellow staining. Her cornea was transparent. Both pupils were equal and round – about 3 mm in diameter. They were sensitive to light. Bilateral eyeball movements were flexible. There were no abnormal secretions from the external auditory canal. There was no tenderness in the tragus and mastoid area. The nasal cavity was unobstructed, and no deviation of nasal septum or abnormal secretions were seen. There was no tenderness in the paranasal sinus areas; chapped lips, with a small amount of bleeding; tongue in the middle, no tremor. There was no congestion in the pharynx, no swelling of the bilateral tonsils, bilateral symmetry of the neck, no jugular vein filling and flaring, no swelling of the thyroid; the trachea was in the middle, and her neck was supple. There was no deformity of the thorax, and both breasts were symmetrical and without deformity. No palpable mass was observed. Bilateral breathing movement was equal, and there was no pleural friction. On percussion, there was a clear sound at the bottoms of both lungs, and no dry or moist rales were heard in either lung. There was no abnormal bulge in the precordial region, and no palpable fine tremor. Percussion showed an enlarged voiced boundary of the heart, with a heart rate of 86 beats/min, regular and strong heart sounds, $A_2 = P_2$. No pathological murmur was observed in any valve auscultation region. The abdomen was flat; no varicose veins were observed in the abdominal wall; the abdomen was soft, and no tenderness and rebound pain was noticed in the abdomen. The liver and spleen were not palpated below the costal margin, and Murphy's sign was negative. The suprahepatic voiced boundary was located in the fifth intercostal of the left clavicle midline. There was no knocking pain in the liver, spleen, and kidney regions; shifting dullness negative, with bowel sounds 4–5 times/min. Mung bean-sized papules were observed scattered around the anus and external genitalia, with a uniform size and no congestion or tenderness. There was no deformity of the spine and limbs; muscle strength and muscle tension were normal, and there was mild atrophy of the limb muscles. The bilateral abdominal wall reflex, triceps tendon reflex, and heel and knee tendon reflex symmetry were normal. Babinski's sign, Kernig's sign, and Brudzinski's sign were negative.

2. Auxiliary examination
Routine blood test: WBC 3.67×10^9/L, N 80.14%, L 14.44%, M 3.34%, Hb 94 g/L, RBC 3.26×10^{12}/L, HCT (hematocrit) 0.279, PLT 66×10^9/L.

Electrolytes: Na^+ 119.3 mmol/L, K^+ 3.2 mmol/L, Cl^- 75.8 mmol/L.

TP positive, anti-HIV positive on preliminary screening. No abnormality found on chest radiograph.

III. Diagnosis and treatment after admission
1. Initial diagnosis
① Syphilis (stage III); ② AIDS; ③ Hypokalemia; ④ Hyponatremia and hypochloroemia.

2. Disease progression
The patient complained of a stomachache at 16:10 and was immediately given a 10 mg intramuscular injection of anisodamine (654-2) and a 5 mg intramuscular injection of

metoclopramide. The stomachache subsided at 17:00. After admission, intravenous gamma globulin was given, together with energy and electrolyte supplementation. At 19:00 on ward round, the patient complained that she had not eaten for a day, and felt obvious nausea and general fatigue. On physical examination, her vital signs were stable, so second-grade care was changed to first-grade care. At 22:50, the patient suddenly experienced cardiac and respiratory arrest. Her blood pressure was 0/0 mmHg, and aortic pulsation disappeared. Artificial extra-thoracic cardiac compression was performed, with one intravenous injection of nikethamide, lobeline, and epinephrine hydrochloride each, and one intravenous injection of nikethamide, lobeline, and epinephrine hydrochloride every five minutes for 30 minutes. The patient's breathing and heartbeat still did not recover, and both pupils dispersed about 1 cm. Her reaction to light disappeared, her blood pressure fell to 0/0 mmHg, and aortic pulsation disappeared. The patient was declared clinically dead at 23:30.

Emergency check: Routine blood: WBC 3.62×10^9/L, N 50%, L 40%, M 5%, abnormal lymphocytes 5%, Hb 84 g/L, RBC 2.94×10^{12}/L, HCT 0.279, PLT 64×10^9/L; three coagulation markers: PT 17.7 seconds, prothrombin activity 53.8%, myocardial enzymes: Lactate dehydrogenase 1,330 IU/L, α-hydroxybutyrate dehydrogenase 1,644 IU/L, creatine phosphokinase 153 IU/L, creatine phosphokinase isoenzyme 35 IU/L, liver and kidney function: AST 300 IU/L, total protein 57.1 g/L, albumin 27.8 g/L, blood potassium 5.71 mmol/L, blood sodium 123.7 mmol/L, blood chlorine 77.8 mmol/L, urea nitrogen 51.3 mmol/L, creatinine 752.4 μmol/L, blood calcium 1.77 mmol/L, blood magnesium 1.39 mmol/L, blood phosphorus 3.42 mmol/L, uric acid 664 μmol/L.

3. Cause of death: Syphilis.

Direct cause of death: Syphilitic heart disease?

Causes of death: ① AIDS; ② Syphilis (stage III); ③ Hypokalemia; ④ Hyponatremia and hypochloroemia.

IV. Lessons learned

The patient began to feel weak one month before admission, with poor general conditions and stable vital signs. She had been a sex worker for six years, with a high risk of sexually transmitted diseases, and was highly suspected of having HIV infection prior to admission. In the emergency check after admission, HIV TP was positive, and the diagnosis of AIDS and syphilis was clear. Symptomatic support treatment was given after admission. On the night of admission, the patient suddenly stopped breathing and her heart stopped. The basic disease syphilis can lead to syphilitic heart disease, and sudden cardiac death can occur. Urgent examination of the significantly increased myocardial enzyme spectrum during the recovery attempt supported this diagnosis. The course of AIDS and syphilis in this patient was long, and she had entered the late stage, which is difficult to reverse clinically. Clinical experience and lessons mainly include improving the monitoring of a patient's condition, detecting changes in good time, and explaining the severity of the disease to the patient's family.

The diagnosis for this patient was clear, and there was a laboratory basis for considering the cause of death as syphilitic heart disease. In recent years, the incidence of sexually transmitted diseases has increased significantly, and people infected with syphilis and HIV are often seen in our department. In this case, the patient had suffered from syphilis and HIV for a long time, and the disease recurred in the absence of regular treatment. The patient's condition was so severe at the time of admission that it could not be reversed. According to the clinical stages of AIDS released by the US CDC, this patient had entered the clinical stage, in which HIV-RNA quantification can be supplemented with patient plasma samples. According to her clinical manifestations, this patient's viral load should be very high, with extremely low immune function. The rapid development of syphilis in this patient was also related to her low immune function. The two diseases (syphilis and AIDS) are overlaid, so the symptoms develop more rapidly than the single disease. The average incubation period after HIV infection is seven years. This patient may have been infected with HIV for less than seven years. The rapid development of the disease may be due to repeated sexually transmitted infections or even the possibility of coinfection with multiple HIV subtypes.

(Wang Yuming)

Intermittent left limb movement disorder for more than eight months, aggravated for one week

I. Medical history

Patient: Male, 45 years old, self-employed. He was hospitalized due to intermittent left limb movement disorder for more than eight months, aggravated for one week.

Eight months earlier, the patient developed left limb movement disorder and progressive aggravation without any obvious causes. However, he had no dizziness, headache, nausea, vomiting, or limb convulsions. He had visited several hospitals and was diagnosed with cerebral infarction. He was treated with anti-thrombosis medication and other drugs, and his symptoms were alleviated. A week earlier, the patient felt a slight left lower limb tic, which spread to the upper limb with numbness in the left upper and lower limbs without obvious causes. There was no nausea, no vomiting, and no blurred vision or abnormality. The patient presented to our hospital today and was admitted for further diagnosis and treatment. There was no history of low-grade fever, emaciation, or night sweats since the onset of the disease.

The patient had previously been healthy. He lived for a long time in the town where he was born, and had no contact with contaminated water. He had no bad habits. His marriage and procreation were age-appropriate, and he had no history of hereditary diseases in his family.

II. Related examinations

Physical examination upon admission: T 36.5°C, P 80 times/min, R 20 times/min, BP 128/80 mmHg. He walked into the ward, but his steps were a little unstable. He had clear consciousness, good mentality, and an active demeanor, and cooperated with the physical examination. There was no palpable superficial lymph node enlargement anywhere on his body. The right bulbar conjunctiva showed mild hemorrhage, but the sclera was not icteric. Both pupils were equal, round, and reactive to light. His hearing was normal. There was no cyanosis of the lips and no swelling of the tonsils. His neck was supple, and his trachea was centered. No obvious palpable abnormality was noted in the heart and lungs. His abdomen was soft, without tenderness or rebound pain. The liver and spleen could not be palpated below the costal margin. There was no edema in either of the lower limbs. The muscle strength and tension of the four limbs were normal, with physiological reflexes present and pathological reflexes not leading out. Klinefelter's sign and Brudzinski's sign were negative.

Test results provided by the other hospital upon admission: Peripheral blood WBC 3.3×10^9/L; routine urine routine and stool normal; biochemical blood ALT 59.4 U/L; B-ultrasound showed fatty infiltration of the liver, a small hepatic cyst, and no obvious abnormality in the liver, gallbladder, pancreas, or spleen. A chest radiograph showed an old lesion in the upper left lung.

III. Diagnosis and treatment after admission
1. Initial diagnosis
Ischemic central nervous system lesions.

> **Thinking prompts:** The patient was a middle-aged man whose illness had spanned more than eight months and seemed to be a chronic process, with the main symptom being left limb dyskinesia. Central nervous system disorders should therefore be considered. Since the patient had no toxemia symptoms such as fever and no manifestations such as headache, nausea, vomiting, or consciousness disorders since the onset of his illness, his condition did not align with common infectious diffuse central nervous system lesions, and tended to have focal lesions. Investigation of the corresponding diseases should be considered.

2. Diagnostic thinking
(1) Ischemic cerebrovascular disease: The patient was a middle-aged male, with no history of hypertension or cardiovascular and cerebrovascular diseases, and insufficient evidence of cerebral infarction. However, after the application of a vasodilator to improve microcirculation, the symptoms were alleviated, meaning that they were related to ischemic cerebrovascular disease.

(2) Intracranial metastases tumor: Intracranial metastases come from malignant tumors in other parts of the body. They can occur from carcinoma, sarcoma, and melanoma. Because the tumors grow quickly and the course of illness is generally short, the brain damage they cause is relatively severe, and the local symptoms are more significant, with a wider scope of involvement. Our patient's general condition was poor. Although the symptoms of increased intracranial pressure appeared early and were significant, the patient experienced a long course of illness from the onset to the time he presented to our hospital, with mild clinical symptoms. Therefore, intracranial tumors were ruled out.

(3) Brain abscess: A pyogenic inflammation and localized abscess caused by the invasion of pyogenic bacteria into the brain, with multiple as well as single occurrences. They include common otogenic and rhinogenic brain abscesses, blood-derived brain abscesses, traumatic brain abscesses, and cryptogenic brain abscesses. Clinical manifestations include systemic and intracranial infection, increased intracranial pressure, and focused symptoms. Generally, the

patient will have a history of fever or intracranial infection first, then the source of infection can be found, such as suppurative otitis media and mastoiditis, cerebral trauma, and infection in other parts of the body. If there no regular anti-pathogen treatment is administered, the inflammatory lesions can spread to the intracranial area, and symptoms of meningeal irritation such as neck resistance can appear. As the symptoms of acute meningitis fade, it is replaced by the formation or increase of a brain abscess, with an increase and aggravation of intracranial pressure. This can lead to the formation of a brain hernia or ruptured abscess, leading to rapid deterioration. The patient in this case had no fever, no local infection, no meningeal irritation sign since the onset, and no low peripheral hemogram, so a diagnosis of intracranial infection and brain abscess was not supported.

(4) Intracranial tuberculoma: A granulomatous lesion in the central nervous system formed after infection with tubercle bacillus. It is common in teenagers and children, and often secondary to tuberculosis in other parts of the body. Clinical manifestations include signs of tuberculosis such as low-grade fever, night sweats, emaciation, and a rapid erythrocyte sedimentation rate. The symptoms of intracranial hypertension and localized brain damage are more prominent, manifested as headache, vomiting and papilledema, hemiplegia, and aphasia. Symptoms of cerebellar damage such as nystagmus and limb ataxia can also be found. Although our patient's chest radiograph showed an old lesion in the upper left lung, there were no clinical signs of tuberculosis or symptoms of intracranial hypertension. Therefore, intracranial tuberculoma can be ruled out.

(5) Cerebral toxoplasmosis: This can be primary encephalopathy or part of systemic toxoplasmosis, and is more common in immunocompromised patients such as those with AIDS. Clinical manifestations include meningitis, diffuse encephalopathy, epileptic seizures, intracranial space-occupying lesions, or mental abnormality. The course of illness is often progressive and recurrent. The patient in this case had left-limb dysfunction, and a mild clinical course. There were no typical epileptic seizures. The patient did not keep pets such as cats and dogs. Therefore, the diagnostic basis for cerebral toxoplasmosis is insufficient.

(6) Ectopic damage from schistosomiasis: More common in patients with acute schistosomiasis. When a patient suffers from a large number of cercarial invasions, the larvae will overflow the normally parasitic inferior mesenteric vein and migrate to the lungs and brain, causing ectopic damage. Cerebral schistosomiasis is either acute or chronic. The former is seen in patients with acute schistosomiasis, with encephalitis as the main symptom, while the latter occurs 3–6 months or several years after infection, and is either epilepsy type or brain tumor-like type. Epilepsy is characterized by localized seizures. It can also begin with localized convulsions and develop into grand mal. The patient in this case had no history of contact with contaminated water, and no hepatosplenomegaly was discovered during the physical examination, so there was no evidence of schistosomiasis infection. However, relevant tests should be noted in differential diagnosis.

(7) Occlusive cerebral arteritis: Usually occurring in patients with subclinical infection or mild illness of some serotypes of leptospirosis, who are suffering from repeated paralysis,

aphasia, or cranial nerve damage 2–3 months after infection, with facial nerve damage being the most common, as well as epileptic seizures or mental retardation. There was no epidemiological data for the disease in this case, and the clinical manifestations were not consistent.

3. Further diagnosis and treatment

Although the diagnosis was still unclear, through the above analysis of the patient's existing symptoms, there was a possibility of cerebrovascular ischemic lesions. Symptomatic treatment was required first, and necessary related examinations had to be conducted promptly. Symptomatic treatment included 500 ml of low-molecular-weight dextran administered intravenously once a day, 20 ml of Mailuoning intravenously dropped once a day in 250 ml of 5% glucose solution, oral administration of 40 mg of Ginkgo biloba extract (Ginaton) three times a day, and 500 μg of mecobalamin three times a day. Consultation from the Department of Neurology was requested, and the patient's condition was closely observed, with special attention paid to the presence of intracranial hypertension symptoms such as headache, nausea, vomiting, and blurred vision. The patient was asked to stay in bed or do a few activities within the scope of the ward.

After the patient was admitted to hospital, he completed the following examinations: An HIV antibody test, agglutination-lysis test, brain toxoplasma antigen antibody test, and Schistosoma japonicum antigen antibody tests. They were all negative, and his erythrocyte sedimentation rate was normal. A PPD (5TU) skin test was negative. However, multiple examinations of the peripheral hemogram revealed that the proportion of eosinophils was slightly high. Parasitic infection was highly likely, and the possibility of intracranial infection was high. Routine, biochemical, cytological, and cysticercus cellulosae antigen and antibody tests of the patient's cerebrospinal fluid were sent for examination after a lumbar puncture, and the results showed that the number of cerebrospinal fluid cells had increased slightly to 38×10^6/L, and the protein content had slightly increased. Eosinophils were visible in the cytological classification of cerebrospinal fluid, and cysticercus cellulosae antigens and antibodies were positive.

The patient had a history of eating low-quality pork, so a diagnosis of cerebral cysticercosis was suggested.

In order to understand the patient's intracranial lesions, a cranial CT examination was performed. The results showed that there were a few scattered low-density saccular shadows and high-density punctiform and nodular shadows in the right frontal lobe. An enhanced scan showed annular, punctiform, and nodular enhancement in some low-density areas, with occasional punctiform calcification. At this point, the diagnosis of cerebral cysticercosis was confirmed.

4. Ward-round analysis on the seventh day after admission

The patient's clinical symptoms in this case were very atypical. The common epileptic symptoms of cerebral cysticercosis never occurred, and only manifested as a movement disorder of the limbs on one side. Moreover, the clinical symptoms improved after the application of a cerebrovascular dilator, leading to an easy misdiagnosis of an ischemic cerebrovascular disease like cerebral infarction. A possible explanation for the clinical manifestations in this case was the mechanical compression or blockage of blood vessels by the cysticercus cellulosae body, as well as the stimulation of the vascular wall by the antigenic substances released by the body, causing inflammation of the small intracranial vessels, followed by narrowing of the lumen and even transient occlusion.

Depending on its clinical manifestations, cerebral cysticercosis is either brain parenchyma type, ventricular type, leptomeningeal type, spinal cord type, ocular type, or heart type: ① The brain parenchyma type is the most common, with the main symptoms of epilepsy, increased intracranial pressure, and mental disorder. Changes to ischemic cerebrovascular disease can also occur. It is usually caused by inflammatory obstruction of the basal arteries of the brain, with small basal endarteritis as the main form and small lacunar infarction as the clinical manifestation. ② The second most common type is the ventricular type, which is caused by parasitic cysticercus in the ventricle. When the patient's head position changes, severe vertigo, vomiting, respiratory and circulatory dysfunction, and consciousness disorder suddenly appear, which is called Bruns syndrome. ③ Ocular type and heart type are relatively rare. The former is often a single cysticercus, and can occur in any part except the crystal. The retina and vitreous body are more common locations. It does not always affect the vision. Patients can sometimes perceive a scalable shadow. Heart type cysticercosis can cause palpitations, chest stuffiness, precordial discomfort or pain, or heart failure and death. There may be manifestations of arrhythmia on the electrocardiogram.

In the treatment of cysticercosis with antiparasitic drugs, local cysticercus death causes an inflammatory reaction and tissue edema, which can lead to severe clinical symptoms. Ocular type cysticercosis can cause blindness, and heart type can induce serious arrhythmia or heart failure. Therefore, before the commencement of antiparasitic therapy, B-ultrasonography of both eyes and fundoscopic examination should be routinely performed to exclude ocular cysticercosis. Myocardial enzyme spectrum examination, an electrocardiogram, and two-dimensional echocardiography should be performed at the same time to exclude cardiac cysticercosis.

In order to prevent inflammation of the brain tissue induced by epilepsy in patients with cerebral cysticercosis, first give 20% mannitol in a 250 ml intravenous drip and 5–10 mg dexamethasone in an intravenous injection, once a day for three days before the start of antiparasitic treatment.

Praziquantel is the main drug used in antiparasitic therapy. The medicine can pass through the cyst wall of cysticercus and has strong and rapid insecticidal effect. In order to avoid an aggravated reaction from treatment or other serious neuropsychiatric symptoms caused by the death of a large number of worms in a short time, we suggest long-term treatment with a small dose, specifically 50 mg/(kg·d), divided into three, with a treatment course of 15 days. During the administration of praziquantel, the patient in this case was instructed to stay in bed and not to move about, and special care was given. To prevent epilepsy and cerebral edema, 10 mg/time prednisolone was given three times a day, and drugs for the prevention of epilepsy were added for three days after the pathogen treatment.

5. Therapeutic effect

After receiving the antiparasitic treatment mentioned above, the patient's symptoms improved. On re-examination of the routine blood test, the white blood cell count was slightly high, the proportion of neutrophils was normal, and the proportion of eosinophils had decreased. Routine urine results were normal. Multiple microscopic stool examinations revealed no parasitic eggs. Liver and kidney functions and electrolytes were all normal. Re-examination of the ECG showed normal results. Re-examination of the cranial CT scan, compared with the first CT slice taken on hospital admission, showed that the low-density saccular shadow was reduced in the original lesion site compared with before, and there was no strengthening effect of the saccular shadow on the enhanced scan, and no edema around the lesion. The patient's cerebrospinal fluid could not be re-examined because he refused to undergo another lumbar puncture. On the twenty-seventh day of hospitalization (three days after the antiparasitic treatment), the patient was in a good general condition, without any discomfort; free movement of limbs, stable walking, no dizziness and headache, sleeping well, with normal urination and defecation. He was discharged and sent home to rest, and was asked to come to the hospital for re-examination every 2–3 months, with the above treatment repeated 2–3 times.

IV. Follow-up

Three months later, the patient returned to our outpatient department. After giving a detailed medical history and undergoing a physical examination, he was confirmed to be in good general health, and was able to do housework without any physical issues. The second antiparasitic treatment was planned, so the necessary per-treatment examinations were arranged.

V. Lessons learned

The clinical manifestations of cerebral cysticercosis are diverse, and the onset priorities vary, so diagnosis is often difficult. The patient in this case was diagnosed with cerebral infarction eight months earlier in another hospital, and a definitive diagnosis was made about one week after admission, which also reflects the difficulty of diagnosis. However, after careful review and analysis of the diagnosis and treatment process in this case, it should be understood that a definitive diagnosis can be made in a timelier manner if the following two points are noted:

1. Do not be confused by typical clinical symptoms and a positive response to treatment: The clinical symptoms in this case and the response to the Thrombus Scavenger suggest a diagnosis of cerebral infarction. However, there were no underlying cardiovascular or

cerebrovascular diseases in this case. Further imaging did not reveal pathological changes consistent with the diagnosis, so other etiologies could be considered, and the correct diagnosis was made.

2. Prioritize routine examination and abnormal results: In this case, a high proportion of eosinophils in the peripheral blood was found in multiple routine blood tests after admission, and parasitic infection was suspected. From this, further examination was conducted, and the diagnosis was confirmed. At present, there is an objective tendency to place great store in personal experience and overly rely on advanced instruments and equipment while neglecting routine examination methods in clinical work. Extensive experience tells us that some routine examinations (including routine blood tests) are still an important basis for finding clues and diagnosing diseases, which should not be ignored or forgotten.

Antiparasitic treatment must be holistic. For cerebral cysticercosis, if the possible damage to the brain, eyes, and heart caused by an inflammatory reaction during treatment is not fully considered, it will often lead to more serious consequences than not using antiparasitic treatment at all. That is to say, the so-called gain does not outweigh the loss, which is totally against treatment objectives and principles of medical ethics. In fact, the concept of holistic treatment has universal significance. The human being is an organic whole. A certain drug or treatment measure targeting a certain pathogen, a certain lesion, or a certain diseased organ will have systemic effects. Making a comprehensive analysis of these effects and weighing up the pros and cons to achieve effective treatment of the disease, and as far as possible to reduce adverse reactions, should be among the basic skills that every clinician must master.

(Zhou Donghui & Huang Zuhu)

Headache, chills, and fever for three weeks

I. Medical history

Patient: Male, 35 years old, Han, a highway construction engineer. He was hospitalized with headache, chills, and fever of unknown origin for three weeks on 10 January 2008 in Chengdu.

> **Thinking prompts:** ① Nature of fever: For FUO patients, the fever type may often prompt diagnosis of a disease. For example, afternoon hot flashes with night sweats suggest tuberculosis, and persistent high fever suggests typhoid fever. ② Accompanying manifestations of fever: For example, obvious respiratory symptoms may indicate that the disease is in the respiratory tract; significant weight loss is suggestive of an infectious or non-infectious consumptive disease; the absence of a clear predisposition to systemic localization of organs may suggest systemic disease. ③ What drugs were taken: If standardized treatment with a certain drug was effective or ineffective, it can help to identify some diseases. On the other hand, fever in some cases may be partly drug-related (drug fever). ④ Epidemiological history: For infectious diseases, epidemiological data can often provide key diagnostic clues.

About a month earlier, the patient developed a headache and physical discomfort. He took his own analgesic and antipyretic drugs for the treatment of common cold, which relieved his pain slightly. Three weeks earlier, he developed an aversion to cold, and chills and fever began to appear. His body temperature was 39°C–40°C, especially in the afternoon. The fever was irregular, but accompanied by chills, which resolved spontaneously. Sweating stopped when the fever was gone. The fever lasted for several hours, and varied in length from day to day. He felt tired after the fever subsided. His headache and body pain were aggravated during high fever. His appetite was poor. For nearly two weeks, he passed loose yellow stool once or twice a day, with no pus, blood, or abdominal pain. Ten days earlier multiple outbreaks of herpes occurred on the skin of his mouth and lip. An antibiotic transfusion at a local hospital for more than ten days was ineffective (drug unknown).

The patient had previously been healthy. He had received a hepatitis B vaccination, and denied any history of blood transfusions or surgery.

II. Physical examination and auxiliary examination

1. Physical examination

Body temperature 39°C, pulse 90 beats/minute, respiration 20 breaths/minute, blood pressure 106/66 mmHg. Normal development, moderate nutrition, acute feverish expression, clear consciousness, cooperation, mental fatigue, no congestion of conjunctiva, no icteric sclera, no rash or hemorrhagic spots on skin mucosa, one soybean-sized lymph node palpable on each side of the neck and groin, both soft and active, and no tenderness. Skin herpes on upper lip, partial scab, and no other abnormality found in facial features; supple neck without resistance, no thyroid enlargement, trachea in the middle. There were no obvious abnormalities in the heart and lungs, and the rhythm of the heart was strong and regular. No pathological murmurs were heard in any valve area. There was no tenderness in the flat and soft abdomen, and no palpable mass. The liver and spleen were not palpable below the costal margin. No mobile voiced sound was found, and no pathological reflex was elicited.

2. Auxiliary examination after admission

Routine blood: White blood cells 3.95×10^9/L, red blood cells 3.9×10^{12}/L, hemoglobin 121 g/L, platelets 98×10^9/L, neutrophils 70%, lymphocytes 15%, monocytes 14%, and eosinophils 1%.

Liver and kidney function and urination and defecation routine normal.

No obvious abnormality in the ECG report.

B-ultrasound: Hepatosplenomegaly (mild).

> **Thinking prompts:** The causes of FUO are either infectious diseases or non-infectious diseases. During physical examination, look for relevant signs that can prompt the diagnosis, as well as the basis for the existence of localized organ damage. For example, a rose rash suggests typhoid fever, meningeal irritation suggests central system infection, metastatic suppurative lesions suggest septicemia, and systemic lymphadenopathy suggests lymphoma.

III. Initial clinical analysis after admission

1. Characteristics of the patient

① The patient was a middle-aged man who had previously been in good health. He fell ill in winter, with a relatively slow onset and high fever of unknown origin for three weeks. ② His fever occurred every day, especially in the afternoon, with an aversion to cold and chills; the fever lasted for an indefinite period, and subsided on its own. The symptoms of systemic poisoning were not serious; the total white blood cells and the proportion of neutrophil classifications were not significantly increased, and no obvious evidence for organ system positioning was found in clinical manifestations. However, the lymph nodes could be palpated in the bilateral neck and groin. ③ No relevant positive clues were found in the preliminary routine examination for common causes of infectious diseases after admission. ④ He worked as a highway construction engineer, often in fields.

2. Differential diagnosis

Thinking prompts: In the differential diagnosis of patients with FUO, the clinical thinking should include both infectious and non-infectious diseases, and should not be limited to infection.

(1) Infectious diseases: In this case, the following are common infectious diseases that first need to be identified:

1) Tuberculosis: One of the most common diseases with long-term fever. The fever generally peaks in the afternoon, often with night sweats. The poisoning symptoms in ordinary patients are not serious; the hemogram is generally normal, the erythrocyte sedimentation rate is fast, and the purified protein derivative (PPD) of tuberculin test is positive. In severe cases, the liver and spleen may be slightly enlarged. Patients with pulmonary tuberculosis may have a cough and shortness of breath; extrapulmonary tuberculosis has different clinical manifestations, but localization characteristics can be suggested according to the various diseased organs. For example, headache and vomiting (which can be projectile) are clinical manifestations of tuberculous meningitis with meningeal irritation and cerebrospinal fluid changes. Lymph node tuberculosis or liver tuberculosis manifests as lymph node enlargement or hepatomegaly, and a histopathological examination is often required to confirm the diagnosis.

2) Typhoid fever and other Salmonella infections: Clinical features include slow onset, a gradually increased body temperature, and persistent high fever for several weeks after one week, accompanied by a relatively slow pulse, a rose rash visible on the trunk, and an indifferent expression. Most patients have mild splenomegaly. The blood leukocytes are low, and the eosinophils decrease or disappear. The definitive diagnosis depends on a positive result of a Salmonella culture in the blood or bone marrow. If the Widal test is positive, it is diagnostically significant in combination with clinical manifestations. Typhoid fever and other Salmonella infections can be distinguished according to the agglutination titer of O and H antibodies.

3) Sepsis: High fever is one of the main clinical manifestations, but the poisoning symptoms in patients with sepsis are serious. In cases caused by pyogenic bacteria, the total blood leukocyte count and the proportion of neutrophils are significantly increased, while in cases caused by Escherichia coli, the total blood leukocyte count may be normal, but the neutrophil classification is increased. On physical examination, always search for a rash, primary lesions, or migratory purulent lesions. The diagnosis depends on the blood culture result. If antibiotics have been used before blood collection, it may cause difficulty in bacterial culture and growth, and may interfere with timely clinical diagnosis.

4) Malaria: Occurring in malaria-endemic areas and during the onset season (summer and autumn). Many malaria patients present with periodic chills and fever accompanied by varying degrees of sweating and often splenomegaly. The total white blood cells in the peripheral blood are normal or decreased. After multiple episodes, patients show obvious anemia. Plasmodium can be found on the peripheral blood smear.

5) AIDS: The infection rate and incidence of HIV have increased in China in recent years. Therefore, HIV infection screening has been included in clinical routine for FUO patients.

The following diseases are less likely, so they can mostly be ruled out.

6) Hemorrhagic fever with renal syndrome: The peak of incidence is from November to January of the following year. In clinic, there are three main symptoms (fever, bleeding, and kidney damage) and five clinical stages (fever, hypotension and shock, oliguria, polyuria, and recovery). There was no significant renal impairment in this patient.

7) Kala-azar: Caused by Leishmania, with no obvious seasonality. The clinical manifestations include long-term fever with varying heat types, and double-peak fever. Hepatosplenomegaly is obvious, and elderly patients present with splenomegaly with hypersplenism, complete blood reduction, extreme reduction of leukocytes, and obvious anemia. In this case, the patient's poisoning symptoms were not serious, but he was weak and emaciated. An amastigote of Leishmania donovani can be found in the bone marrow smear. Immuno-serological tests are positive for Leishmania antibodies.

8) Acute brucellosis: Also known as undulant fever, and caused by the transmission of Brucella infection to humans from cattle and sheep. It is more common in pastoral areas, and can develop in all seasons. The onset is relatively slow, with varying heat types, of which the remittent type is more common. Undulant fever is characterized by an aversion to cold, chills, hyperhidrosis, and arthralgia. If it invades the central nervous system, Brucella meningitis may occur, manifesting as headaches, vomiting, and neck stiffness. This patient had no history of contact with cattle or sheep.

9) Leptospirosis: Occurring in summer and autumn, in patients who have had contact with contaminated water. It is mainly manifested as fever, head and body pain, and fatigue. Patients have bulbar conjunctival congestion, inguinal lymph node enlargement, apparent tenderness of the gastrocnemius muscle, and increased white blood cell and neutrophil counts.

(2) Non-infectious diseases

1) Malignant tumors: ① Malignant lymphoma: Patients usually complain of long-term high fever. Diagnosis is difficult in the absence of superficial lymph node enlargement in the neck and elsewhere; in some cases, the diagnosis is not confirmed until postmortem examination. A lymph node biopsy helps with diagnosis. ② Malignant histiocytosis: Clinical manifestations include high fever, which may be continuous, remittent, or irregular fever, accompanied by hepatosplenomegaly, enlarged lymph nodes, reduction of the complete blood, and possible bleeding symptoms. It is sometimes easily misdiagnosed as kala-azar. However, malignant histiocytosis is a dangerous disease with severe poisoning symptoms and poor prognosis. The average course of the disease is 2–4 months. Diagnosis is often confirmed by aspiration of the

bone marrow, lymph node, or liver. ③ Leukemia: The clinical manifestation of some leukemia patients is fever, but the white blood cells in peripheral blood are lower, and there is no obvious abnormality in classification, that is, so-called aleukemia. A definite diagnosis depends on bone marrow examination.

2) Connective tissue diseases: This group includes various diseases, such as rheumatic fever, systemic lupus erythematosus, polymyositis, and polyarteritis nodosa. Except for fever as the prominent clinical manifestation, these diseases have various clinical manifestations, which will not be described in detail here. The reader should recognize the range of thinking from the above data so as to correctly conduct differential diagnoses and analyses of patients with FUO.

3) Others: ① Adult-onset Still's disease (AOSD): An allergic syndrome characterized by fever, rash, joint pain, and a marked increase in white blood cells and neutrophils, which is similar to sepsis, but without obvious symptoms of toxemia, and negative for repeated blood cultures. Antibacterial treatment is ineffective, while glucocorticoids are effective. The diagnosis of AOSD often uses the rule-out method. After completely excluding infectious diseases, if glucocorticoids can be used effectively, this disease can be considered. ② Drug fever: There is a close causal relationship between fever and the use of certain drugs; other drug-related manifestations such as a rash may be present at the same time.

3. Initial diagnosis
FUO.

IV. Treatment after admission
1. Initial treatment plan
Given that fever due to infectious diseases is usually more acute, once confirmed, infectious diseases can mostly be treated effectively, so timely diagnosis and treatment play a crucial role in prognosis. Fever caused by non-infectious diseases involves malignant tumors and connective tissue diseases. Diagnosis can sometimes be difficult, and the common causes of infectious diseases often need to be ruled out before the diagnosis of non-infectious diseases can be clarified. In addition, several non-infectious diseases with fever as the main clinical manifestation (such as AOSD and connective tissue disease) often need to be treated with corticosteroids, which requires the prior exclusion of infectious factors.

Therefore, when arranging further examination plans for this patient, we should first start with common infectious diseases (such as tuberculosis, typhoid fever, sepsis, and malaria), and perform chest radiograph, blood culture, stool culture, and urine culture (after the third week of the disease course, the positive rates of blood culture for typhoid fever and Salmonella infection decrease, while those of stool culture and urine culture increase), Widal test, tuberculin skin test, erythrocyte sedimentation rate, and primary screening test for HIV antibodies.

During this period, if patients have no obvious symptoms of infection poisoning, offer a general infusion and symptomatic support, but avoid administering anti-infective drugs and antipyretics in order to understand the fever type. Note any changes of signs in clinical observation, and look for relevant indications.

2. Results of laboratory examinations and special examinations

No abnormality was found in the chest radiograph report. Blood culture was performed once, and no bacterial growth was seen. The Widal test and tuberculin skin test were negative, and the erythrocyte sedimentation rate was normal. A blood smear was routinely tested once for Plasmodium and was reported as negative, with a negative initial screening test for HIV antibodies.

The patient still had an irregular fever every day, sometimes lasting more than ten hours before coming down on its own. His headache was aggravated during the fever.

> Thinking prompts: ① Although the diagnostic basis for infectious diseases had not been found, the above preliminary results were not enough to rule out infectious causes. This was because the course of the disease was just over one month, the sensitivity of detection reagents is inherently insufficient, and patients with typhoid fever and Salmonella infection may also show false negativity to the Widal test. No abnormality was found on the chest radiograph. Even if the tuberculin skin test is negative, the possibility of tuberculosis cannot be ruled out. The presence of extrapulmonary tuberculosis lesions should be investigated. In addition, the possibility of other infectious diseases should not be ignored, and further in-depth inquiry and collection of epidemiological data should be conducted. ② The above preliminary negative results for infectious etiology screening also suggested that the search for non-infectious etiology should be intensified.

3. Further inquiry into medical history

The patient had been working on road reconstruction projects in Africa for six months before the onset of illness. He often went back and forth to the construction site and worked in cities, denying the history of visiting prostitutes. He returned home two months ago. The local climate is hot, and there is a malaria epidemic. He had taken malaria prevention drugs, but the name of the medication was unknown. Before going abroad, the patient had a comprehensive physical examination, and the results were normal.

4. Diagnosis & treatment plan for the next stage

(1) Africa has a high incidence rate of malaria and AIDS; it is hot in all four seasons, and there is a malaria epidemic throughout the year, so blood smears should be checked for plasmodium; HIV antibodies should be repeatedly tested for, to rule out false negativity. Meanwhile, blood collection should be continued for bacterial culture to seek evidence of typhoid and Salmonella infection.

(2) Bone marrow aspiration: Bacterial cultures, smears, and biopsies should be performed to examine the bone marrow and look for abnormal cells to understand the possibility of malignant hematological diseases.

(3) Preoperative preparation of liver biopsy should be performed (checking the coagulation function, performing routine blood tests, and communicating with the patient and their family before surgery), as well as investigating the possibility of liver tuberculosis, malignant hematological disease, and lymphoma.

(4) Ask the hematology department for a consultation, and discuss the possibility of arranging a biopsy of the cervical lymph nodes to investigate lymphoid nuclei, lymphoma, and malignant hematological diseases. Closely observe daily clinical changes in patients, and look for relevant signs. Temporarily avoid giving anti-infective drugs and antipyretics, but physical cooling should be implemented when the fever is high.

5. Results of in-depth re-examination

Two blood cultures were negative, and another blood smear showed no evidence of plasmodium. Bone marrow examination showed a series of active erythroid hyperplasia, and the patient's condition gradually worsened, with a moderate enlargement of the spleen, aggravated anemia, and positive urine protein. His headache became even worse, and he was agitated; episodes of projectile vomiting, no obvious resistance in the neck, pathological reflex not elicited. In order to screen for central nervous system infections such as tuberculous meningitis, a lumbar puncture was performed on the patient after the use of a dehydrating agent, which revealed clear cerebrospinal fluid with normal pressure and no abnormalities in routine laboratory tests.

6. Clinical analysis

The patient had worked in Africa for six months before the onset of the disease. Although it was winter in Chengdu at the time of the onset, in Africa it was hot, and malaria was prevalent. Malaria cannot be ruled out for this patient, especially falciparum malaria. The examination of plasmodium in his blood smear was significantly affected by the timing of blood collection, and the individual technical experience of the maker and observer of the smear. Therefore, the blood smear test had to be re-examined. Focus was placed on blood collection during periods of chills and high fever. In order to avoid missed detection of plasmodium, both thick and thin blood smears were sent for examination. However, because the patient reported having taken malaria prevention drugs, members of his family were asked which drugs were prescribed at his unit. Apart from differential diagnosis, if malaria is diagnosed through a blood smear examination of plasmodium, knowing what anti-malarial drugs were used will be helpful for drug selection in anti-malarial treatment.

At the same time, we should continue to closely observe daily clinical changes in patients, looking for new clues to differential diagnosis, and preventing and controlling the aggravation of the disease, especially the possibility of a dangerous attack of falciparum malaria. Therefore, routine blood tests and urine tests must be repeated, blood pressure monitored, and 24-hour urine output recorded. Note the patient's consciousness, cervical muscle resistance, and pathological reflex.

7. The report after the implementation of the above diagnosis and treatment plan was confirmed

It was learned from the patient's unit that he had taken chloroquine for malaria prevention during his time working in Africa. Meanwhile, the laboratory reported that the ring-like body and gametophyte of Plasmodium falciparum had been found in the thick blood smear.

8. Clinical diagnosis

Falciparum malaria, possibly a chloroquine-resistant strain.

V. Treatment after diagnosis

In the treatment of malaria, the most important step is to kill the plasmodium in the red blood cells. Pernicious episodes or serious complications of falciparum malaria should be avoided. Antimalarial treatment was given immediately, with a combination of artemether and primaquine regimen. Artemether was administered orally at a total dose of 640 mg. The drug was taken over seven days, once a day, with 80 mg each time, and the first dose was doubled. Primaquine was also administered as a total oral dose of 45 mg, as 22.5 mg for two days. Because the course of the disease had been nearly a month, and the patient's headache and irritability worsened, he was immediately given 20 mg intravenous dexamethasone to control the deterioration of his condition and the occurrence of cerebral malaria, and clinical changes were closely monitored. After the anti-malaria treatment was started, the patient's condition improved significantly, and the high fever gradually subsided. No fever occurred the next day. After the anti-malaria treatment was completed, the patient recovered and was discharged from hospital.

The basis for administering Dexamethasone was that most severe episodes are caused by Plasmodium falciparum, because the proliferation and development of Plasmodium falciparum schizont are mostly carried out in visceral capillaries. In addition, nodular protrusions appear on the infected erythrocyte membrane, which are liable to adhere to each other and cause obstructions in the visceral capillaries, leading to severe visceral damage. Brain-type is the most common severe attack, and usually occurs a few days after the onset of chills and fever. In a small number of patients, the onset can also be similar to encephalitis, manifested as severe headache, vomiting, irritability, delirium, coma, convulsions, and twitching. Physical examination shows neck stiffness, and pathological reflection may be positive. Because the course of this patient's illness had been nearly one month, and because he failed to receive timely anti-malarial treatment due to unclear diagnosis, he suffered high fever, gradually aggravating headache and irritability, and projectile vomiting. Although signs such as neck stiffness and positive pathological reflex had not occurred, some degree of brain tissue damage may already have occurred. Administration of dexamethasone helped to control inflammation and edema in the brain tissue.

VI. Follow-up

Falciparum malaria does not generally recur, but it may recrudesce. Recrudescence refers to the fact that the plasmodium has not been completely eliminated, but has re-multiplied after a period of time, resulting in the reoccurrence of symptoms. Incomplete treatment is a common cause of recrudescence. It usually occurs a few days to months after the initial episode, and can happen more than once. Recrudescence is often milder than the initial onset. Within about six months (rarely more than a year), the parasites are completely eliminated by the host's immune mechanism, and the patient eventually recovers. Chloroquine-resistant strain infection is especially prone to recrudescence. Therefore, the anti-malarial drugs selected for patients with falciparum malaria should not only be efficient, sensitive, and effective, but also guaranteed to achieve adequate doses and treatment courses, with increased follow-up contact with patients. This patient remained healthy throughout the year of follow-up.

VII. Lessons learned

The patient in this case – who was susceptible due to having no immunity from living in a non-malarial area – was hospitalized in Chengdu in Sichuan Province in January 2008 due to FUO. At that time, it was winter in Chengdu. In the process of making a diagnosis, the receiving doctor often ignored the identification of malaria and failed to inquire from an epidemiological perspective in order to obtain relevant clues, thus failing to perform relevant tests when formulating a diagnosis and treatment plan. This was one of the reasons why the patient failed to obtain an early diagnosis. In fact, Africa as a whole is in an equatorial, tropical, and subtropical climate zone, with more than 95% being hot year-round, and malaria-endemic. Although the patient's work in Africa before the onset of the disease was known through gathering further medical history, the doctor had an insufficient understanding of epidemic infection with drug-resistant plasmodium strains (mostly resistant to chloroquine). Hence, he was confused by the fact that the patient reported taking malaria-prevention drugs, and remained focused on the differential diagnosis of AIDS and other diseases rather than the possibility of drug-resistant plasmodium infection.

Although the doctor in charge also arranged blood smears for the examination of plasmodium, he did not insist on the collection of blood during the period of chills and high fever, nor did he request thick and thin blood smears. Plasmodium falciparum has high density in the viscera and bone marrow. Although bone marrow aspiration was arranged for this patient clinically, according to the reporting doctor, the main purpose of submission was to investigate hematological diseases through bacterial culture and examination of bone marrow. The examiner was not asked to smear for plasmodium, thus delaying its early detection.

After that, through repeated inquiries about the patient's medical history and in-depth clinical analysis, the direction of the investigation was clarified, the method of blood collection for plasmodium examination was improved, and the diagnosis of falciparum malaria was finally established. Despite prompt adjustment of the treatment regimen and the use of sensitive and highly effective anti-malarial drugs, which led to a recovery, the course of the disease was prolonged. It was a fluke that the patient did not suffer dangerous attacks or other serious complications during the exacerbation of his disease. Important lessons should be learned.

Malaria is the most widespread and harmful parasitic disease in the world today, and is one of the most prominent global public health problems. Forty percent of the global population lives in countries and regions at risk of malaria. Over 90% of cases are found in Africa, with the rest mainly occurring in India, Brazil, Afghanistan, and Southeast Asia. In China, the malaria epidemic is still serious in the mountainous areas of Hainan, the border areas of Yunnan, and the central provinces that are home to 120 million people. This case was imported, with the patient bringing it back from Africa to an area where malaria was rare. With the rapid increase of population movement after economic globalization, imported malaria has begun to emerge as a major public health problem. Due to developments in transportation, the migration of susceptible people from the foci where they acquired the infection to where they developed symptoms can be completed in 1–2 days across the two hemispheres. Patients can experience both cold and hot weather from completely different seasons (such as tropical countries that are hot all year round, and temperate countries with four seasons, varying depending on the hemisphere). If medical staff in malaria-rare areas are not vigilant, they may neglect to consider the seasonal epidemiological characteristics of infectious diseases, and the actual climatic conditions of the place where patients lived before the onset of illness. As a result, some infectious diseases with obvious seasonal epidemiological signs are not identified, and the diagnosis is often confirmed only in the late stage, thus delaying treatment.

The harm caused by imported falciparum malaria is more serious. The clinical manifestations of patients with falciparum malaria are complex, with irregular episodes and lack of periodicity of tertian and quartan episodes. This is closely related to the biological characteristics of Plasmodium falciparum. Its development in red blood cells is uneven, and the time it takes to leave the infected red cells and invade the next normal red blood cells is different, leading to the diversification of clinical manifestations of falciparum malaria. Some patients use antipyretic drugs to bring down their body temperature due to unclear diagnosis after the onset of disease, and the clinical manifestation of the fever type will be irregular. The lack of necessary epidemiological information can sometimes lead to difficulties in the early diagnosis of such patients. This is because many attending doctors do not have a comprehensive understanding of the clinical manifestations of malaria. There is a misconception that periodic fever is a clinical feature of malaria, and they are not fully aware of the importance of falciparum malaria in the differential diagnosis of FUO.

The prodromal symptoms of patients with falciparum malaria are common. They may suffer aversion to cold during an attack, but most of them do not experience chills. The fever type is often irregular, and some episodes can last for 20-36 hours or more. However, headache, nausea, and vomiting are more common, sometimes with abdominal pain and diarrhea. Anemia and splenomegaly appeared early and obviously in our patient. The white blood cell count and neutrophil granulocytes can be increased during an acute attack, going back to normal after the attack. After multiple episodes, the white blood cell count decreases and the mononuclear cells increase. Patients without immunity can develop a severe attack 5-10 days after the first occurrence.

In this case, the diagnosis of malaria was based on the capture of plasmodium in blood smears under a microscope. It must be emphasized that the blood sample collection time for identifying plasmodium is crucial for the timely diagnosis of malaria. It is advisable to arrange sampling during the onset of aversion to cold and high fever, when the parasite density in the peripheral blood is relatively high and is easily detected. When blood was collected at other times, the parasite density in the peripheral blood was significantly reduced, which may prevent the detection of plasmodium. It is easy to detect in microscopic examination of thick blood smears, so one thick and one thin blood smear should be taken. If a blood test is negative, the blood smear test should be repeated within 2–3 days to prevent missed diagnosis. If negative, a bone marrow smear can be examined for plasmodium. Within general hospital procedures, blood samples are collected from patients early in the morning. If this does not coincide with the stage of aversion to cold and high fever for a malaria patient, the detection rate of plasmodium may be reduced. At present, all-automated hematology analyzers are widely used in major intermediate hospitals, which has led to modernization, but has also brought new problems. Some inspectors rely too heavily on automatic instruments and ignore the basic skills of morphological examination of manual smears. Manual smear examination often focuses on the morphology of the white blood cell system and ignores the observation of mature red blood cells, which can also hinder the detection of plasmodium.

In addition to artemisinin derivatives, plasmodium has varying degrees of resistance to first-line anti-malarial drugs, and some epidemic areas in Southeast Asia even have multiple drug resistance. In most areas, chloroquine is no longer effective as a treatment for falciparum malaria. Therefore, we must note the curative effect when chloroquine is used against malaria. In areas where chloroquine-resistant strains have been found, the drug is avoided as far as possible in patients with severe and malignant malaria.

The following therapies can be used in the treatment of falciparum malaria:

(1) Artemether: Total oral dose 640 mg. Taken once a day over seven days, 80 mg each time, with the first dose doubled.

(2) Artesunate: Total oral dose 800 mg. Taken once a day over seven days, 100 mg each time, with the first dose doubled.

(3) Dihydroartemisinin: Total oral dose 480 mg. Taken once a day over seven days, 60 mg each time, with the first dose doubled.

(4) Pyronaridine: Total oral dose 1,600 mg, taken over three days, twice on the first day, 400 mg each time at an interval of eight hours, once on the second and third day, 400 mg each time.

The four drugs above require additional administration of primaquine in a total oral dose of 45 mg for two days at 22.5 mg each time.

(5) Artesunate tablets + amodiaquine tablets: Total oral dose 12 artesunate tablets and 12 amodiaquine tablets (50 mg per artesunate tablet and 150 mg per amodiaquine tablet), and four artesunate tablets and four amodiaquine tablets each day for three consecutive days.

(6) Dihydroartemisinin piperaquine tablets: Total oral dose eight tablets (each tablet containing 40 mg of dihydroartemisinin and 320 mg of piperaquine phosphate), two tablets in the first dose, and two tablets in 6–8 hours, 24 hours, and 32 hours after the first dose.

(7) Compound naphthoquine phosphate tablets: Eight tablets (each containing 50 mg naphthoquine and 125 mg artemisinin) taken orally, once in total.

(8) Compound artemisinin tablets: Total oral dose four tablets (each containing 62.5 mg artemisinin and 375 mg piperaquine), two tablets for the first dose and two tablets after 24 hours.

Since China's Reform and Opening-up, the number of Chinese people going abroad for tourism, work, business, research, study, and visiting relatives has been increasing. They contract local infectious diseases outside China and bring them home, meaning that cases of these diseases are increasing. In their clinical thinking around the diagnosis of infectious diseases, doctors must inquire whether patients have been abroad before the onset of illness, and consider the possibility of importing some foreign infectious diseases (not only malaria) into China.

Although malaria is clinically characterized by fever with certain regularity, malignant malaria or poly-infection of tertian fever and quartan malaria can cause the fever pattern of malaria to lack periodicity. Young doctors, especially clinicians in non-endemic areas, often make misdiagnoses due to their lack of experience and limited number of malaria cases. However, quarantine departments at the border control points should also raise awareness of epidemic prevention for entry and exit personnel. They should remind travelers to see a doctor immediately if they fall ill or show any discomfort on returning home, and inform medical staff of their travel trajectory.

(Zhao Liansan)

Ulcer on the right eyelid with facial and neck swelling for three days

I. Medical history

Patient: Female, 36 years old, a Uygur farmer from a county in Southern Xinjiang. She was hospitalized because of an ulcer on her right eyelid with facial and neck swelling for three days.

Three days before admission, the patient noticed a few red papules on her right upper eyelid without any obvious inducements, which turned into herpes with slight pruritus. One day later, the herpes was swollen and burst, and a small amount of bloody secretion was exuded, accompanied by slight pain. There was no fever and no other discomfort. The patient did not seek medical treatment. The next day, the swelling of the right upper eyelid expanded to the left eyelid and the right cheek, as well as the right side of the neck and occipital area. When the patient visited a township hospital, anti-inflammatory and symptomatic treatment were conducted (the specific diagnosis and treatment process are unknown). Her condition did not improve, so she was transferred to our hospital.

The patient had previously been healthy, and had no history of infectious diseases or drug allergies.

II. Physical examination and auxiliary outpatient examination

1. Physical examination

Body temperature 37.6°C, pulse 96 beats/min, respiration 21 breaths/min, blood pressure 120/70 mmHg. Well nourished, well developed. Acute facial features, pained expression. She walked into the ward; clear mind, gave the correct answers, and cooperated with the examination. The skin mucosa on her whole body had no yellow stains, and there were no bleeding points·1 or ecchymosis. The superficial lymph nodes were not enlarged anywhere on her body. There was an ulcer of about 0.5 cm on the skin of her right upper eyelid; the right cheek area and right side of the neck, auricular region, and occipital region were significantly swollen. The left eyelid region was involved in the swelling, without obvious tenderness or feelings of fluctuation. It was non-pitting edema. The patient had difficulty opening her right eye. Her neck was supple, and the heart border was normal. No pathological murmur was heard. Percussion sounds were resonant in both lungs; thick respiratory sounds in both lungs, and no dry or moist rales were heard. The abdomen was soft without tenderness or rebound pain, and the liver and spleen could not be palpated below the costal margin. The whole abdomen was percussion-diagnosed, with voiced sounds and bowel sounds. The physiological reflex was present, but the pathological reflex was not elicited.

> **Thinking prompts:** At the first outpatient visit, the patient (a young female farmer) presented with herpes simplex of the upper right eyelid, and a skin ulcer with edema of the surrounding tissues. There was a wide range of involvement, and low-grade fever without other manifestations. A skin infection was preliminarily considered, and a routine blood examination was helpful for judging whether the issue was caused by a bacterial infection.

2. Routine outpatient blood test

WBC 20.6×10^9/L, N 82.5%, RBC 5.6×10^{12}/L, Hb 172 g/L, PLT 307×10^9/L.

A routine blood test showed a significant increase in white blood cells and neutrophils, suggesting that the skin infection of the patient's right eyelid with edema of the surrounding tissues was caused by a bacterial infection. She was admitted to our hospital with a severe facial skin infection.

III. Diagnosis and treatment after admission

1. Medical history

① Young woman, farmer, with upper right blepharal herpes simplex evolving into a skin ulcer with edema of the surrounding tissues covering a wide area – non-pitting edema with low-grade fever and no other clinical manifestations. ② The white blood cells and neutrophils in the peripheral blood were significantly increased. A skin infection was the preliminary consideration.

2. Differential diagnosis

(1) Suppurative dermatitis (impetigo): Pyogenic infection of the skin, mainly caused by Staphylococcus or Streptococcus, which takes the form of scattered blisters in the early stage and then rapidly enlarges, forming a rough surface after ulceration and yellow pus scabs after drying. If the scope of infection is small, it usually shows no symptoms of infectious poisoning such as fever. It usually occurs on exposed parts such as the face and limbs. The manifestations in this case do not align, so it can be ruled out.

(2) Cellulitis: Diffuse suppurative inflammation of the skin or subcutaneous tissue caused by Staphylococcus aureus or hemolytic streptococcus. Clinical manifestations include redness, swelling, pain, and fever on the local skin and subcutaneous layer of the infected part. In severe cases, systemic poisoning may occur. Skin ulceration can form ulcers, gangrene, abscesses, and septicemia. The manifestations in this case do not align, so it can be ruled out.

(3) Cutaneous anthrax: Caused by anthrax bacillus infection. In this case, small papules or maculopapules first appeared on the skin at the site of infection, which then evolved into blisters. The surrounding tissues showed obvious edema. Three to four days later, necrosis appeared in the center of the skin lesion, and a superficial ulcer appeared in the necrotic area, forming black eschars. The edema of the surrounding tissues significantly expanded. It is usually painless, and is typically accompanied by slight pruritus. The initial presentation of this case was consistent with anthrax, which would be more likely if black eschars were to form 3–5 days later. The diagnosis could be confirmed if etiological examination found anthrax bacillus. Xinjiang is an agricultural and pastoral area, and anthrax occurs all year round. Considering the characteristics of skin lesions in this case, the possibility of anthrax should be considered first.

(4) Scrub typhus (tsutsugamushi disease): Clinical manifestations include sudden high fever with a headache and systemic pain, congestive maculopapules, and enlarged lymph nodes. Insect bites first show red maculopapules, and then blisters form. The lesions gradually necrotize in the center and form black eschars with a slightly elevated periphery. There is no pain, pruritus, or exudation. Ulcers form after the eschars fall off – the most important characteristic of the condition. White blood cells are normal or slightly lower. A positive Weil-Felix test (OX_K titer > 1:160) or positive ELISA test for specific IgM antibodies can be helpful for diagnosis. Scrub typhus is caused by rickettsia infection. Rodents are the source of infection, and it is transmitted through the bite of rickettsia-bearing mites. It is mainly prevalent in southern China. Scrub typhus is not common in Xinjiang, and the clinical manifestations are different, so it can be ruled out in this case.

3. Evolution of the disease after admission

After admission, secretions from the skin ulcer were taken and sent for bacterial smear and culture. Since a bacterial skin infection or anthrax was suspected, antibacterial drugs were administered against staphylococcus and bacillus anthracis: Penicillin 6.4 million U/d, divided into two intravenous injections. The patient's body temperature was 37.5°C–38.6°C three days after admission. She was in poor spirits, with a low appetite and no other obvious discomforts. The edema around the skin on her right upper eyelid was slightly alleviated, and an eschar of about 2 cm × 2 cm was formed at the center. A routine blood test showed WBC 16.2×10^9/L, N 85%, and normal hemoglobin and platelet counts. The secretion bacterial smear showed Gram-positive coarse bacillus, and the bacterium was cultured into anthrax bacillus. At this point, the diagnosis of cutaneous anthrax was confirmed.

The patient was treated in isolation in the ward immediately. After five days of treatment with penicillin, her body temperature decreased to normal. There was still facial edema, but it had markedly subsided. The skin lesions on her eyelid were treated with tetracycline ointment and covered with a gauze bandage. After treatment with penicillin for seven days, the patient's body temperature was normal, her appetite had significantly increased, and she was in a normal mental state. The black eschar on the upper eyelid of her right eye eventually fell off, and the wound healed. The facial and neck swelling disappeared, and her eyes opened and closed freely. A re-examination of her white blood cells showed 6.6×10^9/L, N 60%, and her red blood cell and platelet counts were normal.

IV. Lessons learned

This case presented as a maculopapule of the skin, which developed into herpes followed by ulceration, black eschars, and significant edema of the surrounding tissues. There was mild to moderate fever and a marked increase in white blood cells and neutrophils. A smear and bacterial culture showed Bacillus anthracis. This is the typical clinical process of cutaneous anthrax. Treatment with penicillin had a positive effect, and the prognosis was good.

Anthrax is significantly different from a skin infection in appearance, mainly due to the general pyogenic skin infection manifested as red swelling and hot pain on the skin of the infected part. Ulcers form, accompanied by a large amount of purulent discharge. In cutaneous anthrax, the skin at the infected site breaks out in papules or herpes, and then swells and collapses, forming ulcers and eschars. It is painless, without purulent discharge, and non-pitting edema.

Anthrax is a zoonotic disease, which is prevalent in agricultural and pastoral areas. People who come into contact with herbivorous livestock are at the highest risk. If there is a spate of anthrax in an area, residents should be vigilant. Clinically speaking, in such an area, if there is an infection of the skin without redness, swelling, heat, or pain, especially a skin ulcer with no obvious purulent discharge, we should consider the possibility of anthrax. We should take secretions from the ulcer site for inspection as quickly as possible and perform bacteriological examination. The anthrax in this case occurred in the eyelid, where the tissue was loose and the infection was not easily confined. It could easily develop into anthrax septicemia or anthrax meningitis, requiring prompt treatment with antibacterial drugs.

Anthrax is an acute zoonotic infectious disease caused by Bacillus anthracis, which exists in soil and water in the form of spores in the natural environment. Herbivorous animals such as horses, cattle, and sheep are infected by ingesting soil containing anthrax spores during grazing. Anthrax infections in humans are mostly due to the following:

1. Skin contact with infected animals or animal products such as skin, hair, bone, meat, and other products, particularly to damaged skin
2. Eating animal meat containing anthrax spores, leading to gastrointestinal anthrax
3. Inhaling dust containing anthrax spores, leading to pulmonary anthrax (also known as inhaled anthrax)

Today, anthrax infection among herbivores in the United States and developed countries in Europe has decreased significantly, with occasional cases caused by exposure to animal products from developing countries. However, in developing countries and regions such as Asia, Africa, South America, and Eastern and Southern Europe, there are thousands of cases of anthrax infection from wild and domestic animals every year. In 2001, terrorists spread anthrax spores to the United States by mail, infecting 22. Eleven people developed complications from inhaling anthrax, and five people died, indicating that non-anthrax epidemic areas should guard against bioterrorism.

Bacillus anthracis is a Gram-positive bacterium. In its reproductive state, it can form a capsule in the body, and can resist phagocytosis from the host phagocytes. It can form spores under adverse environmental conditions, with strong resistance. It can survive in the natural environment for decades, and is the main source of infection for anthrax-infected organisms. The pathogenicity of anthrax is mainly caused by the capsule and exotoxin produced by Bacillus anthracis propagules. Anthrax exotoxin consists of three proteins produced by pXO1 coding, namely protective antigen (protective antigen, PA), lethal factor (Lethal factor, LF), and edema factor (Edema factor, EF). PA combines with lethal factors to form a lethal toxin, which can cause cell death in tissue. PA combined with edema factor forms edema toxin, leading to tissue cell edema.

Anthrax infection has three clinical types based on the route of infection, namely skin (cutaneous) anthrax, inhaled (pulmonary) anthrax, and digestive tract anthrax. The most common is skin anthrax caused by contact with anthrax spores at the site of skin injury, accounting for 95% of cases of anthrax infection. It usually occurs on exposed skin, and is characterized by the formation of black eschars and slightly elevated non-pitting edema changes in the surrounding area. If treatment is not conducted, the fatality rate is around 20%, but it is less than 1% with antibacterial treatment.

The key to the treatment of each type of anthrax is the early use of antimicrobial therapy. In vitro tests show that Bacillus anthracis is sensitive to drugs such as penicillin sodium, amoxicillin, doxycycline, rifampicin, chloramphenicol, clindamycin, erythromycin, gentamicin, streptomycin, imipenem, cefazolin, linezolid, vancomycin, ciprofloxacin, and levofloxacin, but resistant to broad-spectrum drugs such as cephalosporin C, cefuroxime, ceftazidime, cefotaxime, aztreonam, and compound sulfamethoxazole. At present, penicillin is still the first choice for the treatment of the various types of anthrax in China. For skin anthrax without systemic symptoms, penicillin can be used in a dosage of 1.6 million U/d–3.2 million U/d in two to three intramuscular injections over 7–10 days. While penicillin-resistant strains have appeared in Western countries, there have been no reports of natural resistance of Bacillus anthracis to quinolones. Therefore, European countries recommend ciprofloxacin and doxycycline as first-line drugs for the treatment of anthrax infection.

(Zhang Yuexin)

Continuous fever for a month

I. Medical history

Patient: Male, 56 years old, a veterinarian. He was hospitalized because of continuous fever for a month.

> **Thinking prompts:** Relevant questions should be asked to complete the patient's medical history. Ask about the regularity of fever, accompanying symptoms, evolution, and treatment. Ask about his past medical history, including infectious diseases, epidemic areas, and occupational characteristics.

The patient developed a fever one month ago without any obvious inducements. His body temperature was 38°C–39.5°C with chills and sweating. It rose every afternoon, lasting for about two hours before it spontaneously subsided, with no other uncomfortable symptoms. He visited a local clinic and was treated with cephalosporins for two weeks, with no effect. He came to our hospital for diagnosis and treatment due to his repeatedly rising body temperature. He had a history of anemia and diabetes, and had been taking hypoglycemic drugs for a long time. He denied a history of infectious diseases such as hepatitis and tuberculosis, as well as a history of trauma and surgery, allergies to drugs and food, residence outside his city before and after the onset of illness, contact with contaminated water, and hereditary diseases in his family. He lived in the countryside, and did not eat raw food. There were no recent similar incidences in the people around him. He was a veterinarian with a history of close contact with animals including pigs and poultry.

> **Thinking prompts:** Inquiries should focus on whether there were any symptoms of infected toxemia during the fever period, including changes to appetite, physical strength, weight, and sleep status, in order to confirm whether there was any serious infection anywhere in his body. Focus on asking whether there are standard antibiotic treatments to exclude certain pathogen infections. For anemia, we should focus on asking about rashes, purpura, bleeding points, bleeding, and soy sauce-colored urine, to see if there has been active bleeding and hematological disorders.

This patient had a history of anemia and diabetes, and had taken hypoglycemic drugs for a long time, suggesting a basis of immunologic hypofunction. His occupation as a veterinarian and his history of close contact with animals, including pigs and poultry, suggest the need to exclude animal-derived infectious diseases.

The patient's medical history and treatment were relatively simple and provided few clues. Therefore, in-depth medical history should be gathered, and targeted physical examination should be conducted.

II. Physical and auxiliary examination

1. Physical examination

Body temperature 38°C, pulse 102 beats/ minute. He was conscious, with the appearance of anemia. No erythema or nodules were observed on his skin. No yellow staining was observed in the sclera, and his conjunctiva was pale. His lips were not cyanotic. His oral mucosa was smooth. His superficial lymph nodes were not enlarged. No abnormality was observed in his heart and lungs. There was no tenderness in his abdomen. The liver and spleen were not palpable, the shifting dullness was negative, the four limbs were able to move freely, and there was no swelling or tenderness in the joints, nor positive signs in the nervous system.

> **Thinking prompts:** We narrow the scope of etiology based on an enhanced medical history and physical examination by means of an associated auxiliary examination. A complete anti-nuclear antibody test, an anti-neutrophil antibody test, and a rheumatism test can be performed to exclude autoimmune vasculitis. A tumor marker, chest X-ray, and abdominal and superficial lymph node B-ultrasound examination can be performed as a preliminary screening for tumor-based diseases. Routine blood tests, C-reactive protein, ESR, Salmonella typhi antibodies, cold agglutination test, blood culture, and bone marrow culture tests can be performed to identify bacterial or nonbacterial infections. The patient in this case had symptoms of anemia, so bone marrow tests should be considered to rule out hematological disorders if necessary.

2. Auxiliary examination

Routine blood: WBC 5.5×10^9/L, N 73.8%, L 20.0%, E 0.80×10^9/L, RBC 2.87×10^{12}/L, Hb 89 g/L, PLT 120×10^9/L.

Liver and kidney function was normal.

The complete set of anti-nuclear antibodies, anti-neutrophil antibodies, rheumatism test, and tumor marker test were all normal.

C-reactive protein 130 mg/l. Erythrocyte sedimentation rate 81 mm/h.

Salmonella typhi antibodies (−), cold agglutination test (−), three blood cultures (−), PPD test (−), HIV antibody (−), blood test for plasmodium (−).

Chest radiograph and B-ultrasound examination of the abdomen and superficial lymph nodes were normal.

III. Diagnostic analysis
1. Initial diagnosis
The patient's body temperature exceeded 38.0°C for more than two weeks, and the reason remained unclear, so it should be classed as FUO (fever of unknown origin).

2. Diagnostic thinking

> **Thinking prompts:** The causes of FUO are either infectious diseases, autoimmune diseases, or neoplastic diseases.

(1) Autoimmune diseases: These diseases cause fever in the elderly, and have their own characteristics. Non-specific vasculitis is more common, often involving multiple systems and having various clinical manifestations. However, this case showed no involvement from the skin, oral cavity, and joints, and there was no multi-organ damage. The complete anti-nuclear antibodies, anti-neutrophil antibodies, and rheumatism tests were all normal, so autoimmune diseases were not considered.

(2) Tumor-related diseases: The tumor marker test, chest X-ray, and B-ultrasound of the abdomen and superficial lymph nodes in this patient were normal. However, in elderly men with fever and anemia for one month and no history of chronic blood loss and tea drinking, we cannot completely rule out hematological malignancies. Bone marrow-related examinations can be performed to identify the cause of anemia.

(3) Infectious diseases: The patient is a veterinarian who often comes into contact with animals. Fever occurs regularly, preceded by chills, so infectious disease should be considered. The patient's previous use of cephalosporins was ineffective, and infection by common bacteria was not supported, but infection by mycoplasma, chlamydia, parasites, fungi, and bacteria insensitive to cephalosporins could not be ruled out. If it is an infectious fever, what pathogen can cause it? The following is an analysis of the characteristics of a variety of pathogen infections:

1) Viral illnesses: Viral illnesses usually last no longer than two weeks, but there are exceptions, such as EB virus infection. Certain viruses cause infections of the central nervous system. However, the former is more common in children. The peripheral blood is dominated by lymphocytes, and heteromorphic lymphocytes are common. The latter should have central nervous system manifestations. In addition, long-term fever often occurs due to secondary infection with AIDS, but in this case HIV antibodies (−), so it was not considered.

2) Treponema infection: Spirochete is sensitive to most antibiotics such as penicillin and cephalosporin. This patient used cephalosporin for two weeks and it was ineffective, so it was not considered.

3) Fungal infection: The patient had no history of long-term application of immuno-suppressive agents or broad-spectrum antibiotics, nor a history of drug abuse and surgical blood

transfusion. Although he took hypoglycemic drugs for a long time, no oral leukoplakia was observed, and the chest X-ray was normal, so fungal infection was not considered.

4) Chlamydia, mycoplasma, rickettsia, and parasitic infections: The patient is a veterinarian with a history of close contact with animals. His illness had an early summer onset, which is mosquito season. The possibility of malaria and eperythrozoonosis cannot be ruled out. Peripheral blood and bone marrow smears and Weil-Felix test can be repeated to confirm.

5) Bacterial diseases: The patient's Salmonella typhi antibodies (−), PPD test (−), three blood cultures (−), chest X-ray, and abdominal B-ultrasound examination were normal, but infectious diseases such as deep tuberculosis and drug-resistant typhoid fever could not be completely ruled out because these diseases are insensitive to cephalosporins and all have a long fever course. Diagnostic treatment may be considered if necessary.

> **Thinking prompts:** Based on the above analysis, corresponding examinations can be performed, such as peripheral blood smear, bone marrow aspiration biopsy, and Weil-Felix test. In this case, symptomatic treatment was given.

IV. Ward-round analysis on the seventh day after admission

After admission, no bacterial growth was observed in multiple blood cultures and bone marrow cultures, and routine bone marrow examinations showed active proliferation of granulocyte cells and increased NAP score. A bone marrow biopsy showed normal proliferation of hematopoietic tissue. Wright's-Giemsa Staining of thin sections of peripheral blood and bone marrow revealed a large number of fuchsia Eperythrozoon on the red blood cell surface and in plasma, accounting for about 50%. The patient had a long history of contact with animals, and was diagnosed with Eperythrozoonosis. Doxycycline (0.1 g) was administered orally twice daily.

V. Condition at discharge (fifteenth day after admission)

After three days of treatment with doxycycline, the patient's body temperature decreased and his symptoms disappeared. A peripheral blood smear showed that Eperythrozoon accounted for about 10%. After one week of medication, his body temperature was normal and his symptoms disappeared. A re-examination of the peripheral blood smear showed that Eperythrozoon accounted for about 6%. C-reactive protein and ESR had decreased significantly (43.9 mg/L and 85 mm/h respectively). Peripheral blood WBC was normal, WBC classification was normal, and Hb was 110 g/L. The patient was hospitalized for a total of 15 days.

VI. Follow-up

Doxycycline was continued after discharge and stopped after two weeks. The peripheral blood smear was re-examined, and the Eperythrozoon infection rate was less than 1%. The patient's body temperature was normal one and three months after discharge.

VII. Lessons learned

As its name suggests, human Eperythrozoonosis is a zoonosis caused by Eperythrozoon. Pathogens are parasitic in the blood of various vertebrates, including rodents, poultry, and pigs. The human infection rate of Eperythrozoon in areas of animal husbandry area can reach 87%. However, the incidence is low, with sporadic manifestations and few clinical reports. The main clinical manifestations are fever, anemia, diarrhea, and lymph node enlargement. It lacks specificity, and has not attracted enough attention from clinicians, which causes difficulties for diagnosis. This case started with an etiology of FUO. The scope was slowly narrowed, combined with the patient's epidemiological history of anemia and close contact with animals, and diabetes, which may cause low immune function. Finally, the patient was diagnosed with eperythrozoonosis by a peripheral blood smear, and was treated accordingly, with success.

(Ruan Bing)

Fever, headache, and diarrhea for six days

I. Medical history

Patient: Male, 59 years old, a farmer from Xianning in Hubei Province. He was hospitalized between 2 and 7 September 2005 for fever, headache, and diarrhea for six days.

On 26 August 2005, the patient had a fever of up to 38.5°C two days after herding cattle in the rain, with persistent fever accompanied by chills, headache, slight back pain, poor appetite, nausea, diarrhea, yellow watery stools 6-10 times/day, no vomiting, no abdominal pain, no tenesmus, no runny nose, cough, or expectoration during the onset. He suffered poor sleep, lassitude, and a marked decline in strength. His urine was yellow, and there was no oliguria. He was treated with 4.0 g/d cefotaxime for two days at his local medical clinic for an upper respiratory tract infection, but the symptoms did not improve, and he was sent to our hospital.

He had a 10-year history of gastric disease, and had smoked ten cigarettes per day for 30 years.

> **Thinking prompts:** Generally, febrile illness can either be infectious fever and non-infectious fever. Infectious fever accounts for 50%–60% of the causes of fever, and its pathogens include bacteria, viruses, mycoplasma, rickettsiae, spirochetes, fungi, and parasites. The most common clinical causes of fever are viral and bacterial infections. From the onset of this case, the illness seemed to be triggered by catching a cold in the rain, followed by symptoms of fever and headache. The patient is likely to have a viral infection, especially of the upper respiratory tract. A secondary bacterial infection after the viral infection cannot be ruled out. Local infectious epidemic diseases such as epidemic hemorrhagic fever, leptospirosis, and acute schistosomiasis infection should also be considered. Dengue fever and type B epidemic encephalitis (Japanese encephalitis) should also be considered as differential diagnosis, as the onset of this case was during summer and autumn.
>
> Among the non-infectious diseases, hematopoietic diseases (such as leukemia, malignant lymphoma, malignant histiocytosis, and multiple myeloma), as well as systemic rheumatic diseases (such as systemic lupus erythematosus, multiple dermatomyositis, and polyarteritis nodosa), are common. The above diseases

can also develop due to trigger such as cold. Thromboembolic disorders can also cause non-infectious fever due to tissue necrosis, proteolysis, and necrotic tissue absorption. The age of the patient indicates that neoplastic diseases need to be differentiated. A diagnosis of drug fever and heat stroke can be ruled out because the patient has no recent history of drug use and no heat stroke.

II. Physical examination on admission

T 38.5°C, P 82 times/min, R 22 times/min, BP 88/55 mmHg, poor mental health, no bleeding spots on the skin anywhere on the body. The superficial lymph nodes were not enlarged; the conjunctiva was not congested or edematous; the pharynx was mildly hyperemia, and several scattered palatal bleeding spots were visible on the soft palate. There was no abnormality in cardiopulmonary auscultation, and no tenderness or rebound tenderness in abdomen palpation; no palpable liver or spleen. There was mild percussion pain in both kidney areas. The pathological reflexes and meningeal irritation signs were negative.

III. Auxiliary examination on admission

1. Ancillary examination on the first day of hospitalization (2 September 2005)

Routine blood test: WBC 2.8×10^9/L, N 78.2%, L 17.2%, M 4.6%, RBC 3.73×10^{12}/L, Hb 116 g/L, PLT 25×10^9/L, no abnormal lymphocytes were found.

Routine urine test: Pro (+++), BLD (+).

2. Ancillary examination after admission (4 September 2005)

Routine blood test: WBC 1.5×10^9/L, N 82.9%, L 13.7%, M 3.4%, RBC 3.88×10^{12}/L, Hb 120 g/L, PLT 13×10^9/L.

Peripheral blood smear: A small number of granulocytes showed mildly poisoned particles, and no abnormal lymphocytes were seen.

Stool test: Yellow, thin.

ESR 19 mm/h.

Liver function: ALT 411 U/L, AST 3,000 U/L, A 37.6 g/L, TB 14.6 μmol/L.

Renal function: BUN 6.4 mmol/L, Cr 78.3 μmol/L.

Serum electrolytes: K^+ 3.74 mmol/L, Na^+ 121.55 mmol/L; Cl^- 96.6 mmol/L, Ca^{2+} 1.68 mmol/L.

PT: 30.9 seconds.

IV. Diagnostic analysis

1. Preliminary diagnosis

Based on the patient's symptoms of fever, headache, and diarrhea, combined with decreased white blood cells (leukopenia) and low platelet count (thrombocytopenia) in the routine blood test, routine urine protein (+++), and impaired liver function, the preliminary diagnosis should focus on infectious diseases, followed by diseases of the hematologic and rheumatic systems.

Thinking prompts: The causes of fever, headache, and diarrhea can be systemic diseases and localized diseases. Localized nervous system diseases are either infectious or non-infectious. Among non-infectious diseases, cerebral stroke and neoplastic diseases are not common with fever and diarrhea; among the infectious diseases, epidemic meningitis and epidemic encephalitis B often have obvious symptoms of meningeal irritation or paralysis or coma. Neurological diseases can be largely excluded due to the absence of clinical signs of the nervous system. Instead, systemic diseases with clinical manifestations of fever, headache, and diarrhea should be the focus.

2. Diagnostic thinking

Further analysis of diseases that need to be considered.

(1) Infectious diseases with fever, headache, diarrhea, and elevated liver function ALT and AST indicators: Common viral diseases, such as epidemic hemorrhagic fever, dengue fever, severe acute respiratory syndromes, enterovirus infections.

1) Epidemic hemorrhagic fever (EHF): Given that there are disseminated cases in Hubei Province, EHF cannot be ruled out in the epidemic season. Fever, headache, thrombocytopenia with gastrointestinal symptoms, and palatal petechiae are consistent with the clinical manifestations of EHF. In addition, the short course of the disease, abnormal liver function, and urine protein (++++) suggest that it may be EHF. However, the patient did not have hyperemia or bleeding conjunctiva, and most notably no oliguria, no elevation in the white blood cell count in the peripheral blood, and no anomalous lymphocytes were seen. Therefore, a diagnosis of EHF cannot be established for the time being, until the detection of the pathogen-specific antibody IgM is available for differential diagnosis.

2) Dengue fever: The patient had a fever, headache, diarrhea, decreased leukocytes and platelets in the peripheral blood, and abnormal liver function, which are in line with the clinical manifestations of dengue fever. However, there was no report of dengue fever in Hubei, nor is it an endemic area. Also, the patient had not traveled to tropical and subtropical areas. Dengue fever often causes a rash, bleeding, and swollen lymph nodes, but this patient does not have the above symptoms. Therefore, it is unlikely that he had dengue fever.

3) Severe acute respiratory syndromes: Common clinical manifestations are fever (> 38°C) and coughing; shortness of breath or respiratory distress syndrome, pulmonary rales or signs of lung consolidation, no increment or reduction of the WBC count in earlier blood test. This patient had no obvious respiratory clinical manifestations; further chest X-rays should be performed to rule out severe acute respiratory syndromes.

(2) Diseases with fever, headache, diarrhea, and leukopenia: Common bacterial infections such as typhoid fever and Gram-negative bacilli sepsis.

1) Typhoid fever: The patient had a fever, headache, diarrhea, leukopenia, and abnormal liver function, all of which support a diagnosis of typhoid fever. However, since the absence of roseola (rose rash) and hepatosplenomegaly, the presence of thrombocytopenia and urinary

protein (+++), and the ineffectiveness of antibacterial treatment, a diagnosis of typhoid fever was not supported. Nevertheless, a Widal test is necessary to rule out typhoid fever. Otherwise, blood culture and bone marrow culture should be performed to confirm the diagnosis of typhoid fever.

2) Gram-negative bacilli sepsis: This disease has an acute onset, and often manifests as systemic toxic symptoms such as fever, headache, hepatosplenomegaly, and hypotensive shock. Also, a routine blood test may show a low white blood cell count, and liver and kidney functions may be impaired. However, it mostly occurs in elderly patients with severe underlying diseases, immunocompromised patients, or patients with long-term use of immunosuppressive agents such as glucocorticoids. The patient in this case used to be a physically fit manual worker, and the effect of treatment with cephalosporin was low, so the possibility of Gram-negative bacillus sepsis is not high. Nonetheless, blood culture and bone marrow culture are still needed to rule it out.

(3) Parasitic diseases: Among the parasitic diseases that present with fever, acute schisto-somiasis is the most common in Hubei, followed by trichinosis and paragonimiasis. However, these parasitic diseases often manifest as leukocytosis (increased white blood cells) and apparent eosinophils, which the patient in this case did not have.

(4) Leptospirosis: Leptospirosis may lead to fever, and damage to the liver and kidneys, but this patient had no conjunctival hyperemia, no lymph node enlargement, and no muscular pain; leptospirosis is not endemic to the local area, so the likelihood of developing it is low.

(5) Internal medicine diseases with fever, headache, and leukopenia and thrombocytopenia: These diseases include hematologic disorders such as malignant lymphoma, thrombocytopenic purpura, neutropenia, and malignant histiocytosis. A bone marrow examination is needed for further diagnosis.

(6) Rheumatic system diseases: Examples include dermatomyositis, systemic lupus erythe-matosus, and rheumatic fever. They generally have a slow onset and are predominant among females. They can lead to multi-organ damage, which can be identified by immunological indicators such as autoantibodies.

V. Examination and analysis on the second day of hospitalization
1. Examination results
Epidemic hemorrhagic fever antibodies (−), Widal test (−), antistreptolysin O test (−); chest radiographs show scattered solitary pulmonary nodules of increased density in both lung fields.

2. Further analysis and investigation
(1) The specific IgM antibody of hantavirus, which is the pathogen of epidemic hemorrhagic fever, can be detected on the second day of illness, and a four-fold increase in titer after a week is of diagnostic value. In addition, epidemic hemorrhagic fever often has a typical five-phase clinical course of fever, hypotensive shock, oliguria, polyuria, and recovery. Most severe cases with a fever period of more than five days have obvious renal function impairment. The renal

function of this patient was completely normal, combined with negative EHF-IgM antibodies, so the possibility of epidemic hemorrhagic fever can be ruled out.

(2) A negative Widal test cannot be used as an exclusion criterion for typhoid fever, because it is mostly positive in the second week of the illness; the positive rate is about 50% in the third week, and could rise to 80% in the fourth to fifth week. Therefore, a diagnosis of typhoid fever requires the results of blood and bone marrow cultures.

(3) The diagnostic criteria for rheumatic fever are made up of the primary manifestations of cardiac inflammation, polyarthritis, chorea, subcutaneous nodules, and annular erythema; secondary manifestations are arthralgia, fever, leukocytosis, anemia, and a positive anti-hemolytic streptococcus O test. The patient was elderly, and the clinical manifestations were not sufficient to meet the diagnostic criteria, so rheumatic fever can largely be ruled out.

(4) X-ray chest radiographs of severe acute respiratory syndromes typically show interstitial infiltration with varying degrees of patchy infiltrative shadows or reticular changes in the lungs. From the clinical presentation and X-ray chest findings of this patient and the absence of a local epidemic of severe acute respiratory syndromes, the disease can theoretically be ruled out.

VI. Examination and analysis on the third day of hospitalization
1. Check-up after admission (6 September 2005)
Routine blood test: WBC 1.6×10^9/L, RBC 3.34×10^{12}/L, Hb 103 g/L, PLT 20×10^9/L.

Peripheral blood smear: Granulocytes with mild to moderate toxic particles; multiple small vacuoles can be seen in the cytoplasm of some granulocytes; some granulocytes have degenerated, and abnormal lymphocytes have increased, accounting for 27%.

Both EB virus IgM and IgG antibody tests were negative.

Cytologic examination of bone marrow: Normal growth of bone marrow, and no abnormal genes are found in the gene rearrangement of bone marrow lymphoma.

Negative blood culture and bone marrow culture.

Ultrasound examination: No enlargement of the liver and spleen, no enlarged lymph nodes in the retroperitoneum.

2. Diagnosis and treatment analysis
The patient's bone marrow and blood cultures were negative on the third day after admission, coupled with the presence of heterogeneous lymphocytosis in the peripheral blood. Therefore, the possibility of infection with typhoid and common Gram-negative bacilli is unlikely, but the possibility of viral diseases (infectious mononucleosis caused by EB virus) and hematologic disease (malignant lymphoma) should be considered.

(1) Infectious mononucleosis: Clinical manifestations include fever, lymphadenopathy, angina, hepatosplenomegaly, and a rash. Laboratory examination shows that the white blood cell counts in the early stage are mostly within the normal range or slightly lower. One week after

the onset, the total number of white blood cells (mainly mononuclear cells) increases, and the serological examination shows positive for EB virus IgM or IgG antibodies. This patient had fever and lymphocytosis in the peripheral blood, but no lymphadenopathy and hepatosplenomegaly, and no rash or angina. The EB virus IgM and IgG antibody tests were both negative. Therefore, a diagnosis of infectious mononucleosis cannot be established.

(2) Malignant lymphoma: It often causes fever, accounting for about 31% to 50% of cases, and mostly starts with fever and no other obvious clinical symptoms. The cytologic examination of the patient's bone marrow revealed normal myeloid proliferation and no obvious abnormal lymphocytes; the gene rearrangement of bone marrow lymphoma was not abnormal, so malignant lymphoma can only be used as a differential diagnosis and not as the primary diagnosis.

From the above analysis, the patient had developed acute fever, headache, and diarrhea together with anomalous lymphocytosis in the peripheral blood. However, a diagnosis of infectious mononucleosis and malignant lymphoma cannot be established, so the patient should be considered as having a fever of unknown origin and a high possibility of rare pathogenic infection. He had a fever, headache, diarrhea, and peripheral blood leukopenia with toxic granules and cell degeneration, which should be considered as a leukophagocyte-dominant pathogenic infection.

VII. Treatment

Symptomatic treatment was given to prevent secondary infections. Anti-infection with 4–8 million units of penicillin, 4.0 g/d cefoperazone/sulbactam sodium, 800 mg/d antiviral with acyclovir, supportive symptomatic treatment with recombinant human granulocyte colony-stimulating factor (rhG-CSF) 150 μg/d and plasma and treatment with dexamethasone (10 mg/d for six days) were given.

The patient's condition gradually worsened after admission. On the fourth day, he was suffering from poor spirits, lethargy, visible ecchymosis at acupuncture sites, and bulbar conjunctival chemosis. On the fifth day, he went into a trance with convulsions, neck stiffness (width of one finger), and the Babinski's sign (+). There was no shock or oliguria during the course of the disease. He was discharged against medical advice on the sixth day of hospitalization, and died two days later. Subsequently, two members of his family were admitted to hospital with similar clinical manifestations, providing epidemiological feedback for the diagnosis and treatment of the patient.

VIII. Family members

Family member A: Male, 36 years old, the eldest son of the patient. He had close contact with his father. He was admitted to hospital with fever and headache for five days and diarrhea for two days. Family member A developed fever without apparent cause on 16 September 2005, with a highest temperature of 39.2°C, accompanied by chills, dull forehead pain, and no upper respiratory tract catarrhal symptoms. On 20 September, diarrhea and loose yellow stools occurred 3–4 times; there were no bloody purulent stools accompanied with nausea, and no vomiting; poor sleep, poor spirits, weakened physical strength, poor appetite, and normal urination. He was treated for an upper respiratory tract infection at a local hospital for two days, but the effect was not good. The patient had previously been in good physical health.

Physical examination on admission: T 39.0°C, P 88 beats/min, R 20 beats/min, BP 110/85 mmHg, poor spirits, no cutaneous petechiae; no enlargement of the superficial lymph nodes; no conjunctival hyperemia; mild pharynx hyperemia; no positive signs in the heart, lungs, and abdomen; mild percussive pain in both kidneys.

Outpatient data: Routine blood WBC $1.9 \times 10^9/L$, N 70.7%, L 21.1%, M 8.2%, RBC $4.71 \times 10^{12}/L$, PLT $100 \times 10^9/L$; a small number of granulocytes were seen with mildly toxic granules; no anomalous lymphocytes were seen. After admission, he was examined as follows: WBC $1.3 \times 10^9/L$, N 55.2%, L 39.1%, RBC $4.3 \times 10^{12}/L$, PLT $44 \times 10^9/L$, ESR normal; routine urinalysis: Pro (+++); liver function: ALT 142 U/L, AST 278 U/L, A and TB normal; renal function normal. PT and APTT were normal; blood and stool cultures were negative; bone marrow findings suggested normal hyperplasia; CD4 and CD8 were normal; Widal test (–); chest radiograph was normal. After anti-infection, thymosin α1, Recombinant Human Thrombopoietin (TPIAO), diammonium glycyrrhizinate, and aminomethylbenzoic acid (PAMA), and supportive symptomatic treatments, family member A had a normal body temperature on 25 September. He recovered and was discharged from hospital on 15 October.

Family member B: Female, 57 years old, wife and cohabitee of the patient. She was admitted to hospital for fever, headache, and diarrhea for two days. The symptoms, signs, and laboratory tests were similar to those of family member A. After supportive symptomatic treatment, family member B recovered and was discharged from hospital on 15 October.

IX. Summary and analysis of the three cases

1. Epidemiological data:

No abnormally dead or sick pigs, cattle, sheep, or poultry were found in the local area, nor were there any cases of dengue fever or leptospirosis. None of the three patients had a recent history of traveling or living abroad. Neither the villagers who had come into close contact with the first patient, the medical staff who treated him, nor the patients in the same ward had the disease. Family members A and B had a history of close contact with the first patient (including living and eating together, having contact with his blood and body fluids, and scrubbing his body).

2. Clinical features

(1) The main complaints were fever, headache, and diarrhea; no cough, and no upper respiratory tract catarrhal symptoms. There was proteinuria, but no oliguria and no blood urea nitrogen (BUN) or abnormal creatinine (Cr).

(2) Signs: The highest body temperature was 38.4°C–39.6°C. Along with mild pharynx hyperemia, palatal petechiae can be seen in severely ill patients. On admission, there are no

positive signs in the heart, lungs, and abdomen. Severely ill patients had complicated lung infections and mild percussive pain in both kidneys.

3. Laboratory data
Routine blood tests in the three cases showed a progressive decrease in WBC and PLT, urine protein (+)–(+++), liver function abnormalities, normal blood BUN and Cr, various degrees of abnormalities in serum electrolytes, a negative Widal test, and negative blood culture; bone marrow cytology examination revealed normal hyperplasia, and severely ill patients had cell degeneration and contained toxic particles.

4. Diagnosis
The three patients with a history of close contact and successive onsets had fever, headache, diarrhea, leukopenia (cell degeneration containing toxic particles), and multiple organ damage. The diagnosis was considered as infectious febrile illness with unknown causes – possibly a leukophagocyte-dominant pathogen.

X. Final diagnosis
1. Etiological diagnosis: Blood from the three patients was sent to the National Center for Disease Control for testing, and an etiological diagnosis of Anaplasma phagocytophilum was made.
2. Disease diagnosis: Human granulocytic anaplasmosis.

XI. Lessons learned
Due to the rare onset and atypical clinical symptoms of human granulocytic anaplasmosis, it cannot easily be differentiated from many viral infectious diseases. There are no clinically applicable etiological diagnostic reagents, which makes it difficult to diagnose in an early stage, and poses difficulties for treatment. In addition, there is no epidemic or occurrence of the disease in Hubei Province. The first patient was in a serious condition. His illness progressed rapidly, and he eventually died. The other two patients' conditions were mild, and they were discharged after supportive symptomatic treatment.

Human granulocytic anaplasmosis (HGA) is a tick-borne infection caused by Anaplasma phagocytophilum (formerly known as human granulocytic ehrlichiae) that infects neutrophils in human peripheral blood and leads to fever presenting with leukopenia, thrombocytopenia, and multiple organ dysfunction. Since the first case of human granulocytic anaplasmosis was reported in 1994 in the United States, about 600–800 cases have been reported annually there in recent years. In 2006, a case was found in Anhui Province, and there were suspected cases in some other provinces. The clinical symptoms of the disease are similar to those of some viral diseases, leading to easy misdiagnosis. In severe cases, it can lead to death. Phagocyte anaplasma (Figures 45-1 and 45-2) belongs to rickettsiales, Anaplasmaceae, and the Anaplasma genus.

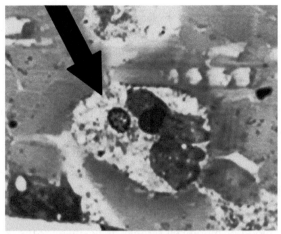

Figure 45-1 Anaplasma inclusion bodies in neutrophils in human blood (× 1,000)

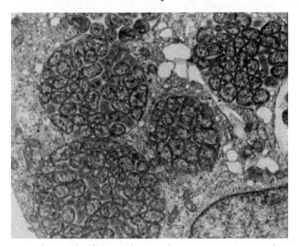

Figure 45-2 Anaplasma inclusion bodies under an electron microscope (× 21,960)

The incubation period of human granulocytic anaplasmosis is generally seven to 14 days (average of nine days). With acute onset, the main symptoms are fever (mostly persistent high fever, which can be 40°C or more), general malaise, fatigue, headache, muscle aches, nausea, vomiting, anorexia, and diarrhea. Some patients also develop coughing and a sore throat. Physical examination shows apathetic expression and relatively slow pulse; a few patients may have superficial lymph node enlargement and a rash. It may be accompanied by damage to multiple organs such as the heart, liver, and kidneys, with corresponding clinical manifestations.

In severe cases, patients may have interstitial pneumonia, pulmonary edema, acute respiratory distress syndrome, and secondary bacterial, viral, and fungal infections. A small number of patients may experience bleeding from the skin, lungs, and digestive tract due to severe thrombocytopenia and abnormal blood coagulation. If they are not treated in time, they may die due to respiratory failure, acute renal failure, multi-organ failure, and disseminated intravascular coagulation.

Laboratory examination of the peripheral blood shows a low white blood cell and platelet count, and increased abnormal lymphocytes. Patients with organ damage have abnormal heart, liver, and kidney function test results. Etiological and serological tests are positive. White blood cell count and thrombocytopenia in routine blood tests can be used as important clues for early diagnosis. In the first week of onset, patients tend to show a reduction in the white blood cell count, mostly $(1.0–3.0) \times 10^9/L$; reduction in platelets, mostly $(30–50) \times 10^9/L$. Abnormal lymphocytes can be seen.

Etiological and serological tests: The serologic indirect immunofluorescence antibody (IFA) test for IgM and IgG antibodies of Anaplasma phagocytophilum are both positive in the acute phase; the IFA test for serological detection of IgG antibodies of Anaplasma phagocytophilum in the recovery phase is four times or higher than in the acute phase; a PCR test of the whole blood or blood cell samples is positive for the specific nucleic acid of phagocytic anaplasma, and sequence analysis confirms that the homology with phagocytic anaplasma is more than 99%; isolated pathogens.

Antibiotics should be used early in treatment to avoid complications. Empirical treatment can be carried out for suspected cases. Hormonal drugs are generally used with caution, to avoid aggravating the condition. Etiological treatment uses doxycycline or tetracycline. When the etiology is unknown, general treatment includes: Bed rest, a high-calorie diet, moderate vitamins, liquid or semi-liquid food, plenty of water, oral hygiene, and skin hygiene. For severely ill patients, sufficient fluids and electrolytes should be supplemented to maintain a good balance of water, electrolytes, and acid-base; those who are weak or malnourished, or have hypoalbuminemia can be given gastrointestinal nutrition, fresh plasma, albumin, and gamma globulin, to improve their bodily functions and immunity.

Prognosis: According to foreign reports, the fatality rate is less than 1%. If treated in time, most patients can have a good prognosis. Severe complications such as sepsis, toxic shock syndrome, toxic myocarditis, acute kidney failure, acute respiratory distress syndrome, diffuse intravascular coagulation, and multiple organ failure can lead to death.

(**Tian Deying**)

Fever with muscle soreness for four days

I. Medical history

Patient: Male, 24 years old, a student from Nanjing. He was admitted to hospital in the afternoon of 27 November 2007, due to a fever with muscle soreness for four days.

Four days previously, the patient experienced fever with aversion to cold, headache, and muscle soreness with no obvious inducements. During the fever there were no obvious chills, but occasional coughing, a small amount of sticky yellow sputum, and no nasal congestion or sore throat. The patient was admitted to a neighborhood hospital that evening, with a temperature of up to 40°C and was prescribed with anti-infection and antipyretic treatments including cephalosporin. His symptoms persisted, and his body temperature remained at 39°C–40°C, so he was sent to our hospital for further diagnosis and treatment. Since the onset, the patient had been in poor spirits with mediocre sleep, but no abnormalities in his urine and stool.

The patient was bitten on the right index finger by a puppy on 30 October. The wound was immediately flushed, and the patient was vaccinated against rabies. He had no history of typhoid fever, hepatitis, tuberculosis, or food or drug allergies. He had recently been home to study for an exam, but had no history of traveling or eating unclean food.

II. Physical examination and auxiliary examination on admission

1. Physical examination

T 40.1°C, P 117 times/min, R 20 times/min, BP 120/85 mmHg. Clear consciousness, low spirits, appearance of hyperthermia, active position, and cooperative during the examination. There was no yellow staining of the skin and sclera, no petechiae or ecchymosis, and no enlargement of the superficial lymph nodes. His neck was soft and non-resistant, and there was a negative hepatojugular reflux sign. The breath sounds in both lungs were slightly coarse, and no dry and moist rales were heard. His heart rate was 117 beats/min with a uniform rhythm. No murmurs were heard in the valve areas. His abdomen was flat and soft with no pressure pain; his liver and spleen were not palpable below the costal margin. There was no percussion pain in the liver and kidney area, and negative shifting dullness. A healing wound was seen on the index finger of his right hand, and a traumatic crust of about 1 cm in diameter was noted on the medial side of the left knee, with no edema in either of the lower limbs.

2. Auxiliary examination

Blood count: WBC 7.1 × 10⁹/L, N 88.4%, Hb 123 g/L, PLT 88 × 10⁹/L.

Routine urine and stool tests were normal; a heterophilic agglutination test was negative.

X-ray chest radiograph (Figure 46-1) showed patchy blurred shadows on the left lower lung, suggesting infection.

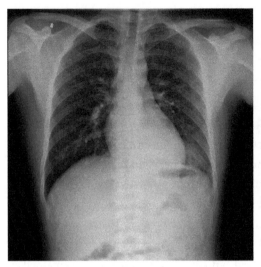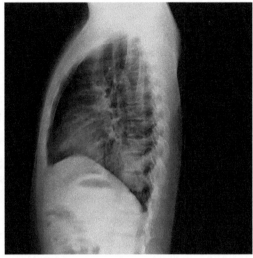

Figure 46-1 The patient's frontal and lateral chest radiographs (27 November) Patchy blurred shadows in the left lower lung

III. Ward-round analysis on admission
1. Preliminary diagnosis of lower left pneumonia

> **Thinking prompts:** The patient was a young male with an acute onset, and a persistent high fever with a mild cough; there was a slightly high neutrophil ratio on routine blood tests. A chest X-ray showed an infectious lesion in the left lower lung, so a clinical diagnosis of left lower pneumonia could be made. However, the etiology could not yet be determined, and the type of pneumonia should be considered.

2. Diagnostic thinking

(1) Bacterial pneumonia: This accounts for 80% of all types of pathogenic pneumonia in adults. With the wide application of antimicrobial drugs, some new features of bacterial pneumonia have emerged, including a change in the pathogenic spectrum, a significant increase in the rate of Gram-negative bacilli in hospital pneumonia, and the predominance of Streptococcus pneumoniae among the pathogens of community-acquired pneumonia, but clinical manifestations tend to be atypical. Bacterial resistance rates have increased, and so-called refractory pneumonia is common, with high mortality rates, especially in children, the elderly, and immunosuppressed patients.

The clinical features are fever, cough, sputum, and chest pain. The sputum properties are indicative of the pathogenic factors – usually rust-colored sputum in typical Streptococcus pneumoniae, pus and blood in Staphylococcus aureus pneumonia sputum, emerald-green pus in Pseudomonas aeruginosa pneumonia sputum, and brick-red jelly-like sputum in Klebsiella pneumonia.

(2) Viral pneumonia: Most patients have a headache, fever, myalgia, and cough with mucopurulent sputum. The most common finding on a chest X-ray is interstitial pneumonia or thickening of the peripheral bronchial walls. The white blood cell counts in routine blood tests are often low or normal; a diagnosis of viral pneumonia is supported by sputum smear findings of sparse bacteria and large numbers of mononuclear cells, or failure to find a possible bacterial pathogen.

(3) Mycoplasma pneumonia: This accounts for about 10% of all pneumonias, and is the most common pathogen of primary atypical pneumonia. The clinical onset is slow, with initial fatigue, headache, sore throat, fever, muscle aches, and loss of appetite. The headache is more pronounced. Two to three days later, there are obvious respiratory symptoms, such as a paroxysmal cough with a small amount of mucus or mucopurulent sputum, sometimes with blood in the sputum. The lung lesions show diverse X-ray manifestations, with early cases showing increased texture and reticulated shadows, which later develop into speckled flaky or uniform faint shadows, deeper near the hilum and more in the lower lobe.

(4) Legionella pneumonia: Most patients develop flu-like symptoms, with discomfort, fever, headache, and myalgia. This is followed by coughing, which is initially sputum-free and later mucus-like. It is characterized by persistent high fever and may be accompanied by relatively slow pulse, and diarrhea is also more common. Unilateral patchy lung segments or large lobar alveolar infiltrates are seen on chest X-ray in the early stages of the disease, and bilateral lesions may appear as the disease progresses, pleural effusion is more common. Peripheral blood WBC is moderately increased, and serum biochemistry is mostly seen with hyponatremia and hypophosphatemia, and there may be abnormal liver function tests and impaired renal function.

3. Further diagnosis and treatment

The clinical diagnosis was first considered to be bacterial pneumonia, based on the patient's medical history, symptoms and signs, and laboratory findings. On the day of hospitalization, he was given Piperacillin and sulbactam sodium to fight infection and Ambroxol (Mucosolvan) for coughing and expectoration.

IV. Further diagnosis and treatment process
1. Progress of disease and treatment in the early stage of admission

On the evening of the day of hospitalization, the patient's body temperature was 40°C, and could not be reduced to normal after antipyretic physical and drug treatment. There was no obvious headache or other accompanying symptoms, but the cough was worse than before with a large amount of yellow mucous sputum. The patient started to have frequent diarrhea with diluted yellow stool.

Physical examination: Clear consciousness, poor spirits, no petechiae or ecchymosis in the skin and mucosa; low-pitched breathing sounds in both lungs with no rales; heart sounds strong and rhythmic, with no murmur; flat and soft abdomen, no pressure pain or rebound pain; the liver and spleen were not palpable below the costal margin; no edema in either of the lower limbs.

Routine blood re-examination: WBC 3.2×10^9/L, N 90.9%, Hb 139 g/L, PLT 76×10^9/L; routine urine test: Urine protein (+), WBC 29.4/μl; blood biochemistry: ALT 17.3 U/L, AST 43.8 U/L, AKP 55.0 U/L, GGT 12.1 U/L, CK 85 U/L, LDH 328 U/L, HBDL 274 U/L, TP 59.9 g/L, A 36.8 g/L, G 23.1 g/L; ESR 10 mm/h, negative Widal test, negative serum hepatitis B virus markers, anti-HIV antibodies, anti-HCV antibodies, and syphilis spirochete antibodies.

On the second day of hospitalization (28 November) at 3:00, the patient experienced irritability, dyspnea, coughing, and coughing with dark red sputum.

Physical examination: BP 110/70 mHg, R32 times/min, P110 times/min. The skin of the extremities was slightly cyanotic; consciousness was clear, both lungs made sputum sounds, which were more obvious in the left lung; the heart rhythm was uniform, and no pathological murmur was heard; the abdomen was flat and soft, and there was no edema in either of the lower limbs. Oxygen was administered immediately, pulse oxygen saturation was measured at 85%, and an electrocardiogram showed sinus tachycardia. Pulmonary infection with left heart failure was considered. The patient was put on non-invasive ventilator-assisted breathing, as well as supportive symptomatic treatment such as 20 mg furosemide, 100 mg hydrocortisone, 200 mg dobutamine + saline at 3 μg/(kg*min) intravenously. The patient had some improvement in dyspnea; there was no cyanosis of the skin of the extremities; pulse oxygen saturation 89%; sputum sounds in both lungs decreased significantly, heart rate 108 beats/min.

From noon onwards on the third day of hospitalization (29 November), the patient was agitated, with open-mouthed breathing at 50–60 breaths/min. With the use of a non-invasive ventilator FiO$_2$ 100%, blood gas analysis pH 7.164, PaCO$_2$ 52.7 mHg, PaO$_2$ 60 mHg and SaO$_2$ around 85%. Since the patient's respiratory failure was aggravated, and the use of a non-invasive ventilator was ineffective, he was treated with mechanical ventilation via tracheal intubation. To reduce the man-machine confrontation caused by agitation, propofol (isoproterenol) was given to sedate the patient before intubation, and a small dose of midazolam was pumped continuously after mechanical ventilation. Furosemide and mannitol were given to reduce cerebral edema by dehydration and diuresis, and intravenous sodium bicarbonate was given to correct acidosis. The patient was in a shallow coma, with equal pupils 2 m. in diameter, reaction to light, 30 spontaneous respirations/min, slightly cyanotic lips, slightly coarse breath sounds in both lungs, extensive moist rales, rhythmic heart rate of 130 beats/min, and poor blood circulation in the extremities.

Routine blood re-examination: WBC 0.8×10^9/L, N 71.7%, Hb 136 g/L, PLT 58×10^9/L. Urine routine test: Urine occult blood (+++), urine protein (+), WBC 28/μl. test troponin T < 0.1 ng/ml, myoglobin 166 μg/L. ALT 73.0 U/L, Cr 36.1 μmol/L, BUN 13.35 mmol/L.

AST 224.0 U/L, Cr 367.1 μmol/L, BUN 13.35 mmol/L. PT 16.6 seconds, APTT 97.6 seconds, TT (plasma prothrombin time) 54 seconds, FIB (fibrinogen) 1.98 g/L. CRP (29 November) 173 mg/L. X-ray chest radiograph suggested severe infection in both lungs (Figure 46-2).

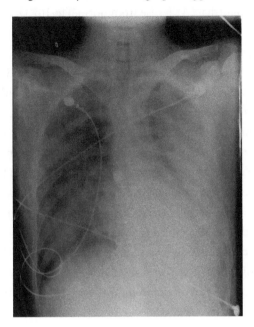

Figure 46-2 The patient's frontal chest radiograph (29 November)
The lesions in both lungs were significantly aggravated, and the left side had become white.

To fight infection and protect vital organ function, antimicrobial drugs were adjusted to 0.5 mg imipenem-cilastatin sodium every six hours, 400 mg moxifloxacin (Bayflor) once daily, and 40 mg glucocorticoid methylprednisolone twice a day by intravenous drip. Symptomatic and supportive therapy such as reduced glutathione sodium (Guladin), diammonium glycyrrhizate, mucosolvan, human albumin, gamma-globulin, and maintenance of the water-electrolyte and acid-base balance were also given.

2. Ward-round analysis on the fourth day after admission

The patient was admitted to hospital with left lower pneumonia. His condition could not be controlled by regular antibacterial drugs combined with anti-infective treatment, so he was placed on continuous mechanical ventilation.

Physical examination: BP 125–135/80–95 mmHg, heart rate 80–90 beats/min, cool extremities, coarse breath sounds in both lungs, audible moist rales, and low breath sounds in the back. The heart sounds were still strong and rhythmic. ECG monitoring showed SaO_2 85%-90%, blood gas analysis: pH 7.364, $PaCO_2$ 39 mmHg, PaO_2 57 mmHg, SaO_2 88%. A chest radiograph suggested no significant improvement of the infection in both lungs from before, with pleural effusion. Routine blood (30 November) WBC 0.7×10^9/L, N 64.8%, Hb 141 g/L, PLT 66×10^9/L.

The process of the patient's illness was reviewed, with the following features: ① Acute febrile onset with muscle aches and cough, and mild transient diarrhea. ② A chest X-ray showed rapid progression of the pulmonary lesions, spreading to both lungs. ③ After treatment with strong antibacterial drugs, the condition did not improve, rapidly progressing to respiratory failure and multi-organ functional impairment. ④ The latest laboratory tests: WBC and PLT in the peripheral blood showed a progressive decrease, suggesting serious damage to the hematological system; biochemical indexes were significantly abnormal (ALT rose from normal to 107 U/L in the latest examination, AST rose from normal to 374 U/L, Cr rose from normal to 352.3 μmol/L, BUN rose from normal to 10.14 mmol/L; CK rose from 85 U/ L to 341 U/L, LDH from 328 U/L to 1,446 U/L, HBDL from 274 U/L to 1,091 U/L) suggesting extensive involvement of bodily tissues and organs. ⑤ Coagulation indicators were significantly prolonged: PT 15.4 seconds, APTT 180.1 seconds, TT 120.1 seconds. ⑥ Progressive increase in CRP: From 173 mg/L to 245 mg/L; progressive decrease in complement: C3 from 0.96 g/L to 0.62 g/L and C4 from 0.577 g/L to 0.0545 g/L, suggesting that disease progression may be associated with abnormal inflammatory response. ⑦ Chest fluid examination: Positive Rivalta test, LDH 3,036 U/L, TP 35.6 g/L, ADA 53.6 U/L. ⑧ Blood, stool, sputum, and bone marrow bacterial cultures were negative; antibody tests for Mycoplasma pneumoniae and Legionella were negative, suggesting that the pathogen may not be a common one, and that the scope of pathogen examination should be expanded. ⑨ Although there was a history of minor skin breakage from pet dog bites, the clinical course could exclude the possibility of rabies. There was no history of contact with wildlife and birds and no recent travel, and there was no epidemiological basis for emerging infectious diseases such as SARS and avian influenza.

Based on the patient's current clinical symptoms, signs, and ancillary findings, the clinical diagnosis was severe pneumonia, acute respiratory distress syndrome (ARDS), and multi-organ functional impairment (MODS). Comprehensive analysis of the disease's rapid progression showed that severe pneumonia was the initiating factor for ARDS and MODS. Based on the patient's clinical features, mycoplasma and legionella pneumonia could be ruled out initially. Although antimicrobial drug treatment failed to control the disease, the patient may have developed sepsis secondary to bacterial infection, and the subsequent release of bacterial toxins and mediators of the organism's inflammatory response may have caused multi-organ functional damage as well as inducing ARDS. Since the patient's onset was late autumn and early winter (the high season of respiratory infectious diseases), there was no clear epidemiological basis, and the possibility of emerging respiratory infectious diseases such as severe acute respiratory syndrome (SARS) and human avian influenza should still be considered. Therefore, further diagnostic and treatment measures are based on continuing antimicrobial therapy, focusing on correcting ARDS and maintaining the function of vital organs, reducing tissue damage from inflammatory mediators, and improving the imbalance of the body's internal environment, as well as collecting blood and respiratory secretions to send to the provincial Center for Disease Control and Prevention (CDC) for etiological detection.

Treatment regimen: Anti-infection with a combination of imipenem-cilastatin sodium, moxifloxacin, and teicoplanin; 500 mg methylprednisolone daily to inhibit inflammatory mediators and increase tissue tolerance; maintenance of mechanical ventilation and continuous chest drainage to improve ventilation and respiratory function; continuous blood purification to remove inflammatory mediators and improve renal function. The patient was treated with granulocyte-macrophage colony-stimulating factor (GM-CSF) to improve granulocyte deficiency and platelet supplementation; high-dose mucosolvan to reduce sputum and cough, low molecular heparin to combat DIC, and supportive therapy such as plasma, human albumin, and globulin, as well as comprehensive treatment measures to correct the water, electrolyte, and acid-base balance.

3. Late progression and diagnosis

On the fifth day after admission (1 December), the patient's condition did not improve after the above treatment. He was in a shallow coma, with both pupils equal in size (about 4 m. in diameter), and a blunted light reflex. He was breathing 16 times/minute spontaneously, with cyanosis of the lips and mouth, coarse breath sounds in both lungs, and a few moist rales. Blood pressure was 125/80 mHg, heart rate was 135 beats/min, with a uniform rhythm. The patient's abdomen was flat and soft, and bowel sounds were absent.

Blood gas analysis: pH 7.474, PaO_2 44 mmHg, $PaCO_2$ 36 mmHg, HCO_3^- 26.4 mmol/L, SO_2 83%. Peripheral blood picture: WBC 5.1×10^9/L, N 88.6%, Hb 105 g/L, PLT 40×10^9/L. CRP 199 mg/L. Renal function: Cr 258.2 μmol/L, BUN 11.94 mmol/L. X-ray examination showed infection in both lungs (Figure 46-3).

Sputum culture was negative. The provincial CDC tested the patient's respiratory samples:

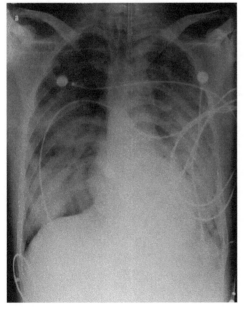

Figure 46-3 Frontal chest radiograph (1 December)
  Both lungs became white, and the lesion was aggravated further.

Positive for H5 and positive for N1 of avian influenza virus nucleic acid. Acinetobacter baumannii, Mycoplasma pneumoniae, Chlamydia pneumoniae, Legionella pneumophila, Streptococcus pneumoniae, Neisseria meningitidis, Haemophilus influenzae, and adenovirus were all negative.

At 01:30 on the sixth day after admission (2 December), the patient's heart rate dropped from 130 beats/min to 88 beats/min, and his blood pressure dropped to about 70/30 mHg. There was no improvement after treatment with hypertensive and cardiotonic drugs, and by 03:40 his heartbeat and spontaneous respiration stopped. The patient died after unsuccessful resuscitation. Respiratory fluid test results from the China National CDC were positive for avian influenza virus nucleic acid H5, and N1 positive. According to the WHO's definition and Chinese diagnostic criteria of confirmed cases of human infections with highly pathogenic avian influenza (HPAI), the patient was a confirmed case of human HPAI.

V. Lessons learned

See Case 47.

(Li Jun & Huang Zuhu)

Fever and cough for two days

I. Medical history

Patient: Male, 52 years old, an engineering technician from Nanjing. He was admitted to hospital on 4 December, with fever and cough for two days.

This man was the father of the patient with human avian influenza in Case 46. A total of 69 people who were in close contact with Case 46 were placed under medical observation. The 52-year-old patient was at the hospital with his son for one day on 28 November. Since 1 December, he had taken oseltamivir (Tamiflu) 75 mg/d as a preventive drug. On 3 December, he developed a low fever, and the dosage of oseltamivir was increased to 75 mg twice a day. Cefradine was added to his treatment, and on 4 December, his body temperature increased to over 39°C, and he was admitted to hospital at 23:30 the same night. After the onset of the illness, he had a mild cough, no headache, no vomiting, no diarrhea, and a mild feeling of fatigue.

He had no recent history of exposure to wild animals or poultry, and no history of travel.

II. Physical examination and auxiliary examination on admission

1. Physical examination

T 39.2°C, R 23 times/minute, P 80 times/minute, BP 118/60 mmHg, clear consciousness, fine mental state. The breath sounds of both lower lungs were slightly diminished, and there were no moist rales. The heart sounds were low and dull; no murmurs were heard in the valves, the heart rhythm was uniform, the abdomen was flat and soft, and the liver and spleen were not palpable below the costal margin. There were no abnormalities in the spine and limbs, and no positive signs in the neurological examination.

2. Auxiliary examination

Routine blood: WBC 6.7×10^9/L, N 81.9%, L 15.8%.

Absolute value of lymphocytes 1.06×10^9/L, PLT: 99×10^9/L, AST 44 U/L.

X-ray examination: Double lower pneumonia (Figure 47-1).

Blood gas analysis: pH 7.48, $PaCO_2$ 27 mHg, PaO_2 59 mHg, HCO_3^- 23.1 mmol/L.

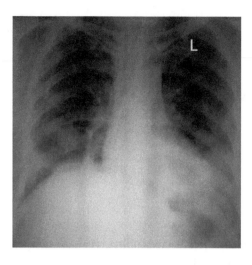

Figure 47-1 The patient's frontal chest radiograph (5 December)
Double lower pneumonia

III. Diagnosis and treatment

1. Preliminary diagnosis

Double lower pneumonia.

> **Thinking prompts:** The patient had a fever and respiratory symptoms; the peripheral blood image showed normal total WBC and a high neutrophil ratio; CT showed double lower pneumonia. Accordingly, the condition was identified as a lower respiratory tract infection. However, the specific etiology still needed to be determined by further examination, and had to be considered from epidemiological and clinical perspectives.

2. Diagnostic thinking

(1) Human avian influenza: The patient had been in close contact with a confirmed case of human avian influenza. The disease developed while under medical observation, and there were clear pulmonary lesions, so the possibility of human avian influenza was extremely high. However, it is believed that human avian influenza does not yet have a pathogenic biological basis for human-to-human transmission, and the few cases of family aggregation that have occurred cannot be identified as such. Therefore, although it cannot be completely ruled out in this case, a diagnosis should be made with great caution, and must rely on definitive etiology evidence.

(2) Other viral pneumonia: The patient was in his 50s, and suffered high mental stress and physical fatigue prior to his illness. He did not have severe respiratory symptoms, and did not have a high total WBC count in his peripheral blood, which did not rule out the possibility of viral pneumonia.

(3) Bacterial pneumonia: The patient had an acute onset and high fever. Although the total WBC in his peripheral blood was not high, the proportion of neutrophils was, so the possibility of bacterial pneumonia could not be ruled out.

3. Initial treatment plan

Based on the above analysis, the following treatment measures were taken: A respiratory specimen was immediately collected and sent to the provincial CDC for nucleic acid testing for the avian influenza virus H5 and N1; the dose of oseltamivir (a drug used to treat the avian influenza virus) was increased to 75 mg three times a day; cefoperazone/tazobactam (Sulperazon) and levofloxacin were given as combined antibacterial therapy; the patient's condition was closely observed.

4. Subsequent treatment course

On the second day of hospitalization (5 December), the patient had T 39.9°C, R 35 times/minute, P 120 times/minute, BP 112/78 mmHg. CT showed an extended intrapulmonary shadow and new lesions in both lung fields.

The same day, the provincial CDC tested the patient's respiratory tract samples, which were positive for avian influenza virus H5 and N1 nucleic acid. The following day, the Chinese National CDC also tested the patient's respiratory tract sample, and found it positive for the H5 and N1 nucleic acids of the avian influenza virus. According to the WHO's definition and Chinese diagnostic criteria, the patient was a confirmed case of human HPAI.

Immediately after diagnosis, the treatment regimen was adjusted to oseltamivir (150 mg twice daily) combined with Rimantadine (100 mg twice daily) for antiviral treatment, levofloxacin 400 mg/d to prevent infection, methylprednisolone (80 mg/d) to inhibit tissue damage by inflammatory mediators, and non-invasive assisted respiration to improve hypoxemia, as well as supportive therapy such as supplementation with human albumin and globulin.

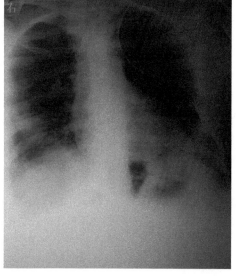

On the third day after admission (6 December), the patient's temperature decreased from 40°C to 38°C, but he had mild diarrhea with 2–3 stools/day without mucus, pus, or blood. Fine moist rales could be heard in both lower lungs on physical examination. There were no red blood cells or pus cells in the routine examination, and WBC and PLT showed a downward trend. An X-ray chest radiograph showed progression of a high-density shadow in the middle and lower parts of both lungs (Figure 47-2). Blood gas analysis showed pH 7.46, PaCO$_2$ 28 mHg, PaO$_2$ 66 mHg, HCO$_3^-$ 21.5 mmol/L (oxygen flow rate 5.5 L/min).

Figure 47-2 The patient's frontal chest radiography (6 December)
There was progression of a high-density shadow in the middle and lower part of both lungs.

Thinking prompts (the third day of hospitalization): Focus on the development of the disease and further treatment measures.

On the third day of hospitalization, the patient was receiving active treatment. Although his hyperthermic state improved, the peripheral blood WBC and PLT continued to decline, the pulmonary lesions were progressing, and the arterial oxygen partial pressure continued to be lower than normal, all suggesting that the disease had not been fully nor effectively controlled and was still on the verge of exacerbation.

In terms of treatment, antiviral, antibacterial, and anti-inflammatory mediators and supportive symptomatic measures are more comprehensive and adequate. As in cases of human avian influenza in other provinces and cities, it is recommended to use infusions of specific immune plasma to enhance the patient's antiviral capacity.

On the fourth day of hospitalization (7 December), 400 ml of human immune plasma treatment with an inactivated H5N1 avian influenza virus vaccine was slowly infused intravenously in two separate infusions (at 01:00 and 05:00), which went smoothly.

In the afternoon of 7 December, blood gas analysis showed pH 7.456, $PaCO_2$ 30.5 mmHg, PaO_2 99 mmHg, SaO_2 98% (oxygen flow rate 4 L/min); an X-ray chest radiograph showed that the original high-density shadow in the middle and lower lungs of both lungs had decreased. The absorption of high-density shadow in the left lower lung was obvious.

On the fifth day of hospitalization (8 December), the patient's body temperature returned to normal and his general condition improved; an X-ray chest radiograph showed that the right lower lung lesions had stabilized, and the remaining lung lesions did not progress significantly; WBC and PLT counts were both on the rise.

In view of the improvement of the patient's condition, the drug dosage was adjusted to oseltamivir 75 mg twice daily and methylprednisolone 60 mg/d.

On the sixth day of hospitalization (9 December), the patient suffered hallucinations, anxiety, and hand tremors. Blood gas analysis: pH 7.404, $PaCO_2$ 30.7 mmHg, PaO_2 76 mmHg, SaO_2 96% (oxygen flow rate 4 L/min). An X-ray examination showed a continued improvement in the absorption of the lung lesions.

Thinking prompts (sixth day of hospitalization): After broad treatment, the patient's condition had obviously improved, and the prognosis was relatively optimistic. However, symptoms such as hallucinations, anxiety, and limb tremors were present, the causes of which had to be analyzed and managed.

The patient had no history of neurological or psychiatric disorders, and there was no other evidence of central nervous system involvement in this illness. The antiviral drugs oseltamivir (a neuraminidase inhibitor) and Rimantadine (an ion channel M2 blocker) currently being administered had been reported as having psychiatric and neurological adverse events. The dosage of oseltamivir in this case was large, so the possibility of drug-induced adverse reactions had to be taken seriously.

Considering that the patient had been on antiviral therapy for more than a week, his condition was stabilizing, and the lung lesions continued to be absorbed according to the X-ray. Therefore, it was decided to discontinue oseltamivir and Rimantadine. Methylprednisolone was reduced to 40 mg/d, and then reduced again to 20 mg/d two days later, being discontinued on 13 December.

On the eighth day of hospitalization (11 December), the patient's hallucinations and limb tremors disappeared; on the ninth day of hospitalization (12 December), blood gas analysis: pH 7.462, $PaCO_2$ 33.2 mHg, PaO_2 91 mHg, SaO_2 96%.

On the tenth day of hospitalization (13 December), routine blood: WBC 8.03×10^9/L, N 66.0%, L 23.0%, absolute lymphocyte value 1.85×10^9/L, PLT 212×10^9/L. An X-ray chest radiograph showed that both lung lesions had been mostly absorbed (Figure 47-3).

On the twenty-first day of hospitalization (24 December), provincial and municipal expert groups agreed that the patient had met the full discharge criteria for human avian influenza cases in China, and unanimously agreed to discharge him for continued recuperation and rehabilitation.

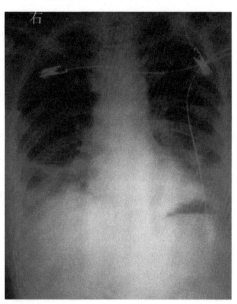

Figure 47-3 The patient's frontal chest radiograph (12 December)
The lesions in both lungs were mostly absorbed.

IV. Follow-up

A month after discharge, the patient came to the hospital for a follow-up examination, and was in a good general condition, with normal blood, liver, and kidney function, and a normal chest X-ray.

V. Lessons learned

1. Timely and accurate diagnosis of the first case of an emerging infectious disease can win valuable time for treatment and preventive control. Clinicians have a great responsibility in the detection and diagnosis of emerging infectious diseases. The first case of human avian influenza in this book (Case 46) was initially diagnosed as left lower pneumonia

on admission to hospital, and was treated aggressively. In cases where strong antibiotics fail and the disease rapidly deteriorates to severe pneumonia of unknown cause, despite the lack of epidemiological evidence, clinicians considered the possibility of emerging infectious diseases such as human avian influenza and sent respiratory samples for testing. This led to a definitive diagnosis before death, and allowed time for effective measures such as controlling the source of infection, cutting off the transmission route, and improving medical observation of close contacts. This shows that clinicians will be able to play a key role in the detection and control of emerging infectious diseases as long as they are always highly alert and sensitive to them.

2. The previous case (Case 46) took a drastic turn for the worse on day five (day two of admission), with both lungs becoming white within a short period of time, and respiratory failure developing rapidly, with multi-system and multi-organ damage. The disease was not reversed despite intensive treatment. It is now believed that the highly pathogenic avian influenza virus (H5N1) can trigger a cytokine storm in the host immune system, with the release of large amounts of cytokines such as IL-10 and β-interferon. This can violently and rapidly damage target organs and cause multi-organ failure by spreading to all organs of the body. Since the immune system is more active in young people, the responses are more intense; the disease progresses more rapidly, and the clinical prognosis is more dangerous. The first case is another example of this. The poor clinical prognosis of young patients with this disease should be noted.

3. The successful treatment of the second human avian influenza case in this book (Case 47) shows that first, the timely diagnosis of the case made early and aggressive etiologic treatment possible. Second, the significant improvement of the patient's condition after human immune plasma treatment with an inactivated avian influenza virus vaccine once again suggests that specific immune plasma treatment may be of great value in the treatment of emerging viral infectious disease. Third, the application of glucocorticoids (such as methylprednisolone) in appropriate amounts and short courses has positive significance for diseases that may cause a strong immune response in the body, such as human avian influenza. Fourth, to master the pharmacokinetic and pharmacodynamic nature of therapeutic drugs, and to make timely detection, accurate judgment and decisive treatment should be given when patients display adverse drug reactions.

4. The second human avian influenza case in this book was related to the first case (father and son). The second case was only with the first patient for one day when he had diarrhea, and none of the other family members and medical personnel who had longer and closer contact with the first case were infected with the disease. Most of the reported family aggregations of human avian influenza have a history of contact with a common infectious agent or are immediate relatives. A more detailed epidemiological investigation failed to confirm that the father and son may have been co-exposed to a suspected infectious agent. The

nucleotide sequences of the two H5N1 avian influenza viruses isolated from the respiratory secretions of the two patients were highly homologous, suggesting that the second patient was infected through close contact with the secretions or excretions of the first patient, and that the same genetic background between father and son determined the high susceptibility of the second case. The scholars concerned believe that this is a possible limited human-to-human transmission of human avian influenza occurring with a specific genetic background. Therefore, in clinical practice, high priority must be given to the disinfection and isolation of chaperones and staff, and stricter isolation and protection measures should be taken for the relatives of patients.

(Li Jun & Huang Zuhu)

Persistent fever for 20 days, with a recurrence of two days

I. Medical history

Patient: Female, 43 years old, a farmer. She was admitted to the hospital on 9 May 2000 with a persistent fever for 20 days with a recurrence of two days.

The patient developed a persistent fever with no obvious inducements 20 days earlier with a temperature above 39°C, accompanied by constipation and loss of hearing, but no rash, coughing and expectoration, or apathy. After five days of persistent fever, she went to her local county hospital, where she was examined and found to have a negative Widal test and a negative blood culture (on the second day of hospitalization). No bone marrow culture was performed, and she was diagnosed with typhoid fever. After six days of treatment with levofloxacin, her body temperature and hearing returned to normal. The patient requested to be discharged from the hospital two days after the fever subsided. Six days after returning home, she once again developed a fever, constipation, and loss of hearing without any inducements, and her body temperature was consistently above 39°C. She did not have a cough or expectoration, nor abdominal pain or diarrhea, and there was no blood in her stool. The local health center gave her Cefalexin (Cephalexin-c IV) for two days, which was ineffective, so she came to our hospital and was admitted to the outpatient clinic with typhoid fever.

The patient had previously been healthy, with no history of diabetes mellitus or a contaminated diet in the past 2–3 months. There were no similar infections in the surrounding area.

> **Thinking prompts:** Fever is a common manifestation of many diseases. When gathering a patient's medical history, we should note the magnitude of temperature change, the remission of the fever, and accompanying symptoms such as coughing, abdominal pain, polyuria, urgent urination, dysuria, and local symptoms. The patient had two fevers before and after admission. We noticed that the amplitude of the temperature change, remission, and accompanying symptoms was similar, suggesting that the two episodes were due to a common cause. So, what caused the disease to recur within a short period of time? The most important reason is

that the pathogen was not completely killed in the first case, and reproduced, i.e., the remission of the previous disease was only self-limited and not the result of proper treatment, or the previous treatment was appropriate but the course was insufficient. Since the patient had no accompanying symptoms such as arthralgias and polymorphic rashes in the two previous fevers, and since the temperature of the previous fever was quickly reduced to normal with levofloxacin, the treatment was thus considered appropriate but insufficient in duration. In addition, infectious (contagious) diseases often require attention to epidemiological information, which includes the causative factors of the disease, the patient's occupation, residence, and environmental health, as well as the three links that cause the spread of infectious diseases (infectious sources, transmission routes, and susceptible populations), and a focus on the transmission routes according to the symptoms when gathering medical history. For example, for fecal-oral transmission diseases such as typhoid fever, we should ask whether the patient eats a contaminated diet; for respiratory transmission diseases, we should ask whether there is a history of contact with other patients or going to crowded places; for insect-borne diseases, we should inquire if there is a history of field work or travel.

II. Physical examination and auxiliary examination on admission
1. Physical examination
T 39.7°C, P 76 times/min, R 16 times/min, BP 112/73 mmHg, clear consciousness, answered questions to the point, no apathy, no enlargement of the superficial skin lymph nodes, no rash, no dry or moist rales heard in either of the lungs, heart rate 76 times/min, rhythmic, no pathological murmur heard; the abdomen was soft without tenderness, no rebound pain; the liver was not palpable below the costal margin; the spleen was 1.5 cm below the costal area; shifting dullness sound (−), no positive signs found in neurological examination.

> **Thinking prompts:** The physical examination should be focused on the patient's symptoms. Fever is a systemic manifestation, and attention should be paid to the presence of enlarged lymph nodes, rashes, and arthralgias. The patient in this case had been diagnosed locally with typhoid fever, and was treated effectively with levofloxacin, so attention should be paid to typical typhoid signs such as a slow pulse, rose rash, and splenomegaly.

2. Auxiliary examination
Blood test: WBC 3.5×10^9/L, N 67%, L 32%, E 3%.
> Liver function: ALT 82 U/L, AST 56 U/L; other liver function indexes were normal.
> CRP: 23 mg/L (reference value < 10 mg/L).
> B-ultrasound examination: Suggesting splenomegaly.
> ESR and chest X-ray were normal.

III. Preliminary diagnosis

Patient was a female farmer; recurrent fever for 20 days, recurrence for another two days, with constipation and loss of hearing, body temperature persistently above 39°C during the first and second instances of fever; initial fever treated effectively with levofloxacin; physical examination revealed splenomegaly and a slow pulse; total white blood cell count in peripheral blood decreased, eosinophilia decreased, and liver function mildly impaired. The preliminary diagnosis was typhoid fever.

> **Thinking prompts:** The patient had two episodes of fever before and after admission, without the trapezoidal ascending and descending process of the body temperature that is typical of typhoid. Other clinical manifestations such as persistent fever, constipation, loss of hearing, slow pulse, and splenomegaly were more typical. Antibiotic treatment was effective at the initial onset, so the clinical diagnosis of typhoid fever seemed clear. However, the following issues should be noted when treating patients like this:
>
> 1. The first major feature of infectious diseases is the presence of pathogens. The highest standard of diagnosis of infectious diseases is to identify pathogens, so we should collect specimens carefully, and avoid over-eager empirical treatment of pathogenic bacteria. That is, blood culture or bone marrow culture should be conducted before antibiotic treatment. Otherwise, bacterial cultures performed after the start of antibiotic therapy are likely to fail to culture the pathogenic bacteria, even if antibiotics that are not sensitive to the pathogenic bacteria are applied.
>
> 2. Treatment with levofloxacin was effective at the time of the initial fever. However, the fever recurred six days after the antibiotic treatment was discontinued, because it was not complete at the time of the initial onset, and the pathogenic bacteria multiplied and invaded the blood again. In any specific treatment of a pathogen, if not thorough, the disease has the possibility of recurrence or re-inflammation. It is harder for antibiotics to kill intracellular parasitic pathogenic bacteria than extracellular pathogenic bacteria. Therefore, the former is less likely to be killed, and the probability of recurrence or re-inflammation is higher. At the same time, in patients with recurrent infectious diseases, we must exclude the possibility of other underlying diseases such as immune deficiency to avoid misdiagnosis.
>
> 3. The pathology of typhoid fever is characterized by a proliferative response of the systemic monocyte-phagocyte system, with lesions of the collective lymph nodes and isolated follicles in the lower ileum. The pathological changes to the intestinal tract in typical typhoid fever go through four phases (medullary swelling, necrosis, and ulceration). They heal in order, with each pathological phase lasting almost a week. Most intestinal complications occur in the ulcerative stage, and intestinal bleeding and perforation occur only after pathological changes to the necrotic stage. Almost three weeks after the onset of her illness, the patient in this case had been

reminded that a contaminated diet could trigger intestinal bleeding and perforation. She was instructed to eat low-fiber food that was easy to digest and produced less gas. Of course, the recurrence of typhoid fever will be less severe than the first attack, with fewer intestinal complications.

4. Cases like this can be treated with a combination of quinolones and third-generation cephalosporins. Cephalexin belongs to first-generation of cephalosporins. The antibacterial spectrum is mainly Gram-positive bacteria, and it is not effective against Salmonella.

5. Infection with S. typhi can cause secondary bacteremia. Only second-time bacteremia causes clinical symptoms. After 2–3 weeks of bacteremia, S. typhi can be excreted through the bile duct, and can be long-term parasitic in the gallbladder. Therefore, typhoid fever is a systemic infection that can manifest as multiple organ damage, such as a slow pulse. It can cause typhoid hepatitis and pneumonia.

IV. Ward-round analysis four days after admission

After the patient was treated with levofloxacin and cefotaxime, her body temperature decreased. Her highest body temperature the previous day was 38.1°C, with no loss of hearing and no abdominal distension. She defecated twice after admission; Widal test: O ≥ 1:80, H ≥ 1:60, typhoid lipopolysaccharide antibody negative. Fourth day blood culture report: Salmonella infection, sensitive to levofloxacin and cefotaxime.

Thinking prompts: The diagnosis of typhoid fever was confirmed by the serological Widal test and etiology. The initial onset of the disease was negative for the Widal test at the local hospital, due to the short duration of the disease and the low antibody titer in the patient. Widal tests are usually positive in the second week of the disease, with the highest rate of positivity in the third to fourth week. Therefore, it is important to review the tests. The Widal test can only be used as a clinical auxiliary diagnosis and not as a confirmatory criterion. However, if the changes to the Widal test are dynamically observed, its clinical diagnostic value will be increased.

The typhoid lipopolysaccharide antibody test is a new serological test for typhoid fever, developed in the past decade or so. It can be positive on day four of the disease, and is more sensitive and specific than the Widal test. However, it can also only be used as a clinical auxiliary diagnosis of typhoid fever; a negative test cannot exclude a diagnosis, while a positive test must be combined with clinical diagnosis.

Identifying the pathogen of an infectious disease is the gold standard for diagnosis. The local hospital in this case could not culture S. typhi at the time of the initial onset, which is related to the application of antibiotics before the culturing. There are a variety of ways to obtain S. typhi, such as from blood, bone marrow, stool, urine and bile culture, and rose rash culture (from scrapings). The choice of culture specimen must be based on the various phases of the disease, for instance, blood culture for the first week of disease, and stool culture for the third and fourth week. The positive rate in bone marrow culture is the highest and has the longest duration.

Since S. typhi is intracellularly parasitic, antibiotic treatment must be continued until 10–14 days after the fever subsides to avoid recurrence and reduce chronic carriers. Because S. typhi can reproduce in bile and be excreted through the bile duct (making chronic carriers of typhoid a critical hidden source of infection), it is clinically important to eliminate chronic carriers. Detection of antibodies to surface antigens can detect some chronic carriers.

V. Condition at discharge

The patient suffered no discomfort, and continued treatment with levofloxacin and cefotaxime for seven days after the fever subsided. She was discharged with instructions to take oral levofloxacin 0.2 g twice a day for five days instead. During this period, her stool culture was negative twice.

VI. Follow-up

Three months after discharge, the patient was free from discomfort.

VII. Lessons learned

1. The treatment of disease is a process of cooperation between doctors and patients. Clinicians should communicate fully with patients to help them understand the outcome of the disease and increase their compliance in order for the treatment to be a success.

2. A culture of pathogenic bacteria should be performed before antimicrobial treatment. This can increase the culture positive rate, and has important value for diagnosis and differential diagnosis.

(He Jianqin & Li Lanjuan)

Persistent chills and fever for three months, with a recurrence of three days

I. Medical history

Patient: Male, 79 years old, a farmer from Zhejiang Province. He was admitted on 25 March 2005 with persistent chills and fever for three months, with a recurrence of three days.

The patient experienced chills and fever after catching a cold three months earlier with a body temperature rising to 39.5°C, accompanied by a headache. There was no loss of appetite, no coughing or sputum, no abdominal pain or diarrhea, no arthralgia, and no rashes. He was diagnosed with an upper respiratory tract infection at the local county hospital, and his fever gradually subsided after 2–3 days of antibiotic treatment (details unknown). Medication (4–5 days in total) was stopped once the fever subsided.

In the following three months, the patient developed fever four times without obvious inducements. The fevers were two weeks apart, accompanied by chills and loss of appetite, but no other discomfort. The patient immediately went to the local hospital, where routine blood tests showed an increased white blood cell count and an increased neutrophil ratio. Antibiotic treatment was given (details unknown), and the medication was discontinued after his temperature returned to normal as a result of 4–5 days of treatment. Blood culture was performed twice during the treatment period (both after antibiotic treatment), and no bacterial growth was found. Three days earlier, the patient once again developed a fever with no inducements, with a temperature of 40°C and a headache. There was no generalized pain and stiffness, and no subcutaneous bleeding spots. He was transferred to our hospital for a definitive diagnosis because of recurrent fever.

The patient had been in good health, with no history of diabetes, hypertension, drug allergies, or surgery; he did not eat a contaminated diet, and had no contact with raw meat, raw milk, or lamb. He denied contact with patients of similar diseases, and there was no family history of hereditary disease.

> **Thinking prompts:** The patient's chief complaint was recurrent fever, happening six times in three months. When gathering medical history, as well as asking about

the occurrence, development, and remission of symptoms, special attention should be paid to any symptoms related to diseases that can cause periodic fever, such as malaria and lymphoma. Due to the long duration of fever, if it is an infectious disease, it is often related to recurrence, so we should note the patient's occupation, lifestyle, eating habits, and living environment. We should pay particular attention to a history of antibiotic treatment. Standardized antibiotic treatment depends on whether the dose and course of treatment are adequate. Both aspects are important, and the absence of one will preclude the expected curative effect. In addition to treatment history, if a patient suffers from recurrent fever, we must also note whether there is an underlying immunodeficiency disease such as AIDS, and whether there is any long-term application of corticosteroids in the patient's medical history.

II. Physical examination and auxiliary examination on admission

1. Physical examination

T 39.3°C, P 106 times/min, R 18 times/min, BP 123/79 mmHg, clear consciousness, answering questions to the point; no enlargement of the superficial skin lymph nodes, no rash, no boils; normal and even temporal artery pulsation, no bulging temporal artery. No dry and moist rales were heard in either of the lungs, H 106 times/min, rhythmic, no pathological murmur. The abdomen was soft, with no pressure pain, and no rebound pain; the liver was 1 cm below the ribs, the spleen was 2.5 cm below the ribs, shifting dullness (−); no positive signs were found in the neurological examination.

> **Thinking prompts:** Based on the medical history above, if the fever is caused by a bacterial infection lasting more than 2–3 weeks, there are often migratory lesions. Physical examination should focus on finding the localized foci of the infection. Because of the long duration of the fever, systemic lymph nodes and subcutaneous nodules are also the focus of the search. Physical examination of the heart and related auxiliary examinations are often overlooked. However, subacute infective endocarditis and mucinous cardiac tumors can also cause prolonged fever, and should also be examined closely. Neglecting dental caries may lead to long-term fever in the elderly, so careful whole-body physical examination is very important.

2. Auxiliary examination

Routine blood: WBC 12.9×10^9/L, N 78%, L 21%, E 1%, RBC 2.98×10^{12}/L, Hb 9.7 g/L.

   Liver function indicators were normal.

   CRP: 46 mg/L.

   ESR, ANA, ANCA, and chest X-ray were normal.

   B-ultrasound examination: Suggesting hepatosplenomegaly.

III. Ward-round analysis on admission

1. Preliminary diagnosis

Elderly male patient; recurrent chills and fever for three months, with a recurrence of three days; hepatosplenomegaly; increased peripheral blood leukocytes and increased neutrophils. Preliminary diagnosis: FUO.

2. Diagnostic thinking

The diagnostic thinking around FUO has been mentioned in several cases. Please refer to the relevant sections.

Fever is either infectious or non-infectious forms. The likelihood of non-infectious fever increases with the duration. This patient was 79 years old, and his fever lasted for three months with hepatosplenomegaly. It was noted as a non-infectious fever.

(1) In cases of non-infectious fever, the following diseases should be considered:

1) Tumor-associated fever: Solid tumors can lead to fever from tumor necrosis and/or ectopic hormone syndrome. A diagnosis is easier to make when combined with ancillary examinations (ultrasound, CT, and endoscopy) for comparison. Hematologic tumors are often non-solid, among which leukemia is relatively easy to diagnose (a routine bone marrow examination is sufficient to identify or exclude it). However, lymphomas that do not cause lymphadenectasis often do not have specific clinical features, and can manifest as simple fever (periodic or persistent), rash, hepatosplenomegaly with hyperagglutinin syndrome, gastrointestinal ulcers, and perforation. However, in lymphoma, the number of white blood cells in the peripheral blood is generally not increased, and may even decrease. Although bone marrow biopsy establishes a diagnostic probability of lymphoma of only 15%–20%, it can be performed. This patient had increased peripheral leukocytes and increased neutrophils, and there was a lack of a definite basis to support lymphoma. Infectious diseases must be ruled out before lymphoma can be diagnosed. Therefore, tumor-associated fever was not considered.

2) Autoimmune diseases: Non-specific forms of vasculitis such as rheumatic polymyalgia and giant cell arteritis tend to occur in the elderly. In addition to fever, the former causes wandering myalgia and stiffness, and sometimes granuloma-like changes can be found in the liver and other organs on imaging; the latter may cause headache, weakened temporal artery pulsation, and temporal artery manifestation. This patient lacked all of these manifestations, so autoimmune diseases were not considered.

3) Endocrine metabolic diseases: These diseases seldom cause fever, or only low fever (as in hyperthyroidism), but almost all metabolic disease crises cause fever (often high), such as hyperthyroid, pituitary, and adrenal crisis. However, these diseases usually have a corresponding medical history and obvious abnormalities in endocrine metabolic examination, so they were not considered in this case.

4) Hematologic disorders such as a chronic acute hemolytic attack: In addition to fever, there is often low back pain, change in urine color, and significant changes to the

blood. None of these changes were present in the patient in this case, so these disorders were ruled out.

The above clinical analysis cannot determine the cause of non-infectious fever, and infectious diseases must be ruled out before diagnosing it. Although this patient had a recurrent fever for three months, the possibility of non-infectious causes was high. However, the fever subsided after the application of antibiotic treatment for each fever, suggesting that the cause was an infection. Blood and/or bone marrow cultures should be performed prior to antibiotic treatment with a view to obtaining the pathogen.

(2) Common infectious diseases that can cause recurrence of the disease:

1) Salmonella infection: Infection due to a contaminated diet – either S. typhi or S. paratyphi infection. The typical clinical manifestations of the former are described in Case 48, while the latter takes the form of paratyphoid A, B, or C. The clinical manifestations of paratyphoid A and B are like typhoid fever, but the roseola rash appears earlier, in greater quantities, and lasts longer. It can have the clinical manifestations of acute gastroenteritis, with mild toxic symptoms, a shorter duration, and fewer intestinal complications. The clinical manifestation of paratyphoid C is more complex. It can be manifested as septicemia-type, typhoid-type, and acute gastroenteritis-type. In addition to chills and high fever, septicemia-type can have migratory septic foci, peripheral blood leukocytosis, and neutrophilia. The disease can be delayed and repeated. The patient in this case was a farmer, with recurrent fever for three months. His fever subsided after anti-inflammatory treatment. Hepatosplenomegaly supports a diagnosis of typhoid and paratyphoid fever, but the patient's leukocytes and neutrophils increased with each attack. Therefore, typhoid and paratyphoid A and B can be ruled, but paratyphoid C cannot. Confirmation of diagnosis requires blood or bone marrow culture.

2) Brucellosis: A zoonotic disease, mainly prevalent in pastoral areas in China, caught by delivering lambs, slaughtering sick animals, milking, and drinking unpasteurized milk. Typical clinical manifestations are recurrent fever, excessive sweating, arthralgia, and hepatosplenomegaly. The patient was not from a pastoral area and did not drink unpasteurized milk or deliver lambs, so brucellosis was not considered.

3) Malaria: Global distribution, but most common in tropical and subtropical regions, and more common in temperate regions. It is transmitted by the bite of Anopheles mosquitoes, so there is a clear seasonality in areas with four seasons. Typical clinical manifestations include periodic chills and high fever, sweating, enlargement of the liver and spleen, and anemia. In this case, the patient's initial onset was in winter, with no obvious sweating. The fever subsided after 4-5 days of antibiotic treatment, so malaria was not considered. If necessary, peripheral blood and/or bone marrow smears can be sent to professionals to look for Plasmodium and perform diagnostic antimalarial treatment if required.

4) Eperythrozoonosis: A zoonotic disease, of which pigs are one of the main sources of infection. People become infected by eating raw meat (e.g., in hot pot), with typical clinical

manifestations such as recurrent fever, hepatosplenomegaly, and anemia. The patient in this case denied epidemiological conditions such as eating raw meat, so it was not considered. If necessary, peripheral blood smears for electron microscopy of red blood cells can be used to look for pathogens.

In conclusion, diagnosis must first exclude infectious diseases or co-infections based on primary diseases (such as other immunocompromised diseases like AIDS and lymphoma). Blood and bone marrow cultures should be conducted immediately after admission, as well as routine bone marrow, immunoglobulin typing, T-cell receptor analysis, and bone marrow biopsy. In addition, serological tests for autoimmune diseases should be performed. No special treatment should be administered for the time being, and temperature changes should be observed to determine the fever type.

IV. Analysis of Ward-round seven days after admission

The patient's temperature remained at 37.6°C–39.7°C for four days after admission. Ice was sometimes used to lower it. Prior to the rise in body temperature, there was an obvious aversion to cold but no chills, poor appetite, poor mental health, and fatigue, but no rash, and no abdominal pain or diarrhea. Bone marrow culture report: Salmonella paratyphi was grown, which was sensitive to levofloxacin and cefotaxime. Combined treatment of levofloxacin and cefotaxime was started on the fourth day of hospitalization. On the second day of antibiotic treatment, the patient's body temperature dropped significantly. His fatigue and malaise improved, and his body temperature dropped to normal on the fourth day of antibiotic treatment. Blood culture at seven days reported no bacterial growth. The Widal test was negative.

> **Thinking prompts:** A pathogen was found in the blood marrow culture, and the diagnosis of Salmonella paratyphoid C (septicemia-type) was clear. Paratyphi C has no O antigen, and cannot stimulate the body to produce O antibodies; the flagellar antigen is less immunogenic, and the body's ability to produce the corresponding antibodies is weaker, making it prone to false negative and false positive results. Therefore, the clinical value of the Widal test is even lower in paratyphoid C. Paratyphoid C is the most common septicemia-type, and has more complications, most commonly pulmonary infections (pneumonia or lung abscesses). It can also have other sites of migratory septicemia lesions, such as liver abscesses, pyelonephritis, endocarditis, and central infections, but causes fewer intestinal complications. The treatment of paratyphoid C is the same as that of typhoid fever, and if an abscess develops, it should be promptly incised and drained. This patient's septicemia paratyphoid C lasted for three months without migratory septic lesions, which was related to the fact that he was treated with sensitive antibiotics at his local hospital every time he had a fever. Also, since each course of antibiotic treatment was inadequate, it led to repeated multiplication of pathogens,

resulting in multiple bacteremia and morbidity. Blood cultures were obtained at the local hospital twice, and both showed no bacterial growth, probably because the timing of specimen collection was not optimal; blood was not collected before antibiotic treatment, and the antibiotic treatment was administered in a hurry, which hampered the definitive diagnosis.

V. Follow-up

The patient was discharged from hospital after 17 days of combined treatment with levofloxacin and cefotaxime. At the time of discharge, he had no fever, no headache, and no coughing or expectoration. He was in better spirits, and his appetite had improved. Three months after discharge, fever had not recurred.

VI. Lessons learned

1. Before diagnosing non-infectious diseases, infectious diseases should be ruled out. The diagnosis of infectious diseases should still take into account the regional and seasonal characteristics of infectious diseases, considering common and multiple diseases first, and then rare and imported diseases.
2. Emphasizing the standardized detection of pathogens and standardized treatment can be a source of clinical experience, which can reduce misdiagnosis and missed diagnosis.

(He Jianqin & Li Lanjuan)

Fever for eight days; palpitations and dizziness for one day

I. Medical history

Patient: Male, 33 years old, a coal mine worker from a county in Guanzhong in Shaanxi Province. He was admitted to hospital at 20:30 on 17 November 2008 with fever for eight days, and palpitations and dizziness for one day.

The patient had developed a fever eight days previously after catching a cold, with a body temperature of 38.5°C, accompanied by mild sweating and loss of appetite. There was no nasal congestion and runny nose, no coughing and sputum, and no nausea, vomiting, or diarrhea. He was treated at a local county hospital and given oral medication for flu, with no obvious effects. His fever persisted for several days, peaking in the afternoon and at dusk, and once reaching 39.4°C. On the fourth day of illness, the antibody for hemorrhagic fever was found to be negative. Since his high temperature did not subside, the patient was admitted to the emergency department of the local county hospital for observation, and was treated with intravenous fluids (details unknown) for four days. His body temperature gradually normalized, and his sweating decreased. He was discharged, and returned home for treatment.

One day before admission, i.e., on the eighth day of the illness, there was no obvious inducement to palpitations, dizziness, and general discomfort. The patient's urine output was significantly reduced, so he went to the county hospital again. His heart rate measured 115 beats/min. His blood pressure was not taken. He was given oral medication and infusion therapy, but his symptoms showed no significant improvement. In the afternoon of the same day, he was transferred to the emergency department of a top-tier hospital in the city, where his blood pressure was measured at 100/90 mHg. His pulse was weak and indistinct, so he was given a fluid infusion – 3,000 ml of balanced salt solution and 500 ml of hydroxyethyl starch via intravenous infusion. His routine blood test showed WBC 36.74×10^9/L, PLT 10×10^9/L, Hb 222 g/L, and anomalous lymphocytes 32%. Urine protein and hematuria were both (+++). After a massive infusion, his blood pressure rose to normal, and he was transferred to the hospital's infectious disease ward at 20:30 that night.

Thinking prompts: The patient was a young male with a fever onset and a history of cold, but no upper respiratory tract symptoms or gastrointestinal symptoms such as nausea and vomiting or diarrhea. This was obviously different from general upper respiratory tract infections, i.e., colds. The illness was treated as a cold for a while, but there was no obvious effect, and the patient's body temperature increased daily to 39°C or more. Since the Guanzhong area in Shaanxi Province is known for epidemics of hemorrhagic fever with renal syndrome, with a peak from November to January every year, the local county hospital tested the patient's serum hemorrhagic fever antibodies on the fourth day of illness, but it was negative. His temperature gradually decreased after four days of continued fluid therapy during the observation period, but his general malaise increased, and there were palpitations, dizziness, and decreased urination. After transfer to a higher-tier hospital, his pulse was weak, and his blood pressure pulse differential was only 10 mmHg, showing typical shock manifestations. At this point, his total white blood cell count was significantly increased, his platelet count was significantly decreased, and his hemoglobin (Hb) was 222 g/L with 32% of the anomalous lymphocytes. Urine protein and hematuria were both (+++), indicating that the patient's plasma exudation and blood concentration were very serious. A clinical diagnosis of hemorrhagic fever with renal syndrome was inevitable.

The patient was given appropriate treatment and placed under observation at the local county hospital, but there were two obvious errors at the time of transfer. First, the patient did not bring his medical records, so it was not clear what his diagnosis was, nor if there were any changes in his condition, as well as clinical monitoring, laboratory test results, and specific treatment at the local county hospital from the fourth to the eighth day before the transfer. This caused issues in the gathering of medical history and treatment at the subsequent receiving hospital. Secondly, the patient had a significantly decreased urine output the day before the transfer, and there should have been closer monitoring of vital signs in the days before, i.e., at the end of the fever period and the hypotensive shock period. If there is hypotension or hypotensive tendencies, local treatment should be given to stabilize the vital signs for 12 to 24 hours before transferring the patient. This type of patient often suffers from shock (even refractory) during transfer, leading to death.

The patient in this case developed hypotensive shock on the ninth day of illness, which was relatively later than most patients with hemorrhagic fever with renal syndrome. Usually, the febrile phase of hemorrhagic fever with renal syndrome lasts only 4–6 days, followed by the hypotensive shock phase in moderate, severe, and critically ill patients. The latter presents with mild or severe hypotensive shock, whereas mild patients may enter the oliguric or polyuric phase directly. It has been documented that hypotensive shock can occur in individual patients after 17 days of fever, but it is rare.

II. Physical examination and auxiliary examination on admission

1. Physical examination

T 37.3°C, P 94 times/min, R 20 times/min, BP 140/90 mmHg, weight not measured. He had a clear consciousness, poor mental health, dozens of pinpoint-sized bright red hemorrhagic spots on his chest and bilateral axillary skin, mild edema of the face and both eyelids, degree II[1] chemosis, and reticular congestion of the oral soft palate mucosa. The respiratory sounds of both lungs were clear, and no dry and moist rales were heard; the heart rhythm was uniform, the heart rate was 94 beats/min, and no heart murmur was heard in the auscultation area of either valve. The abdomen was full, the abdominal wall was soft, and there was mild tenderness in the whole abdomen with no rebound pain. Percussion pain was positive in bilateral renal areas, predominantly on the right side. Preliminary diagnosis after admission: Hemorrhagic fever with renal syndrome, with an overlapping hypotensive shock phase and oliguric phase.

2. Auxiliary examination

Peripheral blood: WBC 18.97×10^9/L, differential leukocyte count was unavailable, PLT remained 10×10^9/L, Hb had dropped to 154 g/L.

Blood biochemistry: AST 248 U/L, ALT 78 U/L, A 34.5 g/L, BUN 13.11 mmol/L, Cr 270.4 μmol/L.

Serum electrolytes: Na$^+$ 124.9 mmol/L.

Peripheral blood: WBC 18.97×10^9/L, differential leukocyte count was unavailable PLT remained 10×10^9/L, and Hb had dropped to 154 g/L.

> **Thinking prompts:** The main manifestations of hemorrhagic fever with renal syndrome in the febrile period are moderate to high fever, flushing of the skin of the face, neck, and upper chest; hemorrhagic spots on the skin of the trunk, especially of the bilateral axillae, the back of the shoulders, and the mucosa of the soft palate, and chemosis; abdominal distension, nausea, vomiting and diarrhea, and percussion pain in the bilateral kidney area. The patient's fever gradually decreased after one week, but his condition did not improve. It worsened, manifested by palpitations, dizziness, and malaise with no obvious inducement, and a significant decrease in urine output. Physical examination after admission revealed that he had a low fever, with a pulse pressure difference of only 10 mHg, hemorrhagic spots on the trunk, degree II chemosis, and percussion pain in both kidney areas. Although there was no typical triple flushing of the skin (face, neck, and upper chest) or triple pain (headache, orbital pain, and lumbago), the clinical diagnosis of hemorrhagic fever with renal syndrome was not problematic in combination with the typical changes in routine blood and urine and renal function tests and epidemiological history (located in an infected area and in the peak season for hemorrhagic fever). However,

---

[1] Degree II is described as 0.5 < Edema Index ≤ 1.0 in *Chin J Clin Neurosurg* 22, no. 3 (March 2017): 168.

the diagnosis must still be confirmed by detecting antibodies for hemorrhagic fever, i.e., anti-Hantaan virus IgM antibodies. A single positive serum can confirm the diagnosis, or a double serum (serum at the first week of onset and after an interval of at least one week). With anti-Hantaan virus IgG antibodies, the antibody titer should be increased at least fourfold to have diagnostic value, and serum hantavirus RNA can also be detected to help confirm the diagnosis.

III. Development of the disease and history of treatment

The patient was admitted to hospital and reported as critically ill, and was given first-degree care. During the first 12 hours of admission (20:00 that day to 08:00 the next morning), a total of 1,500 ml of various types of salt-containing crystalloids, 700 ml of glucose solution, and 200 ml of plasma were infused intravenously; his vital signs were still stable, with blood pressure fluctuating from 130–150/90–100 mmHg, heart rate of 80–95 beats/min; blood oxygen saturation was maintained at 98% or more, under low-flow nasal catheter oxygen (1–2) L/min, and respiration was 20–25 times/min. However, he passed no urine or stool for 12 hours. On the morning of the next day, his hemoglobin dropped to 154–159 g/L, WBC (20.16–21.81) × 10^9/L, neutrophil count (N) 0.485, and platelet count 12 × 109/L. Blood urea nitrogen rose to 19.31 mmol/L and creatinine 277.6 μmol/L.

Considering that the patient had already entered the oliguric phase, treatment was started the day after admission on the basis of stable blood pressure, implementing the basic treatment principles of stabilization, promotion, conduction, and permeation: ① Stabilization = stabilizing the body's internal environment, i.e., limiting fluid intake: 24-hour intake = the previous day's apparent fluid loss (ml) + 500 (in winter when perspiration is low) to 800 ml (in summer or when perspiration is high); a total of 950 ml of sugar-containing crystalloids and 200 ml of salt-containing crystalloids were input during that period. ② Promotion = promoting diuresis, usually using various types of loop diuretics such as furosemide or Sodium Etacrynate, but other strong diuretics can also be used; the patient received 480 mg of furosemide intravenously on the second day after admission. ③ Conduction = if hemodialysis or peritoneal dialysis is not available, conduction treatment can be given. ④ Permeation = various types of dialysis treatment such as hemodialysis, including continuous renal replacement therapy (CRRT).

After the above treatment, the patient had still not passed urine on the second day after admission, but his vital signs were stable, and his blood pressure fluctuated between 130 mHg and 160/80 mHg to 120 mmHg. On the morning of the third day after admission, his blood urea nitrogen rose to 26.23 mmol/L, and creatinine rose to 469.7 μmol/L. Therefore, the first hemodialysis treatment was four hours long, with a net dehydration of 2,000 ml; after hemodialysis, the blood urea nitrogen fell by more than half, to 13.11 mmol/L, and creatinine fell to 323.3 μmol/L; mild hypokalemia and hyponatremia. Treatment medication was added with 6.4 million U/d penicillin to prevent infection. On the third day, a total of 800 mg of furosemide was administered intravenously; 990 ml of urine was excreted throughout the day, 300 ml of dilute stool was passed, and a total of 1,450 ml of fluid was administered, including 250 ml of salt-containing crystalloid fluid. Arterial blood gas was checked, acid-base was approximately normal, and partial pressure of oxygen was high. Blood pressure was 125–150/85–100 mHg, pulse pressure was 40–65 mHg, heart rate was 80 beats/min, and respiratory rate was reduced to 18 breaths/min. The patient was conscious, and no dry and moist rales were heard in either of the lungs.

On the fourth day after admission, furosemide was administered at the same dose as the previous day via intravenous injection, but only 380 ml of urine was excreted throughout the day. The patient's blood pressure was measured to be high, fluctuating from 130–160/80–100 mHg, and his pulse pressure increased to 50–70 mHg. Phentolamine was given intermittently and intravenously, and oral nifedipine was administered at the same time.

On the morning of the fifth day of hospitalization, the patient's routine RBC decreased to 120 g/L, WBC 8.3 × 10⁹/L, N 0.699, platelet count 34 × 10⁹/L; blood urea nitrogen increased to 21.54 mmol/L, creatinine 587.7 μmol/L. A series of coagulation tests showed normal prothrombin time, but fibrinogen degradation products and D-dimer increased, suggesting mild secondary hyperfibrinolysis; a chest radiograph also suggested infectious lesions in both lungs. The patient's blood pressure fluctuated from 160–180/80–100 mHg throughout the day, and his pulse pressure increased to 60–80 mHg. Although a chest radiograph revealed infectious inflammation in both lungs, no fever, coughing, sputum, chest pain, or other respiratory symptoms were observed. No dry and moist rales were heard in either of the lungs during physical examination. There were no obvious abnormalities in peripheral blood leukocytes and neutrophils. In addition to anti-fibrinolytic drugs, 2.0 g ceftriaxone sodium was added twice a day to combat the infection, and hemodialysis was performed for the second time. A total of 3,000 ml was dehydrated during dialysis; the blood urea nitrogen decreased to 7.95 mmol/L and creatinine decreased to 327.2 μmol/L on post-dialysis recheck. A total of 1,050 ml of urine was excreted throughout the day.

On the sixth day of hospitalization (22 November), the patient's renal function improved significantly, and 800 mg of furosemide was still administered in divided doses throughout the day via intravenous injection; 2,060 ml of urine was excreted throughout the day, blood pressure fluctuated from 130–160/75–100 mHg, and pulse pressure was 55–70 mHg. The next day (23 November), blood urea nitrogen rose to 16.64 mmol/L and creatinine 589.6 μmol/L on morning recheck. The peripheral blood platelet count had risen to 131 × 10⁹/L and hemoglobin 132 g/L.

On the seventh day of hospitalization, the treatment was the same as before. A total of 3,470 ml of urine was excreted throughout the day; the patient's body temperature ranged from 36.8°C to 37.2°C, heart rate 78–92 beats/min, blood pressure 140–60/90–100 mHg, and pulse pressure 50–60 mHg. The next day (24 November), the blood urea nitrogen rose to 19.12 mmol/L and creatinine 617.8 μmol/L. Peripheral blood WBC 8.07 × 10⁹/L, N 0.647, platelet count rose to 153 × 10⁹/L, hemoglobin 130 g/L; a routine urine test showed that urine protein had turned negative, and the urine leukocyte quantification was slightly higher, but the urine red blood cell quantification had dropped into the normal range. The patient felt that the nausea and vomiting had disappeared. His abdominal distension had reduced, and he could consume a small amount of semi-liquid food. As for the treatment, monitoring was reduced and the original drug regimen and symptomatic treatment were maintained.

IV. Summary and lessons learned

1. The patient's blood pressure stabilized after emergency fluid resuscitation treatment at the emergency department, and he continued to receive 2,200 ml of fluid and 200 ml of plasma for 12 hours after admission. Thereafter, his blood pressure did not drop again; his heart rate slowed, radial artery pulsation was strong, and the oxygen saturation of low-flow oxygenated blood was normal, indicating the success of the anti-shock treatment.

2. After the patient was admitted to hospital, he quickly moved from the hypotensive shock phase into the oliguric phase, passing no urine for 36 hours after admission, especially after receiving a high dose of furosemide; his blood urea nitrogen gradually rose to 26.23 mmol/L and creatinine rose to 469.7 μmol/L. It was decided that hemodialysis should be performed, and the dosage of furosemide was increased to 800 mg/d.

According to the National Epidemic Hemorrhagic Fever Prevention and Control Program set out by the Ministry of Health in February 1997, the indications for dialysis in the oliguric phase of hemorrhagic fever with renal syndrome are as follows: ① Oliguria for more than five days, or anuria for more than two days, ineffective with diuretic treatment, or slow increase in urine output, increasing severity of uremic manifestations, blood urea nitrogen > 28.6–35.7 mmol/L. ② Hypervolemic syndrome not responding to conservative treatments, with pulmonary edema, cerebral edema, and intestinal hemorrhage; can be administered in conjunction with medication. ③ Combined hyperkalemia (> 6.5 mmol/L), which cannot be relieved by general methods. ④ The disease progresses rapidly after entering the oliguric phase, with early onset of severe consciousness disturbance, persistent vomiting, massive hemorrhaging, and rapid rise of urea nitrogen exceeding 9 mmol/L per day (hypercatabolic type); dialysis should be performed as early as possible, without being bound by the number of days of oliguria and biochemical blood indexes.

The above regulations are undoubtedly of great importance in guiding clinical treatment. However, with the more widespread application of blood purification technology and the improvements in medical conditions in recent years, most scholars have become more lenient in their grasp of the timing and indications of dialysis in the treatment of acute renal failure in hemorrhagic fever with renal syndrome (HFRS), i.e., they advocate for early dialysis, and even early prophylactic dialysis treatment. This is to prevent or rapidly reverse renal failure and avoid serious complications. Other scholars advocate for the early application of continuous renal replacement therapy (CRRT) when available, to correct azotemia as quickly as possible.

The advantages of hemodialysis are high efficiency, short duration, and low price. The disadvantages are that it causes significant disturbances to the body's internal environment, which may lead to more complications. Also, the short-term application of a large amount of anticoagulant (heparin) can aggravate the patient's coagulation disorder, especially for hemorrhagic fever, which is a hemodynamically unstable disease with an abnormal coagulation mechanism. The advantages of CRRT are that it simulates the work of the kidneys and has less impact on the body's internal environment, including hemodynamics and blood osmolality, so it is particularly suitable for patients with cardiopulmonary comorbidities and unstable blood pressure; at the same time, CRRT can partially remove excessive inflammatory factors from the body and allow the implementation of bedside treatment and long-duration therapy; the disadvantages of CRRT are low efficiency and high cost. Therefore, despite the advantages of CRRT, hemodialysis is used much more often, because patients with hemorrhagic fever are mostly from low-income and rural populations.

3. The oliguric phase is the extreme phase of hemorrhagic fever with renal syndrome, which is prone to various serious complications such as massive hemorrhaging, severe infections, heart failure, pulmonary edema and cerebral edema, and acute respiratory distress syndrome. It is mostly seen in patients with improper disposal during hypotensive shock (e.g., excessive amounts of expansion fluid), severe or prolonged shock, or oliguric anuria lasting for more than one week. Massive gastrointestinal hemorrhage can lead to life-threatening shock; massive respiratory hemorrhage can induce circulatory respiratory arrest; intracranial hemorrhage can cause convulsions and coma. Heart failure, pulmonary edema, and ARDS, which mostly occur in the shock phase and hypervolemia phase of oliguria, have poor prognoses. The oliguric phase and early polyuric phase are prone to complications such as pneumonia, urinary tract infections, and septicemia, which often aggravate the condition and cause death.

In this case, due to the timely treatment of shock, no serious complications occurred in the oliguric phase. There was simply mild hypertension, mild bilateral lung infection, and secondary hyperfibrinolysis, and none showed obvious clinical symptoms or signs. After anti-hypertensive, anti-infection, and anti-fibrinolytic therapy, especially for the underlying disease, the patient finally entered the polyuric and recovery phase.

(Bai Xuefan)

Restlessness for four days, with oliguria for three days and fever for 33 hours

I. Medical history

Patient: Male, 49 years old, an employee of a company in Xi'an, Shaanxi Province. He was hospitalized between 19 and 21 June 2008 with restlessness for four days, oliguria for three days, and fever for 33 hours.

The patient had been admitted to our neurosurgery department for cerebral infarction two and a half months earlier (7 April 2008). His condition improved, and he was discharged on 15 May after 40 days of treatment. He stayed at home and rested with mild limb paralysis, and did not go out. Four days earlier, he became irritable and restless, and his family was not concerned because his temperature was normal at first. The following day, he became thirsty and drank 4,000 ml of water, but only urinated about 150 ml throughout the day. His family was still not concerned, and did not send him to hospital for examination. At 01:00 on the third day, he developed chills and fever, and his body temperature reached 39°C. His family mistook it for a cold and treated him with cold and flu tablets, Yinqiao tablets, and amoxicillin, but his body temperature fluctuated from 38°C to 40°C throughout the day. At 01:00 on the fourth day, he suddenly developed nausea and non-projectile vomiting of stomach contents, followed by confusion, no response to calls, cold hands and feet, and blue limbs and lips. He was rushed to the emergency department of our hospital. His blood pressure was measured at 80/60 mmHg, and a small number of bleeding spots were found on the anterior chest skin. A routine blood test showed WBC 14.34×10^9/L, Hb 163 g/L, PLT 23×10^9/L; serum sodium 120 mmol/L; renal function BUN 8.95 mmol/L, Cr 206.6 μmol/L. An electrocardiogram showed atrial fibrillation (the echocardiography report of the previous hospital record was checked for severe mitral stenosis, moderate tricuspid and aortic valve insufficiency, and pulmonary valve insufficiency), and a cranial CT scan showed an old cerebral infarction in the left temporoparietal occipital region. After multidisciplinary consultation, the preliminary diagnosis was as follows: ① FUO (Fever of Unknown Origin) – hemorrhagic fever with renal syndrome to be ruled out; ② Atrial fibrillation; ③ Rheumatic heart disease combined with valve damage; ④ Cerebral infarction (old).

The patient was treated with 250 ml 3% sodium chloride solution, and 1,000 ml balanced salt solution by rapid intravenous infusion and oxygen therapy. His blood pressure rose to 100/60 mmHg, and he was transferred to the infectious disease ward at 09:50 that day.

> **Thinking prompts:** This patient was recovering from a previous cerebrovascular disease. He had been treated at a hospital neurosurgery department for 40 days around 2.5 months before this illness, and was discharged to recuperate at home when his condition improved. His family was not concerned until the morning of the third day when he developed a high fever, when they gave him simple treatment. He went into shock on the fourth day of the illness. On admission to hospital, a preliminary examination revealed an old cerebral infarction and heart valve disease, as well as a marked increase in peripheral blood WBC and Hb, a marked decrease in PLT, and mild renal impairment. The patient lived in the urban area of Xi'an, which has a low incidence of hemorrhagic fever with renal syndrome. June is the high incidence season for the disease. The patient had manifestations of hemorrhagic fever such as high fever (although late detection) and oliguria, but no other etiology was found; the preliminary examination on admission revealed an increase in the peripheral blood WBC and Hb, while PLT was significantly decreased. This was accompanied by mild increased BUN and Cr, so hemorrhagic fever with renal syndrome was ruled out. However, there were inconsistencies with hemorrhagic fever in this case. One was that the oliguria came before the fever, so it was presumed that the patient had had the fever for more than two days. It was not clear whether he had it in the first two days of the disease because his family did not take his temperature. It was also possible that the patient's body temperature was not high at the beginning of the disease, which may have been related to his weakness and slow response to fever. Second, as a rodent-borne infectious disease, the patient should have a clear history of contact with rodents. Direct or indirect contact with rodents cannot be ruled out. However, in this case, the patient was either hospitalized or resting at home due to mild paralysis in the two months before the illness (high-floor resident) and did not go out at all, so it would have been difficult for him to have direct or indirect contact with rodents. Therefore, the mode of infection is worth exploring.

II. Physical examination after admission

The patient's body temperature was 38°C; his pulse was weak at 100 beats/min, uneven in strength; respiration was 35 breaths/min, blood pressure was 100/60 mmHg. Confused consciousness; painful stimuli could still be localized. Small patches of petechiae were seen on the skin of the left elbow fossa venous puncture site, and several bleeding spots were seen on the skin of the anterior chest wall. His eyelids were edematous, and the bulbar conjunctiva was mildly edematous; the pupils were equally large and rounded, and the reflex to light was sensitive. The neck was soft and non-resistant. The breath sounds of both lungs were coarse, and no dry and moist rales were heard. The border of cardiac dullness did not expand. The patient's heart rate was 120 beats/min, with absolute arrhythmia and varying intensity of the first heart sound. A grade 3/6 low-pitched, rumbling-like mid- to late-diastolic murmur could be heard in the apical region, which was limited and non-conducting. The abdominal muscles were slightly tense; there was no pressure pain throughout the abdomen; the liver and spleen were not palpable below the costal margin, the muscle tone of the right limb was slightly high, and the hemiplegia test was positive. The knee tendon reflex, Achilles tendon reflex, and abdominal wall reflex were symmetrically present.

III. Diagnostic analysis

1. Preliminary diagnosis

① Hemorrhagic fever with renal syndrome, with three overlapping phases of fever, hypotensive shock, and oliguria; ② Atrial fibrillation; ③ Rheumatic heart disease combined with valve damage; ④ Cerebral infarction (old).

> **Thinking prompts:** The diagnosis of hemorrhagic fever with renal syndrome is based on three symptoms and five phases, namely short-term fever and triple pains as the main symptoms of infection and poisoning, congestion (triple red), exudation and bleeding as the main signs, and manifestations of kidney damage. Typical patients should have five phases (fever, hypotension (shock), oliguria, polyuria, and recovery), and atypical patients should have polyuria (urine volume > 3,000 ml/d). Fever withdrawal and severe illness are the characteristics of this disease, and have diagnostic value. The diagnosis of mild or atypical cases often requires laboratory tests.
>
> The clinical manifestations of this disease are more distinctive after entering the hypotensive shock or oliguric or polyuric phases, and diagnosis should not be a problem. Therefore, diagnosis (especially early) refers to the diagnosis of patients in the febrile phase. For this reason, we should be familiar with the various clinical manifestations of the febrile period, such as acute onset of high or moderate fever, obvious headache, flushed skin on the face, neck, and upper chest, petechiae on the bilateral axillae and mucous membrane of the soft palate, and chemosis. Moderate or severe chemosis is the most characteristic or unique clinical manifestation of the disease and should be kept in mind.
>
> In this case, the patient presented with high fever and oliguria before admission to the hospital. On physical examination, there was increased body temperature, tachypnea, shortness of breath, decreased blood pressure, hemorrhagic spots or petechiae on the skin and mucous membrane of the soft palate and the bulbar conjunctiva, as well as the classic manifestation of hemorrhagic fever, chemosis, so it was consistent with the preliminary diagnosis of the emergency department, but the confirmation of the diagnosis of hemorrhagic fever still depends on testing positive for hemorrhagic fever antibodies.

2. Differential diagnosis

> **Thinking prompts:** The diagnosis is not difficult in typical patients, and the obviously staged process can be identified after entering the oliguric or polyuric phase, and specific serum antibodies can be easily detected. Therefore, the diagnosis of this disease should be differentiated mainly from febrile diseases such as upper respiratory tract infection, influenza, epidemic encephalomyelitis and septicemia and diseases with hypotensive shock such as acute toxic bacillary dysentery and shock pneumonia.

(1) The febrile phase should be differentiated from the following diseases:

1) Viral upper respiratory tract infection or influenza (flu): The manifestations of both are similar to the febrile phase of hemorrhagic fever with renal syndrome, mostly occurring in the cold winter and spring seasons, with rapid onset, high fever, chills, generalized joint and muscle aches and pains, accompanied by a certain degree of headache. However, the upper respiratory tract infection has a history of cold; influenza should be in the flu epidemic period, so family members or colleagues living together often fall sick at the same time; respiratory symptoms such as nasal congestion, runny nose, sore throat, and light cough are more prominent, and systemic illnesses improve significantly with the reduction of fever; there are few clinical manifestations unique to hemorrhagic fever with renal syndrome, such as obvious headache, lumbearlier flushed skin on the face, neck and upper chest, hemorrhagic spots or even petechiae on the skin of soft palate and axillae, and chemosis. Routine blood and urine tests for upper respiratory tract infections or influenza show normal or mildly reduced white blood cell counts, and no increase in neutrophilia or atypical lymphocytes. Normal platelet counts and marked urine protein (≥++) are rare. If available, anti-Hantaan virus (HV)-IgM can be tested on days 4–5 of the illness, and a negative test result can rule out hemorrhagic fever with renal syndrome.

2) Epidemic cerebrospinal meningitis (ECM): An infectious disease with a high prevalence in winter and spring. The incidence has decreased significantly in China in the past ten years. Most patients have no clear history of exposure. They may present with high fever and aversion to cold and chills after the onset, accompanied by bleeding skin spots, and significantly increased peripheral blood WBC and neutrophils. It is easily confused with hemorrhagic fever with renal syndrome in diagnosis. However, ECM is more common in children, with significant headaches and marked or projectile vomiting. Skin hemorrhages (petechiae) in ECM should be noted mainly in the lower body, and may increase and expand rapidly with the aggravation of the disease (mostly combined with DIC), and even fuse into large purpura. The patient in this case had varying degrees of nuchal rigidity, and the Brudzinski's and Kernig's signs were mostly positive. Peripheral blood picture can sometimes be similar to that of hemorrhagic fever with renal syndrome, but urine protein is not prominent. Cerebrospinal fluid pressure collected from a lumbar puncture can show a significant elevation, and the total

WBC count can be more than 500/μl in routine tests, with polynucleated cells dominating. Protein quantification can also significantly increase, and sugar quantification can be normal or low, showing changes associated with septic meningitis. Differential diagnosis can be made by examining meningococcal antigens or antibodies and anti-HV-IgM when available.

3) Epidemic typhus: Also known as louse-borne typhus. An acute infectious disease caused by lice-transmitted Rickettsia prowazekii, which most often occurs in the winter and spring, with a high incidence of poor sanitation. Rapid onset, continuous high fever, and severe headaches are often misdiagnosed as hemorrhagic fever with renal syndrome. However, epidemic typhus has a natural fever duration of more than two weeks, and may show transient hypotension without exudative signs. Red papules often appear on the fifth day of illness, first on the trunk, then spreading rapidly to the whole body; there may be hemorrhagic rashes, with a larger amount of congested rashes. Renal damage is mild, with only transient proteinuria; peripheral blood WBC count is normal or may be low, and the classification count is mostly normal; urine routine is mostly normal. Diagnosis can be confirmed by a Weil-Felix test with OX_{19} potency of 1:160 or higher, or a fourfold or higher increase in the potency of a double serum. Endemic typhus, which occurs in summer and fall, is similar to hemorrhagic fever with renal syndrome, and should be differentiated. For both forms of typhus, the test for IgM antibodies to hemorrhagic fever should be negative.

4) Typhoid fever: An acute infectious disease caused by S. typhi infection through the gastrointestinal tract, mostly occurring in the summer and autumn. The fever period is long, mostly without hypotension. Bleeding and urine volume changes are rarely seen. The toxic symptom is continuous high fever. It must be distinguished from hemorrhagic fever with renal syndrome occurring in summer and autumn. A typical typhoid fever patient should present the characteristic "typhoid face" – a pale, indifferent expression, with a relatively slow pulse. A dozen pale rose-red rashes 2–4 mm in diameter may appear on the lower chest and upper abdomen on the sixth or seventh day of illness, and mild splenomegaly may be found in physical examination. In contrast, the patient in a typical case of hemorrhagic fever with renal syndrome may have a drunken appearance, i.e., the face and bulbar conjunctiva are congested and flushed. On examination, the rash in hemorrhagic fever should be a hemorrhagic spot rather than the congested rash of typhoid fever. The WBC count (especially eosinophils) in peripheral blood tests for typhoid fever should be normal or reduced, which is distinctly different from that of patients with hemorrhagic fever with renal syndrome. Widal tests and the increasing potency of antibodies against S. typhi bacteriophage antigen O and flagellar antigen H have diagnostic value. Diagnosis can be confirmed by the presence of S. typhi in blood, feces, or bone marrow culture.

5) Leptospirosis: An acute systemic infectious disease caused by various types of pathogenic Leptospira. Leptospirosis usually occurs in summer and autumn, with high fever, aversion to cold and chills, headache, and a drunken appearance. It is easily confused with hemorrhagic fever with renal syndrome, which develops in summer and autumn. However, leptospirosis is associated with exposure to infected water, high fever, and significant fatigue,

accompanied by gastrocnemius muscle strain and generalized lymph node enlargement. Common pulmonary hemorrhage and diffuse alveolar hemorrhage may lead to characteristic clinical manifestations such as varying degrees of dyspnea, respiratory distress, and hemoptysis. Atypical lymphocytes are rare. If the blood culture is positive, the diagnosis can be confirmed.

6) Septicemia: Often accompanied by a primary lesion, chills and hyperthermia, and heavy systemic toxic symptoms, but no exudative signs. Blood picture shows bacterial infection, and atypical lymphocytes are rare. Positive blood culture can confirm the diagnosis.

(2) The hypotensive shock period should be differentiated from the following diseases:

1) Acute toxic bacillary dysentery: Occurring in summer and autumn and in children, mostly with a history of unclean diet. The onset of the disease is rapid, with high fever, chills, malaise, or convulsions; toxic shock, respiratory failure, or coma may occur rapidly. Routine testing of fecal specimens collected through rectal examination or diagnostic enema is useful for diagnosis. Early fecal culture may provide a confirmatory basis for diagnosis, but it usually takes 3–7 days and does not help in the early differential diagnosis of the two diseases. Compared with toxic bacillary dysentery, the course of hemorrhagic fever progresses slowly, with hypotensive shock mostly occurring on the fourth to sixth day of illness (rarely within 24 hours) and with more obvious hemorrhagic tendency and renal damage. Laboratory tests can show a significant increase in atypical peripheral blood lymphocytes and a decrease in platelet count, and routine urine tests can show significant proteinuria; if the serum anti-HV-IgM antibody is positive, the diagnosis of hemorrhagic fever may be confirmed.

2) Shock-type pneumonia: Likely a history of cold, with respiratory symptoms such as coughing, sputum, chest pain, and shortness of breath at the beginning, and hypotensive shock occurring on the second to third day of the disease, without obvious signs of exudation and bleeding. Blood tests and routine urine tests show no increased rates of atypical lymphocytes, and no decreased platelet count or severe proteinuria. An X-ray chest radiograph and serum anti-HV-IgM test can help to confirm the diagnosis.

3) A tendency for severe bleeding is a differentiation from acute leukemia and allergic and thrombocytopenic purpura.

4) Hemorrhagic fever with predominant renal damage should be differentiated from renal diseases such as primary acute glomerulonephritis, acute pyelonephritis, and nephropathy.

5) Surgical acute abdominal disease should be ruled out for a small number of patients with severe abdominal pain and obvious signs of peritoneal irritation.

IV. Diagnosis and treatment after admission

After admission, the emergency examination came back positive for anti-Hantaan virus IgM antibodies, 31.7% prothrombin activity, urine protein (+++), and hematuria (+++). The preliminary diagnosis was made as before, and the patient was reported to be critically ill according to the initial diagnosis of hemorrhagic fever with renal syndrome (hypotensive shock phase), and vital signs (mental status, temperature, blood pressure, respiration, and heart rate) were monitored every two hours. The patient was given balanced saline solution, plasma, and albumin to expand the volume, intravenous drips of a small amount of dopamine and m-hydroxylamine, and nasal catheter oxygen 2–4 L/min. A consultation with cardiovascular medicine and neurology was also requested to assist diagnosis and treatment. A total of 5,900 ml of various crystalloid and colloid solutions, including 20 g of albumin solution, 1,000 ml of hydroxyethyl starch, and 40 ml sodium chloride solution (706 plasma substitute), 250 ml of 20% mannitol, and one dose each of hydrocortisone and dexamethasone, were administered intravenously during the first 24 hours after admission, but were not applied or used in sufficient amounts due to a shortage of plasma and albumin. By the evening of the same day, the routine blood WBC was 9.55×10^9/L, Hb had decreased from 163 g/L at admission to 128 g/L, and the platelet count was only 13×10^9/L. The patient's blood pressure was stable at 110–130/80–90 mHg; his heart rate fluctuated at 115–130 beats/min; respiration was constant at 34–35 breaths/min, the oxygen saturation of his blood was 95%–100% under the condition of oxygen inhalation. Routine blood tests were performed at 01:00 the day after admission, with WBC 19.46×10^9/L, Hb 69 g/L, platelets 37×10^9/L, serum potassium 4.60 mmol/L, sodium 121.9 mmol/L, and chloride 88 mmol/L. A total of 350 ml of urine was excreted on the first day after admission.

Treatment on the second day of hospitalization remained the same as the previous day. A total of 2,680 ml of fluids, including 200 ml of fresh plasma and 500 ml of hydroxyethyl starch, and 40 ml sodium chloride solution, were administered throughout the day, but the patient still had a rapid heart rate, low blood pressure, and shortness of breath. In the afternoon, due to unstable blood pressure, vasoactive drugs (dopamine and m-hydroxylamine) were slowly injected intravenously.

At 06:00 on the third day of hospitalization, the patient's respiration became more urgent and agitated. His blood pressure dropped to 80/50 mmHg; his heart rate was 75 beats/min, respiration was 37–45 breaths/min, and oxygen saturation was only 75%–85%. After consultation with the professor on duty, the oxygen flow rate was increased to 6–8 L/min, and 5 mg of dexamethasone was administered intravenously twice. The drip rate of vasoactive drugs was increased. The blood gas showed severe acidemia, pH 7.18, metabolic acidosis, PCO_2 14.6 mHg, base deficit −12 mmol. 125 ml of 5% sodium bicarbonate was immediately administered intravenously, and 150 ml of additional sodium bicarbonate was administered. 200 ml of fresh plasma was also transfused. The relevant departments were contacted to propose tracheal intubation, and in view of the patient's atrial fibrillation and difficulty tolerating his cardiac function condition, tracheotomy and ventilator-assisted respiratory therapy were prepared. However, because the family decided to discontinue treatment, the patient was finally resuscitated and discharged automatically at noon on the third day. At 12:30 before discharge, the patient was in cardiac arrest but still breathing.

V. Summary and lessons learned

The diagnosis of hemorrhagic fever with renal syndrome could be confirmed in this patient because positive anti-Hantaan virus IgM antibodies were detected. There were also multiple complications, especially an old cerebral infarction and rheumatic heart valve disease. The patient had several features: ① He was a middle-aged male with an old cerebral infarction and rheumatic heart valve disease prior to hemorrhagic fever, with a weak constitution. ② On admission, he was in the overlapping phases of fever, hypotensive shock, and oliguria, and his condition was critical. ③ On the day after admission, his blood pressure could not be stabilized even after adequate fluid resuscitation in the form of anti-shock treatments such as volume expansion therapy. On the third day, shock and respiratory failure reappeared, resulting in a life-threatening condition.

The main problems in recovery and treatment were:

1. Inadequate monitoring: Basic vital signs such as blood pressure, heart rate, respiration, body temperature, and the mental status of patients in shock should be monitored at least once every hour or every 30 minutes. When available, the patient should be sent to the intensive care unit (ICU) for consultation and treatment, or to critical care.

2. Low colloidal fluid application on the first day after admission: The choice of crystalloids or colloids for fluid resuscitation in septic shock remains highly controversial internationally, and several studies on fluid selection in infectious shock have shown no difference in the prognostic impact of the clinical use of crystalloids or colloids on patients. Saline and albumin are equally effective in patients with severe infections and infectious shock. However, most experts still believe that colloids have a higher osmolarity than crystalloids, and are better able to maintain intravascular volume, making them a more desirable volume expanding agent for the treatment of infectious shock. Plasma or fresh plasma is preferred among colloid fluids. The patient in this case was only transfused 20 g of albumin plus 1,000 ml of 706 plasma substitute on the first day after admission for objective reasons, which was obviously insufficient.

3. The use of vasoactive drugs and positive inotropic drugs is debatable: In recent years, norepinephrine and dopamine or dobutamine have been advocated both internationally and in China in the treatment of infectious shock, especially of the high-drain, low-impedance type. It is generally accepted that the initial treatment of infectious shock should be aggressive early goal-directed fluid resuscitation. Even in conjunction with volume resuscitation, the use of vasoactive and/or positive inotropic drugs to increase and maintain perfusion pressure in tissues and organs should be considered, supplemented by low-dose glucocorticoids when necessary. Commonly used medications include dopamine, norepinephrine, vasopressin, and dobutamine.

Dopamine – a first-line vasoactive drug in the treatment of infectious shock – combines the excitatory effects of dopaminergic and adrenergic α and β receptors, exhibiting varying receptor effects at specific doses. Small doses of dopamine act mainly on dopamine receptors (DA) and have a mild vasodilatory effect. Moderate doses are dominated by β_1 receptor excitation, which increases myocardial contractility and heart rate, thereby increasing myocardial work and oxygen consumption. High doses of dopamine, on the other hand, are dominated by α_1 receptor excitation, and show significant vasoconstriction.

Norepinephrine has a dual effect, namely the excitation of α and β receptors. Its strong excitatory effect on α receptors improves tissue perfusion by elevating mean arterial pressure (MAP); its moderate excitatory effect on β receptors increases the heart rate and cardiac work, but the increase in heart rate and myocardial contractility is partially offset by its effect on venous refill and the right heart ventricular pressor receptor, thus reducing myocardial oxygen consumption. Therefore, it is also considered as a first-line vasoactive drug for the treatment of infectious toxic shock.

Dobutamine has strong β_1, β_2 receptor and moderate α receptor excitatory effects. The positive inotropic effect of its β_1 receptor can increase the cardiac index by 25%–50%, and can also increase the heart rate by 10%–20% accordingly. The β_2 receptor effect can reduce pulmonary artery wedge pressure, which can improve the right-side heart ejection and increase cardiac output. Overall, dobutamine increases both oxygen delivery and consumption (especially in the myocardium) and is therefore generally used in the treatment of infectious shock in patients whose cardiac function has not improved after adequate fluid resuscitation. In cases of combined hypotension, a combination of vasoconstrictive drugs is appropriate. Several studies in recent years have reported that for patients with septic shock whose volume-resuscitation response is not satisfactory, norepinephrine in combination with dobutamine improves tissue perfusion and oxygen delivery, increases coronary and renal blood flow as well as creatinine clearance, and reduces blood lactate levels in patients with infectious shock who have suboptimal volume resuscitation, without exacerbating organ ischemia.

In conclusion, hemodynamic monitoring tools for patients in shock at domestic infectious disease clinics or most specialty infectious disease hospitals (especially for the monitoring of cardiac function and oxygen kinetics and oxygen metabolism) are still largely absent. Therefore, the monitoring of the various types of shock, the stages of shock development, and the evaluation of therapeutic efficacy are still relatively backward, and there is a lack of experience in the use of various types of vasoactive drugs and positive inotropic drugs. Only further measurements of the parameters reflecting cardiac preload and volume responsiveness, cardiac output (CO), and microcirculation and tissue oxygenation, in addition to the monitoring of basic vital signs, can provide targeted guidance for the treatment of various types of infectious shock, including the use of vasoactive drugs and positive inotropic drugs.

4. In the morning of the third day of hospitalization, the patient's condition deteriorated sharply, showing the second stage of shock with severe metabolic acidosis and respiratory failure. His life could not be saved in the end, despite the best efforts to resuscitate him, including some objective conditions (his family failed to cooperate).

(Bai Xuefan)

High fever with a red and swollen lymph node for two days

I. Medical history

Patient: (Pediatric) four years old, a herder's daughter. She was admitted to hospital for hyperthermia with a red and swollen lymph node for two days.

The patient developed general discomfort and high fever, accompanied by headache, dizziness, body aches, and fatigue two days earlier and was taken to the local township health center by her family for diagnosis and treatment. A diagnosis was not made. General symptomatic treatment was given, but the effect was not good, and she was transferred to a higher-level hospital for treatment.

II. Physical examination

Body temperature 39°C, pulse 120 times/min, respiration 30 times/min, blood pressure 100/60 mmHg. Drowsy state, facial features of acute illness, pained appearance, flushed face. A red and swollen lymph node (about 2 cm in size) was palpated in the right axilla, adhering to the surrounding tissues, immobile, and with obvious pressure pain. A 0.5 cm × 0.5 cm scar was seen 6 cm below her right breast area. Her neck was soft and non-resistant. No positive cardiopulmonary signs were found. Her abdomen was soft. Her liver and spleen were not palpable below the costal margin, and the bowel sounds were normal. Bilateral Babinski's sign was negative, as were Kernig's and Brudzinski's signs.

III. Diagnosis analysis and medical history supplement

The course of the patient's illness is characterized by the following:

(1) Rapid onset and short duration
(2) High fever with severe systemic toxemia
(3) Enlarged lymph nodes with adhesions to surrounding tissues, immobile, and obvious pressure pain
(4) Skin damage
(5) Ineffective general symptomatic treatment

Thinking prompts: Based on the above features of the patient's medical history, first consider the possibility of bacterial infection, such as possible purulent infection due to skin damage, involving inflammatory enlargement of local lymph nodes. Further questions should be asked about the cause of the skin damage and the manifestations before the onset. Routine blood tests and blood cultures should also be done.

Follow-up history (cause of skin damage): The patient's mother reported that the girl had come into contact with the family's sheepdog, which had eaten a dead marmot two days earlier.

Thinking prompts: The patient had an acute onset, high fever, a red and swollen lymph node, and a clear history of contact with a sheepdog that had eaten a dead marmot, so detailed questions should be asked about the details of the contact, whether there was a history of flea bites, and the condition of the dog that had eaten the marmot. This epidemiological information is helpful in determining the presence of endemic or natural epidemic origin diseases, especially plague. Because the child had a high fever with a headache, dizziness, and drowsiness, attention should be paid to signs and symptoms of septicemia and infections of the central nervous system.

After gathering detailed medical and epidemiological history, we learned that local herders had found several dead marmots, and that sheepdogs often took them near to the herders' yurts to gnaw on them. The patient had often played with the sheepdogs before the onset of her illness, and had also been exposed to the dead marmots themselves. We immediately contacted the local Center for Disease Control and Prevention (CDC) to report the case and ask about a local plague epidemic. The CDC informed us that the area was a source of plague, and there had been several outbreaks of inter-rat and human varieties. At this point, it seemed highly likely that the patient was infected with plague bacteria, and laboratory tests had to be performed as quickly as possible to confirm the diagnosis. Meanwhile, the patient's contacts had to be isolated and quarantined.

IV. Auxiliary examinations
1. Routine examination results
Routine blood: White blood cells and neutrophils significantly increased.
   Routine urine: Possibly proteinuria or hematuria.

2. Pathogenic examination
For suspected plague cases, a rapid and effective hemagglutination test or ELISA should be selected to detect specific antigens or antibodies. The patient's blood, sputum, or lymph node puncture fluid should be smeared and bacterial cultured, as a positive result can confirm the diagnosis. At the same time, smears and bacteriological cultures of dead marmots or sheepdogs with contact (lymph node puncture fluid, blood, visceral tissue, or suspension) should also be

taken. These specimens can also be subjected to animal inoculation tests, and the diagnosis can be confirmed if the manifestations of plague are present and plague bacilli are found in the inoculated animal specimens.

3. Other tests

Liver and kidney function should be checked to determine whether they (and other organs) are involved. A pulmonary X-ray should be taken to see if there is any involvement from the lungs.

> **Thinking prompts:** Routine blood tests and bacterial cultures are among the most commonly used clinical laboratory tests, especially for febrile patients. Increased white blood cells and neutrophils can be used to initially determine strong evidence for bacterial, fungal, rickettsial, and spirochete infections. A positive bacterial culture or serologic test (i.e., an etiological test) of blood or bodily fluids is direct evidence of the pathogenic infection that is being diagnosed.

V. Diagnosis and treatment

A series of tests were performed after admission. The patient's venous blood and sputum specimens were negative for bacteriological tests on the day of onset and four days after the disease, when no lymphatic puncture fluid was taken. The plague bacillus was isolated from all five dead local marmots. After admission, a dynamic detection of serology (hemagglutination test) showed a gradual increase in the antibody titer of Yersinia pestis, from 1:20 on the first day of hospitalization to 1:40 on the second day, 1:80 on the third day, and 1:160 on the fourth day. The local CDC also took blood from ten sheepdogs caught in the infected area to perform an indirect hemagglutination test, and the average titer of the hemagglutination test antibody was positive (1:235). Based on the epidemiological investigation, clinical signs and symptoms, and laboratory findings, the outbreak was confirmed as glandular plague caused by bites from infected fleas from the patient's contact with a dead marmot or infected sheepdog.

Treatment: Once the patient was suspected of plague, she was immediately placed in isolation. She recovered after three weeks of active treatment with streptomycin. By this point, she had been diagnosed and treated promptly and effectively.

VI. Lessons learned

The following points are worth noting: ① The patient was a rural child; the main characteristics of her illness were acute onset, manifested by high fever and heavy systemic toxic symptoms (with drowsiness). ② Physical examination revealed enlarged lymph nodes and a broken scar on the skin under her right breast area, suggesting that this was the source of the infection. ③ Increased leukocytes and neutrophils confirmed pathogenic bacterial infection. ④ The local area was a natural source of plague, and has had epidemics of animal and human varieties. The patient had a clear history of contact with dead marmots and sheepdogs that had eaten them. This should remind clinicians to ask about the epidemiological situation when diagnosing infectious diseases, which can be extremely helpful in the diagnosis of plague. ⑤ Timely collection of human and contact animal specimens for etiology tests is essential to confirm the diagnosis of plague. The patient's negative blood and sputum cultures and antibody levels increasing day by day suggested that Yersinia pestis infection was limited to the lymph nodes and had not yet caused septicemia or pneumonic plague. A lymph node puncture smear and bacterial culture at that time would have been helpful in making an early diagnosis of glandular plague. This has very important clinical and epidemiological implications for the treatment of the patient and the control of the epidemic. ⑥ Although the patient was highly suspected of having plague, because of high fever, headache, and enlargement of the lymph nodes, differential diagnosis should also be made with septicemia and acute lymphadenitis, and emphasis should be placed on the choice of laboratory tests.

The examination for Yersinia pestis should include blood or body fluid examination of the patient, and laboratory examination of local dead marmots, sheepdogs, and rat fleas. The main methods of etiology examination include the following: ① Serological examination of plague: The indirect hemagglutination test for the serological detection of plague was first used in 1951 by Amies. This method was recommended by the WHO in 1956 as one of the routine serological tests for plague, and is a method for detecting plague-specific antibodies. Due to the high specificity and sensitivity of the method, it has been widely used around the world. Reverse hemagglutination assay, or reverse indirect hemagglutination assay (RIHA), is a method that sensitizes red blood cells with plague-specific antibodies, and is used to detect the corresponding antigen. The method is sensitive and specific, and can detect the bacterium directly, as well as soluble (F1) antigens to make retrospective diagnosis, which is more successful in the detection of spoiled specimens. The radioimmunoprecipitation assay (RIP) detects trace amounts of plague F1 antibodies. These methods are still in use in China. ② Lymph node aspiration fluid, blood, cerebrospinal fluid, and sputum for smears and bacterial cultures. Positive results can confirm the diagnosis. ③ The detection of plague-specific nucleic acid sequences by PCR has the advantages of specificity and sensitivity, but care should be taken to avoid false-positive results caused by contamination.

(Zhang Yuexin & Lu Xiaobo)

High fever for one day with chest pain and hemoptysis

I. Medical history

Patient: A young Kazakh herdsman living in the northern Tianshan Mountains of Xinjiang. He was admitted to hospital with high fever for one day, with chest pain and hemoptysis.

In summer, the patient felt unexplained general discomfort, dizziness, headache, fever, and sore throat after waking up in the morning. He went to the local health clinic and was given 0.5 g of oral oxytetracycline and 0.25 g of injectable analgin, which were ineffective. His condition continued to worsen, with chest pain, coughing, and foamy sputum with red blood streaks.

II. Physical examination

Temperature 39.8°C, pulse 108 beats/min, respiration 28 beats/min, blood pressure 90/60 mHg. Appearance of acute illness, shortness of breath, tonsils II° enlarged, no enlargement of the superficial lymph nodes, diminished breath sounds in both lungs, flat and soft abdomen; liver and spleen were not palpable. There were no other abnormal findings. The patient was in good health and had no history of tuberculosis.

> **Thinking prompts:** Questions after clinical reception: ① What has caused the fever? ② What lesions are suggested by chest pain, coughing, and hemoptysis? ③ Which further tests should be performed? ④ What other medical history should be obtained? ⑤ What is the diagnosis and how should the patient be treated?
>
> Fever is one of the most common clinical symptoms after a pathogen infects an organism. If the acute onset of fever is accompanied by general discomfort, headache, dizziness, and sore throat, the possibility of bacterial, viral, and fungal infections is most likely. Blood cells can be tested and classified immediately, which can preliminarily determine whether it is a bacterial, fungal, or viral infection. In general, if the white blood cell count and neutrophil percentage are significantly increased, it is more likely to be a bacterial, fungal, spirochete, rickettsial, or pathogenic infection, while if the white blood cell count and neutrophil percentage

are decreased, it is more likely to be a viral infection.

This patient presented with chest pain, coughing, sputum, and hemoptysis on the day of fever, suggesting that the infection was in the lungs and that hemorrhagic lesions of the respiratory tract tissue were present. In young people with a sudden onset of high fever, symptoms of infection poisoning, respiratory symptoms, and hemoptysis, we should consider common respiratory diseases such as bacterial pneumonia, bronchiectasis, and tuberculosis. Respiratory symptoms with alternative causes should also be considered, such as cardiac failure, multi-organ shock failure, pulmonary anthrax, pneumonic plague, and pulmonary hemorrhagic leptospirosis.

The patient in this case was a young herder from the mountainous region of Xinjiang, with previous good health and no history of heart disease that would suggest heart failure. There were no shock manifestations, so multi-organ shock failure could be ruled out. Bronchiectasis could also be ruled out, as there was no recurrent cough or yellow pus in the sputum. There was no history of tuberculosis or symptoms of tuberculosis poisoning such as afternoon hypothermia and wasting. There was no leptospirosis epidemic in Xinjiang.

In addition to bacterial pneumonia, diseases related to the patient's occupation should be considered. In particular, both anthrax and plague can cause primary lung infections. The manifestations are cough, chest pain, coughing up bloody pus in the sputum, shortness of breath, cyanosis, and some moist rales at the bottom of the lungs. Symptoms and signs are not commensurate. Systemic poisoning symptoms are extremely serious.

III. Additional medical history and diagnosis

Additional medical history: The patient had been grazing marmots with two colleagues two weeks before the onset of his illness, and had skinned the dead marmots five days earlier. One of his colleagues developed general malaise, high fever, headache, chest tightness, cough, hemoptysis, and staggering gait two days earlier, and died without treatment. The other companion also presented with similar symptoms.

Thinking prompts: From this epidemiological history and analysis of these clinical manifestations, all three people showed the same symptoms (high fever, headache, dizziness, cough, and hemoptysis), and all have been in contact with dead marmots. This showed that it was not general bacterial pneumonia, but a contagious animal-derived infectious disease.

Immediate contact was made with the local CDC to report the three cases and to inquire about any outbreaks of plague and anthrax in the Tianshan Mountains in Xinjiang. We learned that the local area was a natural source of plague, but not anthrax. At this point, it was highly likely that the case was primary pneumonic plague. Blood, sputum, and pharyngeal secretions were immediately collected from the patient and his deceased colleague, and were sent for bacteria culture. The following day, the results came back: Yersinia pestis, confirming the diagnosis of primary pneumonic plague. Due to limited conditions at the local health clinic, a routine blood test and chest X-ray were not performed.

IV. Treatment

Strict isolation measures were immediately implemented for these two cases of suspected primary pneumonic plague and their contacts. Immediate rehydration with symptomatic supportive therapy and antimicrobial therapy was given. Antimicrobial treatment with streptomycin 1 g each time, two times/day, intramuscular injection; oral tetracycline, 0.75 g to 1 g each time, four times/day. Since aminoglycosides and tetracycline antibacterial drugs are sensitive to Yersinia pestis, the combination of drugs for pneumonic plague is superior to antibacterial drugs alone. Both patients' body temperatures normalized and the symptoms disappeared after five and six days of treatment, respectively. Blood and sputum cultures were taken on days six, nine, and 12, and were negative. The patients were released from isolation and discharged on day fifteen.

V. Lessons learned

For young herders with a sudden onset of high fever with severe toxemia and respiratory symptoms and a clear history of exposure to dead marmots in plague endemic areas, the possibility of pneumonic plague should be considered. In these three cases of primary plague, except for one patient who died without timely treatment, the other two survived due to timely treatment with antimicrobial drugs. Although there were no conditions for further laboratory tests in pastoral areas, analysis by virtue of epidemiological history and clinical presentation played a key role in making the correct diagnosis and offering timely treatment.

Once plague is diagnosed, it should be handled in accordance with the treatment for Class A infectious diseases and the Emergency Plague Plan. Strictly isolate patients and keep the sickroom free of rats and fleas. Patients' excreta should be strictly and thoroughly disinfected before dumping. Medical and nursing personnel should wear protective isolation clothing, protective gloves, and masks as required when entering the infected area or coming into contact with patients. Immediately report any outbreaks to the local CDC and health administration. Conduct an epidemiological survey of inter-rat plague in the area. Isolate the patient until the swollen lymph nodes disappear, and then observe them for five to seven days. In areas that are natural sources of plague, enhance publicity and education for herdsmen, and conduct plague vaccinations. Immediately report cases of sudden, unexplained deaths of animals such as marmots and wild rats to the local health administration and CDC. Do not touch the carcasses of dead animals to avoid being infected.

(Zhang Yuexin & Lu Xiaobo)

Fever and generalized rash for seven days

I. Medical history

Patient: Male, 12 years old, from Wuqing County in Tianjin. He was hospitalized between 4 and 12 March 2006 with fever and generalized rash for seven days.

The patient developed a fever with no apparent cause seven days earlier, with a temperature fluctuating from 38.5°C to 39.5°C. A rash appeared on his face and chest, initially as a macule resembling a mosquito bite, followed by papules and herpes with mild itching and no pain, which was not taken seriously. He was treated with penicillin, Qingkailing, and ribavirin for four days at a local clinic, but his symptoms were not reduced. He was admitted to the local county hospital where he was treated with Shuanghuanglian and ribavirin for three days, but the treatment was not effective. The rash increased day after day, and was densely distributed on his face and trunk, and less so on his extremities, accompanied by diarrhea and dilute watery stools 3–4 times a day, with a headache, cough, decreased appetite, and persistent high fever. He was transferred to our hospital.

The patient had previously been healthy, with no history of food and drug allergies. Epidemiological history: Varicella was present in the hospital in the town where the patient lived.

> **Thinking prompts:** The patient complained of fever and rash. Many infectious diseases are accompanied by these symptoms, and are called rash infections. A rash can either be on the skin (exanthem) or the mucosa (enanthem). The time and sequence of the appearance of the rash is an important reference for diagnosis and differential diagnosis. For example, a varicella rash occurs on the first day of the course of varicella and rubella, on the second day for scarlet fever, on the third day for smallpox, on the fourth day for measles, on the fifth day for typhus, and on the sixth day for typhoid. The varicella rash is mainly distributed on the trunk; the smallpox rash is mostly distributed on the face and extremities. Measles has a mucous membrane rash that first appears behind the ears and on the face, and then spreads to the trunk and extremities. All have their own features, and should be investigated carefully. Self-perceived symptoms of the rash should also be asked about, such as the presence and extent of pruritus. If the rash is contact dermatitis, eczema, or urticaria, the pruritus is heavier, which helps to identify it.

During the examination, attention should be paid to the morphology, nature, size, number, color, edge, boundary, shape, surface, base, content, location, distribution, and arrangement of the rash. When palpation is performed, note the presence of tenderness (is it firm or soft?) and the presence of Nikolsky's sign. Blisters often occur on normal-looking skin. If the blisters are gently pushed and pressed with the fingers, can their walls be expanded and can they be enlarged? If normal-looking skin is pushed and rubbed slightly, can the epidermis be peeled off, or do blisters appear soon after rubbing (Nikolsky's sign?) Clinically, skin diseases that are positive for Nikolsky's sign include herpetic epidermolysis bullosa atrophica drug eruption, scald-like staphylococcal skin syndrome, pemphigus, epidermolysis bullosa, and familial chronic benign pemphigus.

Asking about the course of treatment (including the medications used, dosage, and efficacy) can help determine the cause of the fever and rash. If antibiotics are ineffective, then a bacterial infection may be considered less likely. If fever and rash manifest after taking certain drugs, the possibility of drug eruption should be considered. In infectious diseases, epidemiological information plays an important role in the diagnosis of infectious diseases, and for any disease, the first inquiry should be the epidemiological history. Vaccination history and past history help to understand the patient's immune status. Allergy may also present with fever and rash. Therefore, attention should be paid to the history of allergy.

II. Physical examination and auxiliary examination on admission
1. Physical examination
T 39.5°C, clear consciousness, apatheia; had to be carried to the ward. Cooperated with the examination; face, trunk, and extremities were covered with herpes, locally fused, with translucent apices, clear herpes fluid, top coated with methyl violet, and obvious swelling of the face, with a negative Ney's sign. The eyes could not be opened, and clusters of herpes could be seen on the lid conjunctiva, oral mucosa, external auditory canal, perianal area, scrotum, and perineum. There was no abnormality in cardiopulmonary auscultation. The liver and spleen could not be palpated under the ribs. There was no pressure pain throughout the abdomen, and pathological signs were not elicited.

2. Auxiliary examination
Routine blood test: WBC 7.0×10^9/L, N 87.2%, E 3.5%, PLT 214×10^9/L.

CRP 65 mg/L.

Routine urine, routine stool, heart, liver and kidney functions, electrolytes, ECG, chest X-ray, urological ultrasound and cardiac ultrasound were all within normal range.

III. Treatment after admission
1. Preliminary diagnosis
There was an epidemiologic history of disseminated varicella at the hospital in the area where

the patient resided. There was an acute onset, short history, fever, and herpes all over the body including on the mucous membrane and skin, so the first consideration was varicella.

> **Thinking prompts:** The patient had a fever and rash, which are seen in both infectious and non-infectious diseases. The presence of papules and herpes in children should indicate possible papular urticaria, which is a non-infectious disease. This patient had more and larger herpes and severe clinical symptoms, which did not correspond to the typical varicella presentation. It had to be differentiated from epidermolysis bullosa drug eruption in non-infectious diseases. This patient's rash was special. Although macules, papules, and herpes were all present, herpes was the main manifestation. Viral infections such as varicella, herpes simplex, smallpox, hand, foot and mouth disease, and herpes zoster can all have herpes manifestations and should be differentiated.

2. Differential diagnosis

(1) Papular urticaria: Papular urticaria is common in children and adolescents, and is mostly caused by bites from certain arthropods such as mosquitoes, fleas, mites, midges, and bedbugs. It can also be caused by digestive disorders and allergies to certain foods. The rash is characterized by red papules with small blisters at the top and no red halo, appearing in batches, centrifugally distributed, mostly on the lower back, abdomen, both lower limbs, not involving the head and mouth; generally, no fever or other systemic symptoms. The clinical manifestations of this patient are not consistent with it, so it was ruled out.

(2) Epidermolysis bullosa-type eruption: A serious drug eruption, often caused by sulfonamides, antipyretic and analgesic agents (salicylates and aminopyrine), antibiotics, and barbiturates. The onset of the illness is rapid, with severe symptoms of systemic toxicity. The rash appears as diffuse purplish red or dark red patches, often starting in the axillae and groin, and rapidly spreading to the whole body, with significant tenderness, followed by flaccid blisters of varying sizes at the erythema, which can become eroded when rubbed slightly, or can form large areas of epidermal necrosis and loosening, with a positive Nikolsky's sign. The necrotic epidermis is grayish red over the erosion, leaving a painful exfoliated surface. There is an increased percentage of eosinophils in laboratory tests. The patient in this case had taken a variety of drugs, including the antibiotic penicillin, so epidermolysis bullosa-type eruption was considered, but he had a fever and rash before taking medication, and the herpes did not show obvious erosion or rupture. Nikolsky's sign was negative and eosinophils were normal, so it was not consistent with the manifestations of the disease, so it was ruled out.

(3) Smallpox: Smallpox patients have generally not been vaccinated against it, and have been exposed to it. There can also be macules, papules, herpes, and scabs in sequence. However, the rash appears after 3–4 days of fever and is distributed centrifugally, mostly on the head, face, and extremities, with a denser and larger rash, mostly round, with a depressed center, deep within the skin, and firm to the touch like a small bean. There is hyperthermia with severe

toxemic symptoms. So far, there have been no cases of smallpox in China. The patient's latent period was short, and the rash appeared on the day of fever, with concentric distribution. These symptoms were not consistent with smallpox, so it was ruled out.

(4) Hand, foot, and mouth disease (HFMD): Most often seen in children under four years of age. Enteroviruses that cause HFMD include enterovirus 71 (EV71) and certain serotypes of group A coxsackie virus (CoxA) and echo virus (Echo). The rash is centrifugally distributed, with painful rice grain-sized scattered herpes on the oral mucosa; there are rice grain-sized herpes on the palms of the hands or feet, with less fluid in the blisters and no scab formation. This patient's symptoms did not match, so it was not considered.

(5) Herpes zoster (shingles): Usually seen in adults who have had varicella in the past, with herpes arranged in clusters, distributed along the peripheral nerves of the skin on one side of the body, asymmetrical, and with localized pain. This patient's symptoms were not consistent with this, so it was ruled out.

(6) Varicella: Based on the patient's fever and rash manifestations, varicella was initially considered. Clinicians proposed to administer varicella antibodies for further clarification after admission.

3. Hospital admission

The patient had dense laminar herpes, with translucent pulp, a large amount of exuding pulp, thick walls, and almost no normal skin between the rashes. It was seen in the oral mucosa, bulbar conjunctiva, perianal area, scrotum, and perineum, and had critical clinical manifestations with high fever, cough, diarrhea, apatheia, and decreased appetite.

Laboratory tests: Neutrophils were significantly elevated, showing signs of mixed infection, and severe varicella was considered in combination with the above manifestations.

Severe varicella is most often seen in pediatric patients with malignant diseases and impaired immune function, and long-term use of various cancer drugs and adrenal cortical hormone. Detailed medical history should be taken to understand the cause of severe varicella.

Severe varicella can lead to varicella hepatitis, acute liver failure, interstitial myocarditis, and nephritis, so clinicians proposed to perform heart, liver, and kidney function tests, routine urine and chest X-ray, an electrocardiogram, and an abdominal ultrasound after admission for further clarification. Varicella comorbidity includes primary varicella pneumonia and encephalitis. Varicella pneumonia is more common in adults than children. The severity of the disease varies from mild inflammation and rapid regression on an X-ray in mild cases to being fatal in severe cases, manifested by high fever, coughing, chest pain, hemoptysis, shortness of breath and cyanosis, and dry and moist rales in both lungs. An X-ray may reveal obvious inflammation of the lungs, and in cases of secondary bacterial infection, the condition may be aggravated and sometimes death may occur. Attention should be paid to this. During ward rounds, inquire about corresponding symptoms. Detailed lung auscultation and chest X-ray examination should be performed to be alert to its occurrence. The incidence of varicella encephalitis is less than

1 per 1,000, mostly in children aged 5–7 years. It often occurs between the end of the first and second week of the rash. The clinical manifestation and cerebrospinal fluid status are similar to general viral encephalitis, with a fatality rate of about 5%, with central nervous system sequelae in a few cases. During ward rounds, talk with the patient and examine their nervous system.

Patients should be isolated upon admission to avoid transmission to others. The skin should be kept clean and the nails trimmed, and scratching blisters should be avoided to prevent secondary infection. During the fever and rash period, the patient should take bed rest, drink more water, and consume nutritious, easily digestible food such as milk, eggs, fruit, and vegetables. They should avoid spicy food, fish, and shrimp.

The treatment in this case was a 0.75 g acyclovir injection every eight hours by intravenous drip, three million U/d interferons via intramuscular injection for antiviral therapy, and an intramuscular injection of gamma globulin to improve immune support therapy. The hemogram suggested the possibility of mixed infection, and the patient had a greater amount of larger herpes, so infection had to be prevented. Ceftriaxone sodium (2.0 g/d) was given in an intravenous drip. The patient had a high fever and decreased appetite, so rehydration, electrolyte replenishment, and timely correction of the water-electrolyte balance were closely monitored. Local treatment with helium-neon laser irradiation and topical antiviral and antipruritic symptomatic treatment with topical interferon spray were given.

4. Ward-round analysis on the fifth day after hospitalization

Laboratory tests results: Herpes simplex virus (HSV) type I and II antibodies were negative, CMV antibodies were negative, varicella antibodies IgM were positive; liver function: ALT 65 U/L, AST 56 U/L; cardiac function and renal function, and routine urine tests were normal. ECG, chest X-ray, and abdominal ultrasound were normal.

Follow-up medical history: The patient was given a small dose of glucocorticoid at the primary care clinic at the beginning of his illness due to persistent high fever, leading to the spread of the virus, which was aggravated by co-infection with bacteria. Mild liver damage was considered to be related to viral infection.

The day after treatment, his body temperature began to decrease, and on the morning of the fifth day of hospitalization it dropped to normal. The herpes did not increase and gradually dried up. The patient was eating more than before. Rehydration was stopped but other treatments continued.

5. Condition at discharge

After treatment, the child's body temperature was normal, and herpes fluid was gradually absorbed. On the seventh day, acyclovir was discontinued. After eight days of comprehensive treatment, all herpes had formed scabs, a small amount of which had fallen off. Routine blood and liver function results were normal.

IV. Follow-up

At the follow-up visit after two weeks, all the scabs on the patient's body had fallen off and there were no scars. He was back at school.

V. Lessons learned

When the etiology is not clear and high fever occurs with rash-producing illnesses such as measles and early varicella, remember not to rush to reduce fever and use glucocorticoids, as this may aggravate the patient's condition. Regarding the use of hormones in patients with varicella, high doses given early in the course of the disease may cause aggravation and be detrimental to the patient, especially during the latent period. Later in the course of the disease, when the rash forms scabs and no new rash appears, or when treating critical cases such as severe laryngitis, varicella pneumonia, or varicella encephalitis, corticosteroids can be applied without the risk of spreading the lesion.

To prevent the transmission of varicella, patients should be isolated until the rash has scabbed over. Children who have been in contact with varicella patients should be isolated and observed for three weeks. Those who are particularly frail can be injected with gamma globulin within four days of contact.

(Cao Wukui)

Eye pain and headache for four days, and herpes on the right frontal and nasal tip for three days

I. Medical history

Patient: Male, 43 years old, from Tianjin. He was hospitalized from 1 to 7 May 2006 with eye pain and headache for four days, and herpes on the right forehead and nasal tip for three days.

Four days before admission, the patient developed right-sided ocular pain and discomfort, lachrymation, and severe and persistent right-sided headache and dizziness without nasal congestion, with no obvious cause. He went to an external ophthalmology clinic and was diagnosed with conjunctivitis. He was given topical levofloxacin ophthalmic solution and oral amoxicillin, with no relief. One day later, multiple erythema, clusters of blisters and papules without crusting, and pruritus appeared on the right side of his forehead, hairline, and tip of his nose, without fever. Two days later, due to aggravated dizziness and nausea, the patient went to the emergency department of an external hospital and was given a Xingnaojing injection (XNJi) and ranitidine, which did not relieve his symptoms. An ophthalmology consultation was held at the same time, and keratitis was considered. Acyclovir eye drops were given for topical application, but the patient's condition still did not improve, so he was referred to our hospital.

The patient had previously been healthy, with an unknown history of infectious diseases, and no history of food and drug allergies.

Thinking prompts: Eye pain, headache, dizziness, and a rash were the main complaints in this case. Because patients are often unable to give a full and detailed medical history, questioning is required to complete the picture. The steps below can be followed:

1. Eye pain is an ocular stimulus symptom. Others include eye redness, photophobia, and lachrymation, which should be asked about. Ocular stimulus symptoms are commonly seen in conjunctival inflammation, corneal inflammation, trauma, acute iritis, and glaucoma. Note specialist eye examinations.

2. The main points of inquiry for headache and dizziness are as follows: ① Headache characteristics such as urgency, location, timing and duration of attacks, degree, nature, and factors that provoke, exacerbate, and relieve it; ② The presence of associated concomitant symptoms such as insomnia, anxiety, nausea, vomiting (whether projectile or not), dizziness, vertigo, syncope, sweating, convulsions, paresthesia or motion abnormalities, mental abnormalities, drowsiness, and disturbance of consciousness; ③ History of relevant site diseases such as infections, hypertension atherosclerosis, craniocerebral trauma, tumor, psychosis, epilepsy, neurosis, and abnormalities of the eyes, ears, nose, and teeth; ④ Occupational characteristics and history of toxic exposure; ⑤ Treatment history and responsiveness.

Combined with the clinical manifestation of right-sided ocular pain accompanied by a headache, and in addition to the possible ophthalmogenic factors, local extracranial lesions such as sinusitis and trigeminal neuralgia should be considered. Therefore, it is necessary to ask about the basic characteristics of the headache, such as nature and location, and whether there is nasal congestion. If projectile vomiting is present, the case needs to be differentiated from intracranial diseases such as epidemic encephalomyelitis. The disease may present with signs of meningeal irritation, so neurological examination should be noted.

Rashes include both subjective and objective symptoms. Subjective symptoms include itching, pain, a burning sensation, and numbness. Objective symptoms, i.e., skin lesions, also known as rashes, are lesions of the skin mucosa that can be detected visually or by touch, mainly in the form and changes of the rash. If the rash is due to allergies, then the patient's history of drug and food allergies is quite important, and should be inquired about. The rash was one of the patient's main manifestations in this case, and its appearance and characteristics should be noted in detail during the physical examination.

II. Physical examination and auxiliary examination on admission
1. Physical examination

T 36.5°C, multiple erythematous spots on the right forehead, hairline, and nasal tip, clusters of blisters and papules on the surface, no pustules or blood blisters; right eye congested, right preauricular and submaxillary lymph nodes enlarged with pressure pain. Binocular vision: Right eye visual acuity 0.5, corrected to 1.0 with small aperture glass and 1.0 in the left eye. The conjunctiva of the right eye was a mix of congested and edematous; the conjunctiva of the upper and lower eyelids was congested, papillary hyperplasia and follicle formation were visible, aqueous discharge was visible in the conjunctiva, scattered punctate infiltrates were visible on the cornea, anterior chamber (−), the pupil was equal in size and round, the reflex to light was present, lens (−), fundus (−), the mobility of the eye was approximately in place;

the intraocular pressure and orbital pressure were normal. There was no pressure pain in the facial nasal sinus area. The neck was soft and non-resistant. The cardiac border was not large, there was no bulge in the precordial region, and no pathological murmur was heard in the auscultatory area of either valve. The meningeal stimulation sign was negative, as were the pathological signs.

> **Thinking prompts:** Blood tests were performed based on a complete history and physical examination to understand the changes in the blood and to assist in identifying the cause of the rash. Because blisters are most often seen with viral herpes infections, herpes virus antibody testing and scraping of herpes lesions are required. The infection may damage the heart, liver, and kidney function. Abdominal color doppler ultrasonography should be performed.

2. Auxiliary examination

Blood count: WBC 5.8×10^9/L, N 54.4%, L 41%.

HSV type I and II antibodies were negative, CMV antibodies were negative, and varicella antibodies IgM were positive.

Liver function was normal; heart function and kidney function, and routine urine were normal. Color doppler ultrasonography of the abdomen was normal.

III. Diagnosis and treatment after admission

1. Preliminary diagnosis

The patient had severe right-sided migraine with herpes manifestations, multiple erythematous spots, clusters of blisters and papules visible on the right side of the forehead, hairline, and tip of the nose, and manifestations of right-sided conjunctivitis and keratitis, so the diagnosis of ocular herpes zoster was considered.

> **Thinking prompts:** The coexistence of unilateral conjunctivitis and keratitis in patients can be due to infectious factors. In combination with the unilateral herpes and clear herpes fluid and the predominantly lymphocytic blood picture, a viral infection was considered. Viral herpes combined with conjunctivitis and keratitis can be considered in addition to herpes zoster, such as herpes simplex viral blepharitis and herpes simplex keratitis. Herpes can also be seen in bacterial infections such as impetigo, so it should be differentiated. Unilateral headache is significant, and can also be differentiated from trigeminal neuralgia.

2. Differential diagnosis

(1) Primary trigeminal neuralgia: In addition to local pain, primary trigeminal neuralgia rarely shows herpes, keratitis, and conjunctivitis, so it can be ruled out.

(2) Pustules: Also known as infectious pustules or yellow water sores, occurring mostly

due to cocci infection. Most cases occur in summer and autumn, the patients are mostly children aged two to seven years old. It occurs on exposed areas of the skin, such as the face and extremities. The rash is a cluster of pustules of soybean size or larger, or first blisters that turn cloudy and purulent. The typical blister fluid is a half-moon shaped and cloudy, surrounded by inflammatory redness. The blister wall is thin, and prone to erosion from scratching. Later there are honey-yellow scabs, which are itchy, slightly painful but do not scar. The lymph nodes nearby are enlarged. More severe cases may be accompanied by fever and other systemic symptoms. Individual recurrent attacks may cause secondary nephritis, and herpes fluid bacterial culture will be positive for Staphylococcus or Streptococcus. The patient's presentation was not consistent with this, so pustules were ruled out.

(3) Herpes simplex blepharitis: The symptoms of viral herpes simplex blepharitis are relatively mild, with a tingling and burning sensation at the onset of the disease, and no significant neuralgia, which can cross the midplane line and develop in both eyes. The lesions are mostly confined to the mucosa-skin junctions such as the lid margin, mostly on the lower lid; the blisters are small and scattered, with relatively clear and transparent fluid inside. They dry up and crust over in about one week, leaving no trace after shedding, but are prone to recurrence. Most patients have follicular conjunctivitis as a complication, and a few develop chronic blepharitis. In this case, the patient's presentation was not consistent with this, and herpes simplex blepharitis was ruled out.

(4) Herpes simplex keratitis: Herpes simplex keratitis is generally not accompanied by herpes on the forehead and upper lid skin; painless skin sensitivity increases, eye pain is not intense, and corneal infiltrates are often located in the center, branching and expanding at the terminal, with epithelial defects. Herpes simplex keratitis was ruled out in this case.

(5) Herpes zoster: Herpes zoster is caused by the varicella-zoster virus. The first infection manifests as varicella, and later the virus can be latent in the posterior spinal root ganglion for a long time. When the body's resistance decreases, immune function is weakened. With some triggering factors, the varicella-zoster virus can become active again, grow, and multiply, and spread along the peripheral nerves to the skin, resulting in a rash known as herpes zoster. This is most common in middle-aged and elderly people. Sensory allergy and neuralgia often appear 1–2 days before the herpes zoster rash appears. The rash is initially erythematous, followed by clusters of non-fused millet to mung bean sized papules, mostly distributed along a peripheral nerve, arranged in a band, occurring on one side of the body, and not exceeding the midline. Ocular herpes zoster is a special type. Ophthalmic branch involvement is most common when the virus invades the trigeminal nerve. Clusters of blisters may occur on the scalp, forehead, and eyelids of the innervation area of the affected side with congestion, swelling, and severe pain. If the cornea is involved, ulcerative keratitis may form when the blister breaks, which can lead to blindness due to scar formation. Severe cases can cause panophthalmitis, encephalitis, and even death. When the nasal branch of the ophthalmic branch of the trigeminal nerve is invaded, blisters often appear on the side of the nasal bridge and the tip of the nose. The patient in this case had an acute onset with

conjunctivitis and migraine as the first manifestation, followed by multiple erythema, and clusters of blisters and papules on the right side of the forehead, hairline, and nasal tip. Keratitis was found, so this diagnosis was considered clinically. Other common sites of herpetic nerve damage are the chest, head, neck, and waist. Herpes zoster is most common in the chest, accounting for about 60% of cases. The rash is distributed along the intercostal nerve, extending from posterior to inferior and ending at the midline, mostly involving two or three intercostal nerve distribution areas, with tingling or burning pain when the rash appears, resembling pleurisy. Herpes zoster of the head, neck, and waist accounts for about 20%. Herpes zoster of the head can also damage the trigeminal nerve, and the rash is distributed on the cheeks, nose, lips, and mouth; facial nerve involvement results in facial palsy, which may not be accompanied by skin damage; III, IV, and V pairs of cranial nerve paralysis can result in extraocular muscle paralysis or eyelid ptosis; herpes zoster can also occur in the cervical, lumbar, and sacral regions. The presence of herpes zoster in the waist and chest accompanied by lumbar abdomen pain should be considered for differentiation from intercostal neuralgia, pleurisy, acute myocardial infarction, and angina pectoris.

3. Treatment plan after admission

The patient was treated with acyclovir antiviral therapy, vitamin B_1 and B_{12} for nerve nutrition, and cyproheptadine 4 mg three times daily for pain relief and symptomatic management. Topical application of acyclovir or ftibamzone ointment on the affected skin. Patients with skin redness and exudation can be treated with magnesium sulfate powder or 3% boric acid as a cold wet compress on the affected area, and acyclovir and levofloxacin eye drops to treat conjunctivitis and keratitis.

4. Ward-round analysis on the fifth day of hospitalization

The patient's rash was unilaterally distributed with erythema, clusters of blisters and papules with pain, and enlarged nearby lymph nodes, which confirmed the diagnosis of herpes zoster. The rash was distributed unilaterally on the forehead and tip of the nose with right-sided keratitis, and the virus was considered to have involved the ophthalmic branch of the trigeminal nerve. The patient had a significant headache, which implies the possibility of encephalitis. We closely observed his body temperature, mental status, and nausea and vomiting. On the second day of hospitalization, the patient developed drowsiness, which was considered to be caused by cyproheptadine, and was relieved after changing to 4 mg once per night.

5. Condition at discharge

After admission and treatment, the rash blisters became smaller, the basal erythema became lighter, the original lesions dried and crusted off, and the conjunctival congestion of the right eye was reduced. However, the patient still experienced paroxysmal scalp pain and complained of blurred vision in his right eye with photophobia, lachrymation, and foreign body sensation. He was referred to another hospital's ophthalmology department for further treatment.

IV. Follow-up

The ophthalmology department at the other hospital continued to give antiviral and anti-inflammatory treatment with local eye drops. The patient's condition improved, and he was discharged after 15 days. At the time of discharge, the conjunctiva of his right eye was slightly congested, and small patches of cloudy opacity were visible in the corneal transparency. After the patient's discharge, his 16-year-old daughter presented with varicella. Since varicella may develop in a person with no history, who is exposed to a patient with herpes zoster, the diagnosis of herpes zoster was clearly correct.

V. Lessons learned

Because of the primary presentation of ocular pain and headache, and the unknown epidemiological history and previous history of varicella, the patient had been seen in multiple departments of ophthalmology and emergency medicine at other hospitals. This condition is prone to misdiagnosis, and delays in diagnosis and treatment and should be taken seriously by young physicians.

In clinical cases of ocular pain and headache combined with herpes, the possibility of a viral herpes infection, should be considered, especially herpes zoster. Also, for older patients who present with chest and abdominal wall pain and breath-holding manifestations, although herpes manifestations are present at the same time, pain and breath-holding manifestations can also occur due to some serious medical conditions such as angina pectoris and myocardial infarction, so differential diagnosis should be performed to prevent missed diagnosis. Ocular herpes zoster can be combined with keratitis, and corneal herpes can break down to form ulcers, causing visual impairment or blindness. If secondary bacterial infection occurs, it can lead to serious issues such as panophthalmitis, meningitis, or even death. Therefore, topical treatment with eye drops (including antibacterial and antiviral) should be given along with systemic antiviral treatment.

(**Cao Wukui**)

Fatigue and lack of appetite for more than one year, aggravated by abdominal distension for one month

I. Medical history

Patient: Male, 54 years old, a farmer from Xiangxi in Hunan Province. He was admitted to the hospital on 18 November 1987 due to fatigue and lack of appetite for more than one year, aggravated by abdominal distension for one month.

The patient developed fatigue and lack of appetite in September 1986, which was aggravated by exertion and relieved by rest. In September 1987, the above-mentioned symptoms began to worsen with abdominal distension, low urine output, weight loss, and a gradual increase in abdominal distension. On 28 October, he was admitted to a local hospital, where an ultrasound showed massive ascites, possible subperitoneal fluid accumulation in the right lateral lobe of the liver, and a small, patchy, high-density signal in front of the right hepatic portal vein. He was diagnosed with cirrhosis and ascites, and was given conventional hepatoprotective diuretic therapy, but his symptoms did not significantly improve. He was transferred to our hospital on 18 November.

The patient was previously in good health. He reported no history of hepatitis, blood transfusion or application of blood products, trauma, surgery, or drug allergies. His vaccination status was unknown. He had a drinking habit.

> **Thinking prompts:** The patient had a slow onset with gastrointestinal symptoms such as fatigue, lack of appetite, and abdominal distension as the main manifestations. During the medical consultation, ultrasonography revealed a large amount of ascites. It is easy to assume liver diseases (such as cirrhosis due to hepatitis) and loss of liver function. The first diagnosis of cirrhosis with ascites was made at the local hospital, and symptomatic treatment was given for 20 days. The symptoms did not improve, so we should consider cirrhosis with ascites, possibly combined with spontaneous peritonitis. The infection was not effectively controlled, and the symptoms and ascites did not subside significantly. We should also consider the possibility of ascites due to

causes other than cirrhosis. Therefore, in addition to an abdominal examination, a full physical examination should be carried out, including general nutritional status, and noting the presence of a rash, presence of generalized superficial lymph node enlargement, presence of cardiopulmonary insufficiency, and presence of edema in other areas.

II. Physical examination on admission

T 37.3°C, P 80 times/min, R 20 times/min, BP 120/75 mmHg. Normal development, moderate nutrition, consciousness, poor mental health, able to walk, active position; cooperated with the physical examination. There was no yellowing of the skin anywhere on his body; no liver palm or spider nevus. The superficial lymph nodes were not palpable. There were no positive signs in the five facial features on the skull; the neck was soft, the trachea was centered, and the thyroid was not large. The cardiopulmonary examination was unremarkable. The abdomen was distended, no abdominal wall veins were revealed, and the abdomen was soft with no pressure pain or rebound pain. The upper boundary of the liver was between the fifth rib of the midclavicular line; the liver and spleen were unsatisfactory on palpation, the shifting dullness was positive, and neither of the lower limbs was swollen. There was no deformity of the spine or limbs, and no swelling or pain in any of the joints. There were no abnormalities in the anus and external genitalia. All tendon reflexes were normal, and no pathological reflexes were elicited.

> **Thinking prompts:** Physical examination failed to reveal any positive signs other than obvious ascites. The results of the examination can at least exclude the possibility of ascites due to cardiac insufficiency, systemic malnutrition, or renal disease, because the patient had no obvious signs of cardiac insufficiency and showed no other sites of edema other than ascites. Therefore, efforts should be focused on the search for the cause of ascites. Several liver diseases are common in China, especially viral hepatitis, which should be the focus of diagnosis and differential diagnosis. In addition, ascites can also be caused by infectious factors (such as tuberculosis or parasitic ascites), cirrhosis, and portal hypertension caused by Schistosoma and Clonorchis sinensis, inflammation and obstruction of the lymphatic vessels caused by filariasis. Tumors of the abdominal organs can also cause ascites. Laboratory tests were conducted to address these issues.

III. Laboratory tests on admission

Routine blood tests: Erythrocytes 3.85×10^{12}/L, hemoglobin 135 g/L, leukocytes 11.2×10^9/L, N 0.85, L 0.15, platelets 250×10^9/L.

Routine urine and stool tests were normal.

Liver and kidney function tests: Serum total protein 73 g/L, albumin 35 g/L, ALT 30 U/L,

AST 19 U/L, serum total bilirubin 8.6 μmol/L, conjugated bilirubin 2.4 μmol/L, urea nitrogen 6 mmol/L, blood creatinine 98 μmol/L, uric acid 356 μmol/L.

Prothrombin time (PT) 11.8 seconds, prothrombin activity (PTA) 112%.

ESR: 16 mm/h.

Hepatitis viral marker tests: HBsAg (−), anti-HBs positive, HBV DNA (−), anti-HCV (−), HCV RNA (−), anti-HAV-IgM (−), anti-HIV (−).

Serum parasite antibody test: Schistosoma, Paragonimus, Clonorchis sinensis, Toxoplasma, and Filarial worm, Trichinella spiralis were all negative.

Tuberculosis antibodies (including IgG and IgM) were negative.

Serum AFP (−), carcinoembryonic antigen (−).

Chest radiograph: Normal heart, lungs, and diaphragm.

Abdominal ultrasonography: Smooth liver surface with normal morphology, 12 mm portal vein, 38 mm intercostal thickness of the spleen, normal size and morphology of the pancreas, no lumps. A large amount of ascites.

Routine examination of ascites: Milky white, specific gravity 1.033, positive Rivalta test, cell count $1,200 \times 10^6$/L, N 0.16, L 0.72, interstitial cells 0.12.

IV. Diagnosis and analysis on admission
1. Preliminary diagnosis
The patient presented with fatigue, lack of appetite, and abdominal distension. The examination revealed chylous ascites without viral hepatitis infection, evidence of cirrhosis, or serological evidence of tuberculosis infection or parasitic infection. Therefore, it was a difficult case, with the cause of chylous ascites to be investigated. The main etiologies were as follows: ① Filariasis; ② Tuberculosis; ③ Tumor.

> **Thinking prompts:** The main cause of chylous ascites is lesions of the intra-abdominal lymphatic vessels, or compression and obstruction of the thoracic duct or lymphatic vessels, resulting in rupture of the intra-abdominal lymphatic vessels and leakage of lymphatic fluid. The conditions that can cause these lesions are filariasis, tuberculosis, tumors, and trauma or surgical damage to the lymphatic vessels. This patient had no history of abdominal trauma or abdominal surgery, so the possibility of surgical or traumatic injury to the lymphatics leading to chylous ascites can be completely ruled out. The main differential diagnosis was made for filariasis, tuberculosis, and tumors.

2. Differential diagnosis
(1) The possibility of chylous disease caused by compression of the lymphatic vessels by a tumor: The patient is 54 years old, so the possibility of tumor should be ruled out first. Preliminary laboratory tests showed serum AFP (−), carcinoembryonic antigen (−), and normal chest

radiographs. Abdominal ultrasonography did not reveal any abnormalities in the liver, bile duct, or pancreas, but it was not enough to rule out the possibility of a tumor. Further CT or MRI scans should be performed to examine the abdominal cavity for occupying lesions and lymph node enlargement. The gastrointestinal tract should also be examined with either a barium meal, gastroscopy, or colonoscopy. Of course, performing abdominal lymphography to understand the compression of large lymphatic vessels can also be helpful in ruling out tumors. It is also possible to perform further examination of exfoliated cells in ascites to detect tumor cells, which is also very important for the diagnosis of a tumor.

(2) Tuberculosis: One of the most common causes of chylous ascites. The incidence of tuberculosis has been on the rise in recent years, and this patient was an older farmer with a high probability of developing it. Diagnosing extrapulmonary tuberculosis is difficult, and the possibility of intra-abdominal tuberculosis cannot be completely ruled out in this case, even though the patient had no history of tuberculosis, no manifestations of tuberculosis on the chest X-ray, and negative serum tuberculosis antibodies. A CT or MRI scan of the abdominal cavity, a barium meal, gastroscopy, and enteroscopy are also important for the diagnosis of tuberculosis, as well as further examination of the peritoneum and lymph nodes with ultrasound. A differential diagnosis can also be made by examining the ascites for the presence of tuberculosis bacteria by means of ascites sediment smears, antacid staining, or a tuberculosis bacterium culture.

(3) Filariasis: Although filariasis is now rare thanks to disease control, its lesions are inflammation, hyperplasia, and stenosis of the lymphatic vessels. Therefore, the possibility of filariasis causing chylous ascites is high. If tumors and tuberculosis can be ruled out in this patient, then the diagnosis of filariasis has to be given top priority. The patient was from a filariasis-infected area, and the possibility of infection was present. Eosinophils in the peripheral blood or bone marrow should be checked, and peripheral blood should be collected at night to check for filarial larvae (microfilariae) and also to check for adult filarial worms in ascites.

V. Diagnosis and analysis after admission

The patient did not have a fever during hospitalization. Due to a high volume of ascites and high cell count, 2 g of cefotaxime sodium was given intravenously two times a day. For 20 consecutive days, hydrochlorothiazide, spironolactone, human albumin, ascites release, and ascites reflux treatment were given. The patient's condition improved slightly, but ascites still grew.

Blood tests: A (albumin) fluctuated from 33 g/L to 44 g/L, G (globulin) 26 g/L to 32 g/L, ALT, AST, PT, PTA, and bilirubin were in the normal range, and multiple blood smears were negative for microfilariae.

Blood count: Eosinophil count 66×10^6/L. TB antibodies and all other antibodies were negative. The CT scan, barium meal, gastroscopy, and enteroscopy were all normal, and peritoneal ultrasonography showed no significant thickening.

Six consecutive examinations of ascites: The specific gravity and cell count were similar, and no bacteria, tuberculosis, or fungi were found or grew in the ascites smear and culture. One ascites examination revealed filarial worm residues.

Follow-up medical history: In the 1950s, microfilariae were detected in the patient's ear blood during a medical examination for military conscription, but he was not treated because he felt no discomfort. He was not re-examined. In the early 1980s, another microfilaria was detected, which was also not treated. Therefore, the diagnosis was confirmed as advanced-stage Bancroftian filariasis.

Treatment of filariasis: Insecticide drugs, mainly diethylcarbamazine, are available in varying doses and modes of administration depending on the patient's infection status and tolerance. The dose can be 1.5 g to 4.2 g. It can be administered rapidly and continuously, or intermittently. With the rapid continuous dosing mode, the patient takes the total amount of the drug in a short period of time (1–7 days). For small doses, such as 1.5 g, it can be given in a single dose, or divided over two days. In large doses, the total amount can be divided equally and taken once a day for a week. With the intermittent dosing method, the patient takes 6–7 doses, once a week, and finishes it within 6–7 weeks. The intermittent dosing mode has reliable efficacy and low adverse effects. Insecticidal treatment often requires repeated treatment for three courses with 1–2 months intervals in between.

VI. Lessons learned

The pathological changes of filariasis are mainly inflammatory changes to the lymphatic vessels and lymph nodes. In the acute stage, the main changes are lymphatic vessel congestion, lymphatic vessel wall edema, and eosinophil infiltration. In the chronic phase, the disease is characterized by massive fibrous tissue hyperplasia, hardening of the lymph nodes, fibrosis of the lymphatic vessels, and formation of occlusive lymphangiitis. When the lymphatic vessels are obstructed and the distal ones rupture, various manifestations such as chyluria, chylous ascites, scrotal tunica vaginalis lymphatic effusion, and lower limb lymphedema may occur depending on the site of obstruction. Filaria malayi only parasitizes superficial lymphatic vessels and causes lower limb lymphedema. In contrast, wuchereria bancrofti can parasitize superficial lymphatic vessels, and can also invade visceral or deep lymphatic vessels, causing different clinical manifestations. In this case, the main manifestation was chylous ascites, indicating that the lesion was probably in the intra-abdominal lymphatic vessels, including those in the lumbar trunk, para-aortic lymph nodes, and thoracic duct, and was probably caused by a wuchereria bancrofti infection.

The patient in this case was from a filariasis-endemic area, so the possibility of infection was likely. However, the infection occurred so long ago that when chylous ascites were found and medical history was gathered, the patient did not immediately recall the filarial infection. Due to the time that had elapsed, the worms had died, so the tests for their larvalmicrofilariae were repeatedly negative. In addition, the peripheral blood eosinophils did not increase significantly, which made it difficult to confirm the diagnosis in this case. The patient's treatment history indicates that the detection of pathogens should be repeated several times so as to increase the chance of detection. When the diagnosis and differential diagnosis of the disease can more definitively exclude related diseases, and when the diagnosis of a disease is highly suspected, any opportunity and means of possible discovery of the causative agent should be taken until a definite diagnosis is made.

(Tan Deming)

Recurrent right upper abdominal pain for three years, aggravated by intermittent fever for six months

I. Medical history

Patient: Female, 73 years old, from Sujiatun District in Shenyang. She was hospitalized between 3 and 18 September 2004 with recurrent right upper abdominal pain for three years, aggravated by intermittent fever for six months.

The patient underwent a choledocholithotomy for common bile duct stones with biliary colic seven years ago. She was discharged from hospital after recovering from surgery. Three years earlier, she developed a persistent dull pain in her right upper abdomen again, with paroxysmal aggravation that involved the right shoulder and back, mostly triggered by eating oily food. The pain was relieved at home with several intravenous doses of antibiotics and oral antispasmodics. In the past six months, she had frequent episodes of pain, nausea, and vomiting of stomach contents, with chills and fever, and yellow urine. The treatments mentioned above were not effective.

The patient had no adverse personal habits and no history of other chronic diseases, or drug and food allergies.

II. Physical examination and auxiliary examination on admission

1. Physical examination on admission

T 37.6°C, P 78 times/min, R 21 times/min, BP 135/80 mmHg, normal development, moderate nutrition, pained expression, no bleeding spots on the skin, no yellow sclera, red eyelid conjunctiva, no abnormality in the heart and lungs, flat abdomen; liver and spleen were not palpable below the costal margin, deep pressure pain in the right lower part of the xiphoid process; right upper abdominal rectus muscle was tense, Murphy's sign (+), mild percussion in the liver area. Shifting dullness negative.

> **Thinking prompts:** This patient was an elderly female with a long history of gallstones with biliary colic. She had undergone a choledocholithotomy for stone extraction. Recent attacks were frequent, with mild fever and obvious pressure pain in the right

upper abdomen. It is not possible to exclude biliary tract infection, and we should be alert to complications such as acute suppurative obstructive cholangitis, liver abscess, sepsis, biliary perforation, biliary peritonitis, and infectious toxic shock. Ensure the screening of malignant tumors of the biliary system and digestive system (for bile duct cancer, pancreatic head cancer, and stomach cancer). In addition, her condition should be differentiated from high-level appendicitis, right-sided pleurisy, gastroduodenal perforation, and myocardial infarction.

2. Auxiliary examination on admission
A CT scan of the upper abdomen showed a 23 mm × 17 mm common bile duct stone and a dilated common bile duct above the stone with a diameter of 25 mm.

3. Further examination after admission
Routine blood: WBC 8.7×10^9/L, N 0.909, E 0.005, RBC 3.49×10^{12}/L, Hb 129 g/L, PT 11.3 seconds.

Routine stool and urine were normal.

Liver function: ALT 96 IU/L, GGT 675 IU/L, ALP 278 IU/L, TB 25.3 μmol/L, CB 5.8 μmol/L, A 31.3 g/L, G 31.3 g/L.

Myocardial enzymes were normal, and hematuria amylase was normal.

Abdominal radiograph: No subdiaphragmatic free gas and no fluid levels were seen.

Electrocardiogram and chest X-ray were normal.

III.　Diagnostic analysis on admission
1. Preliminary diagnosis
With a history of gallstones and biliary colic, the patient still had persistent dull pain in the right upper abdomen, with paroxysmal aggravation, and spreading pain in the right shoulder and back, low fever, and yellow urine.

Physical examination: The abdomen had deep tenderness in the lower right xiphoid process, and the right upper rectus abdominis was tense; Murphy's sign (+), and mild percussion pain in the liver area. Routine blood: Increased neutrophil ratio.

Liver function: Glutamic pyruvic transaminase and unconjugated bilirubin were mildly increased, GGT was significantly increased, and a CT scan of the upper abdomen confirmed the presence of common bile duct stones with bile duct dilatation above them. Therefore, a diagnosis of extrahepatic biliary obstruction, gallstones, biliary infection, and infectious toxic liver injury was made. Since biliary obstruction is an important factor in the development of acute septic obstructive cholangitis, surgical treatment should be performed urgently to remove the stones, relieve the obstruction, and reduce pressure on the bile duct.

2. Identification analysis
(1) On admission, the patient was given cefoperazone to fight infection, and 654-2 to stop spasms.

On 4 September 2004, a retrograde cholangiopancreatography with transduodenoscopy was performed. After the stone was localized, a duodenal papillotomy and lithotomy using a Stone Extractor were performed. One brown bilirubin stone measuring 25 mm × 19 mm × 11 mm was removed, confirming the diagnosis of gallstones. Post-operative anti-infective treatment and cholagogue therapy were routinely performed. On the second post-operative day, the patient excreted an 80-cm-long pig tapeworm, including the head and neck segments, in her stool, adding Taenia solium taeniasis to the diagnosis.

(2) In the case of confirmed taeniasis, cysticercosis must be considered as well. Because nearly half of cases of porcine cysticercosis (pork tapeworm infection) are caused by exogenous self-infection and endogenous self-infection routes, about 2.5% to 25% of patients with Taenia solium taeniasis also suffer from porcine cysticercosis. Patients with cerebral cysticercosis are prone to cerebral edema when treated with deworming medication; patients with ocular cysticercosis are prone to blindness. Therefore, for patients with Taenia solium taeniasis, it is necessary to check for specific anti-cysticercus antibodies to determine the presence of porcine cysticercosis before applying anthelmintic treatment. If positive for specific anti-cysticercus antibodies, the patient must have a CT scan of the head, slit lamp, or ultrasound biomicroscopy of the eye, as well as a biopsy of subcutaneous nodules to determine the site of cysticercus parasitism. Stool samples from the patient's family members should also be examined for fecal eggs and larvae.

(3) Predisposing factors: The causes are related to bacterial infection, parasitic infection, and bile retention of the biliary tract.

1) Parasitic infections: In economically backward areas, parasitic infections are still a common cause of gallstones, including liver flukes and roundworms, while tapeworm infections leading to stones are less common. The repeated occurrence of bile duct stones in this patient may be attributed to the entry of Taenia solium eggs through retrograde peristalsis of the small intestine, such as nausea and vomiting, which leads to local inflammation and change in bile composition led to the formation of stones with the eggs as the core. Reasons are as below: ① Stones were first removed by surgical incision seven years ago. Four years later, another stone formed in the common bile duct. It is possible that the Taenia solium was parasitic in the intestine and kept ovulating, which was a constituting factor in stone formation. ② Taenia solium can parasitize the intestine for more than 25 years; without proper deworming treatment, it will not clear up naturally. ③ After the second surgery, the patient was treated with standardized deworming medication, and no stones were found in the common bile duct at a four-year follow-up.

2) Bacterial infection: Bacterial infection was secondary in this patient, especially in the past six months. Frequent episodes of pain, nausea, vomiting with chills and fever, and yellow urine were associated with bacterial infection. Infectious bacteria mainly originate in the intestinal tract, and the most common bacteria are Escherichia coli and anaerobic bacteria. β-glucuronidase produced during infections from E. coli and some anaerobic bacteria and endogenous glucuronidase produced during biliary tract infections can hydrolyze conjugated

bilirubin to produce free bilirubin and precipitate. Unconjugated bilirubin was also mildly increased in this patient. Biliary infection can also affect the liver. A mild increase of glutamic pyruvic transaminase is a sign of toxic liver injury from infection. In severe cases of infection, bacterial liver abscesses can form.

(4) The manifestations of intestinal tapeworm disease: Some patients are asymptomatic. Half of them often suffer vague pain in the upper abdomen; a few may experience wasting, weakness, and hyperphagia. Occasionally there are neurological symptoms such as hypersensitivity, teeth grinding, and insomnia. Diagnosis is mainly based on the presence of excreted tapeworm segments in the feces, and the detection rate of fecal eggs is low. Very few have been reported worldwide with manifestations such as complications of appendicitis, intestinal obstruction, intestinal perforation, obstructive jaundice, megaloblastic anemia, and intestinal bleeding, all of which need to be differentiated from the common causes of their corresponding symptoms.

IV. Ward-round analysis on the fourth day after admission

Although Northeast China is a high-prevalence area for Taenia solium taeniasis, Liaoning Province has a relatively low prevalence. It is rare to see typical cases clinically, and they are more frequent in children and young adults. The patient in this case was an elderly woman who reported that she had not eaten raw or contaminated pork, and had not lived in an infected area. No white banded segments were found in her feces (or had possibly gone unnoticed), so she was not diagnosed and treated for a long time. Clinical symptoms such as abdominal pain, weight loss, dizziness, and weakness were masked by biliary colic symptoms for a long time, and the number of peripheral blood eosinophils did not increase, so it was clinically difficult to consider a diagnosis of Taenia solium taeniasis. The patient's excretion of Taenia solium after papillary sphincterotomy was an unexpected finding. Taenia solium is an anaerobic organism that is usually parasitic in the human duodenum within 50 cm of the proximal jejunum. During the patient's surgery, the tapeworm was paralyzed and lost its adsorption capacity due to the large amount of air in the duodenum and the oxygen contained therein. It was excreted and died on the second day after the surgery.

The patient was given 0.2 g of albendazole three times a day for three days, and no more Taenia solium were excreted. A CT scan of the head, and subcutaneous and ocular examinations did not reveal porcine cysticercosis. Her family members were not infected either.

V. Condition at discharge (sixteenth day after admission)

The patient's body temperature was normal. The abdominal pain and yellow urine disappeared, and her routine blood and liver function returned to normal. She was discharged.

VI. Follow-up

At follow-up, no white banded segments of the pig tapeworm were excreted, and no recolonization of the common bile duct was found.

VII. Lessons learned

Intestinal tapeworm disease is caused by a variety of tapeworms that live in the human small intestine. The most common are pig tapeworm and bovine tapeworm, which are contracted by eating pork or beef containing live cysticercus.

(Liu Pei)

Vague pain and discomfort in the upper and middle abdomen for six months, aggravating and spreading to the whole abdomen for five hours

I. Medical history

Patient: Female, 35 years old, Tibetan, visiting Shenyang on a business trip. She was hospitalized between 7 and 23 April 2006 with vague pain and discomfort in the upper and middle abdomen for six months, which aggravated and spread to the whole abdomen for five hours.

The patient had been suffering from vague pain and discomfort in her upper and middle abdomen for the past six months, unrelated to her diet, without acid reflux or belching. It had been treated as gastric disease for a long time, but the effect was not obvious, and her condition was not taken seriously. The abdominal pain suddenly aggravated after eating a large amount of seafood five hours earlier and spread to the whole abdomen with severe and unbearable pain. The patient liked to eat air-dried beef and lamb or raw meat, and intermittently made short business trips across the country.

She had no history of other chronic diseases, nor drug or food allergies. Normal and regular menstruation. No history of trauma.

II. Physical examination and auxiliary examination on admission

1. Physical examination

T 38.0°C, P 87 times/min, R 22 times/min, BP 125/80 mmHg. Acute pained expression, clear consciousness, no cardiopulmonary abnormalities, flat abdomen, no gastrointestinal type or peristaltic wave; tenderness, rebound pain, and muscle tension in the whole abdomen were obvious; the liver and spleen were not palpable; the borders of pulmonary and hepatic dullness disappeared, shifting dullness (±), and bowel sounds disappeared.

> **Thinking prompts:** The patient was a middle-aged female with a history of chronic gastric disease. The present acute onset was after overeating, with severe pain

throughout the abdomen and clear signs of peritonitis. Common acute abdominal diseases such as acute necrotizing pancreatitis, perforated gastroduodenal ulcer, acute suppurative obstructive cholangitis, perforated acute appendicitis, strangulated intestinal obstruction, and ectopic pregnancy should be considered. Relevant examinations should be performed.

2. Auxiliary examination

Standing abdominal X-ray: A crescent-shaped translucent shadow under both diaphragms was seen.

3. Further examination after admission

Blood count: WBC 16.1×10^9/L, N 0.91, E 0.005, RBC 3.46×10^{12}/L, Hb 124 g/L, PT 12.0 seconds.

Routine stool and urine were normal.

Liver function, cardiac enzymes, blood, and urine amylase were normal.

Electrocardiogram and chest X-ray were normal.

B-ultrasound examination: A small amount of abdominal fluid.

III. Treatment after admission

1. Preliminary diagnosis

The patient seemed to have a history of chronic gastric disease. This time, the disease was triggered acutely by overeating. She had severe pain throughout her abdomen, clear signs of peritonitis, increased total leukocyte and neutrophil ratios in the peripheral blood, increased body temperature, and free gas under both diaphragms on abdominal radiographs. Considering the high possibility of upper gastrointestinal perforation complicated by diffuse peritonitis, perforation repair surgery should be performed urgently.

2. Initial treatment

After admission, broad-spectrum antibiotics, maintenance of the acid-base balance, and nutritional support were applied. Routine preoperative preparation and emergency surgery were performed. Intraoperatively, about 30 ml of purulent exudate was seen in the abdominal cavity, and pus moss and food residues were visible. The stomach and duodenal bulb were examined, and no abnormalities were found. A perforation of about 0.2 cm × 0.3 cm was seen in the jejunal wall about 10 cm from the Treitz ligament. Three white tapeworms, approximately 35 cm in length, were removed from the intestinal canal during the exploration. Due to the long-term irritation of the intestinal wall by the tapeworms, it had become fragile and could not be repaired normally, so only perforated jejunal resection, intestinal anastomosis, and abdominal drainage were performed. The operation was successful. Routine deworming treatment was performed after surgery, and the patient was discharged after the first stage of surgical incision healing. Pathology report: Bovine tapeworm.

3. Ward-round analysis on the seventh day after admission

This patient was a Tibetan who liked to eat air-dried beef and lamb or raw meat. Normally, no white banded segments were found to be excreted in the feces (or had possibly gone unnoticed), and the tapeworm parasite site (upper small intestine) was not easily detected by routine gastroscopy or enteroscopy. The patient's abdominal pain was mistaken as a symptom of gastric disease for a long time, and the number of peripheral blood eosinophils did not increase, so she was not diagnosed and treated for a long time. The emergency surgery was mistakenly performed for a gastroduodenal ulcer causing perforation with peritonitis until the opening of the abdomen (jejunal perforation and gastroduodenal perforation are difficult to differentiate). A routine exploration of the stomach and duodenum did not show any abnormality, and when the jejunal perforation was found during the downward exploration, the surgeon was not alerted and did not think about the cause, and was ready to perform the repair. The diagnosis of bovine tapeworm parasitism was only made when stringy, creeping objects were palpated in the jejunum. Only then was the diagnosis clear: Bovine tapeworm disease, and jejunum perforation with generalized peritonitis.

Small intestine perforation is mostly due to traumatic injuries. Other common causes are malignant tumors, strangulated intestinal obstruction, intestinal necrosis, intestinal ulcers, intestinal tuberculosis, and intestinal typhoid. Different etiologies can affect the choice of surgical procedure. Perforation of the jejunum caused by tapeworms is extremely rare. The jejunum is the best place for tapeworms to live. As the tapeworm continues to grow, those with weak reproductive capacity and low parasitic capacity will be excreted from the body. The remaining tapeworms hook or latch onto the mucosa of the small intestine with small hooks and suckers to absorb nutrients and peristalsis, constantly irritating the intestinal wall and causing local damage and inflammation, which eventually leads to perforation when overeating or consuming harder foods.

CT scans of the head, and subcutaneous and ocular examinations are not necessary for such patients because humans are not suitable intermediate hosts for bovine tapeworms, and it does not cause cysticercosis.

After surgery, the patient was given 0.2 g of albendazole three times for three days of deworming treatment.

IV. Condition at discharge

After taking the medication, the patient did not excrete any more bovine tapeworms. Her body temperature returned to normal, and the abdominal pain disappeared. The results of routine blood examination, abdominal plain film examination, and B-ultrasound examination all returned to normal, and she was discharged.

V. Lessons learned

This is a relatively rare case. Due to the high mobility of bovine tapeworms, patients often have clinical manifestations like abdominal pain or natural discharge of the tapeworm segments. In areas where raw beef is commonly consumed, patients with frequent abdominal pain should be aware of bovine tapeworm.

Although three bovine tapeworms were removed during surgery, it is not certain that all of the adult worms were completely removed from the intestine. Thus, deworming treatment had to be performed.

Bovine tapeworms do not cause cysticercosis in humans, and CT scans of the head, plus subcutaneous and ocular examinations are not necessary before deworming treatment.

(Liu Pei)

Fever for three days, with sore throat and rash for one day

I. Medical history

Patient: Female, four years old, from Tianjin. She was hospitalized between 16 and 26 May 2008 with fever for three days, with sore throat and rash for one day.

The patient developed a fever three days before admission, with a temperature of up to 39.4°C, accompanied by a sore throat. There was no obvious cough or sputum, but a day ago a rash appeared on her back with mild pruritus, which gradually increased and extended to her whole body.

The patient had previously been healthy, with no history of surgery, injuries, blood transfusions, or drug allergies. The patient completed immunizations on time, and her history of exposure to similar cases was unknown.

> **Thinking prompts:** Fever with rash is a common clinical symptom that can be present in many diseases. When taking medical history, the clinician should gain a detailed understanding of the relationship between the time of the fever and the appearance of the rash, as well as the sequence of the rash's appearance. Ask whether the patient has any allergies to certain drugs, and whether he or she took certain drugs before this onset, to exclude a drug rash. Drug rashes often appear after the use of penicillin, streptomycin, and sulfonamides. They are preceded or accompanied by a fever, with irregular rash sequence, and vary in type, number, and distribution. During physical examination, special attention should be paid to the pattern, size, and distribution of the rash, and whether there are changes in the patient's face, whether there are Koplik's spots on the oral mucosa, whether the tongue coating is normal, and the condition of superficial lymph nodes throughout the body. It is also necessary to observe changes in easily neglected areas such as the skin folds in the axillae and groin, and to observe whether there are other foci of infection in the patient, all of which are important for correct diagnosis. Some patients with atypical Kawasaki disease also have similar clinical manifestations. Clinicians should examine the patient's body carefully, especially the auscultation of the heart, and note any

skin changes on the lips, fingers, toes, and perianal area. Early cardiac color doppler ultrasound and C-reactive protein tests should be performed to prevent missed or misdiagnosis. Asking about the patient's previous treatment and the evolution of the disease has the potential to guide the current diagnosis or choice of treatment.

II. Physical examination and auxiliary examination on admission

1. Physical examination

T: 38.1°C, the patient was in a clear state of mind and a fine mental state, and cooperated with the physical examination. The skin on her body and face was diffusely congested and flushed, and a small miliary rash could be seen, which faded when pressed; no normal skin was seen between the rash areas. Pastia's sign was seen in the axillary and inguinal areas. There was no enlargement of superficial lymph nodes anywhere on her body. There was no cranial deformity, no conjunctival congestion, no overflow of pus from the external ear canal, clear nasal cavity, no cyanosis of the mouth and lips, or visible pale circles around the mouth. The pharynx was congested, the tonsils were enlarged bilaterally, purulent secretions were visible, and a "strawberry" tongue was visible. The neck was soft and non-resistant, the respiratory sounds of both lungs were clear; no dry and moist rales were heard. The heart sounds were strong and rhythmic, and no murmur was heard in either of the valve auscultation areas. The patient's abdomen was soft, without pressure and rebound pain, and her liver and spleen were not palpable below the costal margin. Shifting dullness was negative. Physiological reflexes were present, and pathological reflexes were not elicited.

2. Auxiliary examination

Blood count: WBC 17.45×10^9/L, N 86.7%, PLT 314×10^9/L.

C-reactive protein: 65 mg/L.

Pharyngeal swab culture: Suggesting Streptococcus pyogenes infection.

Routine urine, routine stool, and occult blood (BLD), heart, liver and kidney function, electrolytes, ECG, chest X-ray, urinary system ultrasound, and cardiac color doppler ultrasound were normal.

Thinking prompts: Routine blood tests are performed on the basis of a complete medical history and physical examination to suggest viral or bacterial infection initially. Perform routine urine tests to find out whether there is protein and cellular cast in the urine, to infer whether the kidneys are damaged; routine stool plus occult blood test should be performed to ascertain the presence of parasites and red and white blood cells in the stool; a pharyngeal swab culture can identify the causative organism; liver, kidney, heart function, and electrolyte tests can identify the presence of important organ damage; urological color doppler ultrasound can show the condition of both kidneys; cardiac color doppler ultrasound should be performed to check the condition of the coronary artery; a chest X-ray can show abnormalities in both lungs, the heart, and the diaphragm; an electrocardiogram can clarify the condition of the heart.

III. Diagnostic analysis on admission
1. Preliminary diagnosis

The patient had a rapid onset of illness with a fever, sore throat, and rash as clinical manifestations. Combined with a physical examination and auxiliary tests, a preliminary diagnosis of scarlet fever could be made, but it should be differentiated from other eruptive diseases.

> **Thinking prompts:** Fever with a rash is most commonly seen in infectious diseases, but also occurs in autoimmune-related diseases, specific skin diseases, and malignancies. This patient was young, and presented with typical signs and symptoms such as fever, acute isthmitis, rash, perioral pale circles, "strawberry" tongue, and Pastia's sign – many of the symptoms of scarlet fever. The diagnosis was confirmed by a pharyngeal swab culture suggestive of Streptococcus pyogenes infection, and the fact that the patient was admitted to hospital at a time when scarlet fever was rife.
>
> Diagnosis could be difficult for a clinician due to the use of certain antibacterial drugs prior to the patient's visit, a possibly negative pharyngeal swab culture, or the absence of certain typical symptoms or signs in the patient. Therefore, it is necessary to differentiate and diagnose diseases associated with fever plus rash based on their existing experience and knowledge. This will improve the diagnosis rate, reduce the rate of misdiagnosis and underdiagnosis, reduce unnecessary laboratory tests, and save medical resources, thus reducing the economic pressure on patients.

2. Diagnostic analysis

Several common diseases in which fever is accompanied by a rash:

(1) Rubella: Rubella rash appears early, half a day to one day after the onset of fever. It appears on the face, spreading to the trunk and extremities on the first day; the next day, it starts to fade from the face; on the third day, most of the rash fades completely. There is no hyperpigmentation or desquamation after the rash subsides. Systemic symptoms are mild. The lymph nodes behind the ear and behind the occiput are enlarged. However, this patient's rash started two days after the onset of fever and gradually spread across her body. It was still present at the time of consultation, and no enlarged superficial lymph nodes were palpable anywhere on her body, neither of which supported the diagnosis of rubella.

(2) Measles: Measles rash appears within 3–4 days of fever, and the body temperature is higher when it appears. It spreads from behind the ears to the neck, face, trunk, and extremities in three days. The skin between the rash is normal, with pigmentation and fine debris after it has subsided. Systemic symptoms, respiratory catarrhal inflammation, and conjunctival inflammation are more severe. Koplik's spots appeared on the oral mucosa after 2–3 days of fever. However, this patient had a rash two days after the onset of fever, and no normal skin was

seen between the rash, so the symptoms were not consistent with measles. No Koplik's spots were seen in the oral cavity, so measles could be ruled out initially. If clinical differentiation is difficult, the patient's blood can be tested for measles antibodies to clarify the diagnosis.

(3) Acute rash in toddlers: Also known as infantile roseola rash, this is characterized by a high fever for 3–5 days, with the rash emerging from the neck and spreading to the rest of the body after the fever has subsided. The process is complete in one day. The rash consists of light red papules, and is not itchy. It is scattered or fused into patches 2–3 mm in diameter, surrounded by a light red ring, and fading when pressed. It usually subsides after 2-3 days, without desquamation or pigmentation, and the lymph nodes behind the ears and occiput may be enlarged. However, the patient in this case still had a fever at the time of rash, and the lymph nodes behind her ears and occipital area were not enlarged, so infantile roseola rash could be ruled out.

(4) Isthmitis caused by other pathogens/septic bacteria: This cannot be clinically distinguished from pre-rash scarlet fever, and the diagnosis needs to be confirmed by a pharyngeal swab culture, except for Staphylococcus aureus, which can produce a scarlet fever-like rash two days after the onset of the disease. However, septic infections generally do not have a scarlet fever-like rash. In this patient, the pharyngeal swab culture was suggestive of Streptococcus pyogenes infection, and a scarlet fever-like rash was seen all over her body, so other septic bacterial causes of isthmitis could be tentatively ruled out.

(5) Staphylococcus aureus infection: Certain Staphylococcus aureus can also produce Dick toxin and cause a scarlet fever-like rash. The rash starts in 3–5 days, lasts for a short time, and fades quickly; there is no skin desquamation; the systemic symptoms of toxicity are heavy and do not diminish after the rash subsides; there are often local or migratory foci of infection, such as impetigo and boils; Staphylococcus aureus can be cultured in the secretions of the foci. The pharyngeal swab culture from this patient suggested Streptococcus pyogenes infection, which was not consistent with Staphylococcus aureus infection.

(6) Streptococcus pyogenes infection (streptococcal toxic shock syndrome): In the early 1990s, thousands of scarlet fever outbreaks were reported in the Hai'an area of Jiangsu Province, which were identified as Streptococcus pyogenes (belonging to Viridans Streptococci) infections. Young and middle-aged patients were predominantly affected, often with severe symptoms of systemic toxicity. High fever, toxic gastroenteritis and toxic shock, significant soft tissue infection, multi-organ involvement, liver and kidney damage, scarlet fever-like rash, and desquamation may be present, and isthmitis is not obvious. Bacterial culture is required for identification. Outside of China, streptococcal toxic shock syndrome caused by Viridans Streptococci is rare, and occurs in septic patients with severe underlying issues such as tumors, organ transplantation, and immunodeficiency. The patient in this case was a preschooler with few systemic symptoms, and the pharyngeal swab culture suggested Streptococcus pyogenes infection, which was inconsistent with Streptococcus pyogenes infection and could be ruled out.

(7) Certain viral infections: Some viral infections can cause high fever, isthmus of fauces congestion, and a scarlet fever-like rash. For instance, enterovirus infections can appear during

fever or after the fever subsides, with the nature, shape, and distribution of the rash being more variable and possibly recurring. Herpetic isthmitis and viral meningitis, myalgia, and diarrhea are often present simultaneously, whereas the symptoms of upper respiratory tract inflammation are less frequent. For such diseases, detailed observation of the rash characteristics based on medical history, routine blood count, and classification of white blood cells are required. In this patient, an increased percentage of neutrophils in routine blood tests suggested bacterial infection, and a pharyngeal swab culture suggested Streptococcus pyogenes infection. There were no symptoms of gastrointestinal inflammation, so a viral infection could be ruled out.

(8) Infectious mononucleosis: This is caused by EBV infection. Symptoms are moderate or high fever usually lasting 5–10 days, diffuse pseudomembranous tonsillitis, petechiae on the palate, generalized lymph node enlargement, and splenomegaly. About one third of patients develop a rash 4–6 days after the onset of the disease, which is a bright red measles-like rash on the trunk and upper extremities; scarlet fever-like, herpes-like, and erythema multiforme-like rashes are rarely seen. The lymphocytes are increased, and there is a large number of anomalous lymphocytes, accounting for more than 10% of the total white blood cells. Infectious mononucleosis is characterized by fever, pseudomembranous tonsillitis, generalized lymph node enlargement, and a large number of anomalous lymphocytes. The peripheral blood neutrophilia in this patient suggested bacterial infection, so infectious mononucleosis could be tentatively ruled out.

(9) Viral hemorrhagic fever: This includes epidemic hemorrhagic fever and dengue hemorrhagic fever. The main clinical features are fever, hemorrhage and rash, shock, oliguria, and renal failure. The fever is mostly bimodal or persistent. Patients with epidemic hemorrhagic fever have flushed, congested skin on the face, neck, and upper chest, eye conjunctival hyperemia, and a drunken appearance, with hemorrhagic spots and ecchymosis visible on the skin mucosa. Patients with dengue hemorrhagic fever have scattered petechiae and ecchymosis on the extremities, face, axillae, and soft palate, and may have erythema, maculopapular rash, and a wheal rash, which was not consistent with this case.

(10) Scarlet fever-like rash: This can occur after a belladonna overdose, or when taking scopolamine preparations, aminopyrine, phenobarbital, ampicillin, or cephalosporins. The diagnosis of drug rash can be based on a clear history of drug use before the rash, sudden onset of the rash, uneven distribution, and increased total white blood cell count and eosinophils. This patient's medical history showed that she was not taking any medication before the onset of the disease, and the blood eosinophil percentage was normal, meaning that scarlet fever-like rash caused by medication could be ruled out.

(11) Kawasaki disease: Currently, there is no gold standard for the diagnosis of Kawasaki disease; it relies mainly on certain clinical symptoms for diagnosis: ① Persistent fever for more than five days; ② Conjunctival congestion in both eyes; ③ Flushing, dryness, and cracking of the lips and mouth, "strawberry" tongue, and diffuse congestion of the oropharyngeal mucosa; ④ Acute non-purulent cervical lymph node enlargement; ⑤ Polymorphic erythema or scarlet

fever-like rash; ⑥ Erythema and hard swelling on the palms and feet in the acute stage, and membrane-like peeling on the ends of the fingers and toes starting 10–15 days after the onset of the disease.

This patient lacked the characteristic manifestations of Kawasaki disease, with no abnormalities detected on cardiac auscultation. A cardiac color doppler ultrasound was normal, so the condition could be ruled out.

IV. Diagnosis and treatment after admission

Based on the patient's symptoms, signs, and laboratory tests, a clear diagnosis of scarlet fever was made. The disease is an acute respiratory infectious disease, and needs to be treated in isolation.

Anti-infective penicillin was the preferred clinical treatment. A penicillin skin test was given on the day after admission, and a skin test (−). Then, 600,000 units of penicillin were given intravenously by drip three times a day based on kilogram weight. On the third day of treatment, the patient's peripheral rash mostly subsided, and the routine blood WBC was 16.07×10^9/L, N 10.81×10^9/L, and PLT 523×10^9/L. Considering the possibility that the course of penicillin was insufficient, the patient continued with the original treatment.

On the fifth day after admission: WBC 12.86×10^9/L, N 8.94×10^9/L, PLT 511×10^9/L. Pharyngeal swab culture (−) was checked. The patient's condition was better than before, but she had to be monitored for complications such as purulent otitis media, sinusitis, toxic myocarditis, glomerulonephritis, rheumatic fever, and arthritis. Her cardiac, hepatic, and renal functions, chest X-ray, electrocardiogram, and ultrasound examination of the urinary system were normal, so the above complications were not considered.

The patient will not be immune to the disease for life. There is a possibility of recurrence or reinfection, and the treatment plan should be adjusted according to the changes in the disease during treatment. Hematologic changes should be observed, and a regular review of pharyngeal swab cultures should be used to evaluate the efficacy of antibiotics. Those who are allergic to penicillin can be treated with erythromycin, lincomycin, cephalosporin, or rifampin. If acute complications occur, prompt measures should be taken for symptomatic support treatment. If a septic lesion occurs before penicillin treatment, the dose can be increased; if it occurs after treatment, other antibiotics should be considered; complications of rheumatic fever can be treated with anti-rheumatic treatment; complications of glomerulonephritis and arthritis can be treated accordingly.

V. Condition at discharge

The patient was in a good general condition, and did not complain of discomforts such as a cough, sore throat, or fever. Physical examination: Body temperature was 36.3°C; the peripheral rash had subsided; no desquamation was seen; the pharynx was slightly congested, the bilateral tonsils were I° enlarged, and no purulent secretions were seen. No abnormalities were heard in the heart and lungs, the abdomen was soft, no pressure pain, and the liver and spleen were not palpable below the costal margin. The patient was on antibiotics for ten days, and her condition stabilized. Re-examination of routine blood: WBC 8.09×10^9/L, N 4.83×10^9/L, PLT 528×10^9/L, pharyngeal swab culture (−).

VI. Follow-up visits

After being discharged from hospital, the patient was advised to maintain a reasonable diet and rest. Oral amoxicillin 0.25 mg was to be continued three times daily for four days. The anti-infection treatment resulted in a normal temperature. Three days after discharge from hospital, a large patch of peeling skin appeared on her hands and feet. The pharyngeal swab culture was repeated after three days of drug withdrawal to determine whether the potential pathogenic bacteria in the pharynx had been completely eliminated. The patient's pharyngeal swab culture (−) was obtained three days after discontinuation of the drug, and blood and urine tests were normal two weeks after discharge.

VII. Lessons learned

This was a typical case of scarlet fever, and the correct diagnosis was easy to make by combining the patient's medical history, physical examination, and laboratory tests. In clinical work, it has been found that the disease can occur throughout the year, with more incidences in temperate regions, during winter and spring, and in individuals from five to 15 years old. In recent decades, the clinical manifestations of scarlet fever have become milder, and the clinical manifestations of sepsis and poisoning have decreased significantly. The reasons for this are thought to be the widespread use of sensitive antibiotics and the prolonged external environmental effects that cause streptococcal mutations, as well as the early application of antibiotics that cause streptococci to be quickly suppressed or killed, reducing the occurrence of complications.

VIII. Prevention

1. Isolate patients: Medical observation of contacts for seven days. If a patient is identified, report the infectious disease outbreak to the nearest health epidemic prevention station, and isolate him/her for seven days after treatment or pharyngeal swab culture (−), especially in children's institutions.

2. Reduce exposure: Try not to go to public places during an outbreak, or go there as little as possible.

3. Treatment of close contacts: Frail and immunocompromised people with a history of close contact with the patient can take oral amoxicillin for prevention, usually for 2–3 days. An injection of 1.2 million units of long-acting penicillin can end the outbreak and prevent the occurrence of rheumatic fever and glomerulonephritis.

4. Treatment of carriers: Temporarily transfer the carrier from the children's institution and give penicillin for ten days. Wait for the pharyngeal swab culture (−) before returning to work at the original setting.

(Cao Wukui)

Fever and cough for two weeks

I. Medical history

Patient: Male, 14 years old, a student. He was hospitalized with fever and cough for two weeks.

The patient developed a fever two weeks ago after catching a cold. His body temperature fluctuated greatly in the morning and evening, up to 40°C, with intermittent fever, no discomfort after the fever subsided, no chills, profuse sweating, no night sweats, and wasting. He had an occasional cough, little sputum, vague chest pain, no headache, vomiting, and no frequent or urgent urinary. No abdominal pain and diarrhea. No rash and gum bleeding since the onset of the disease. B-ultrasound showed enlarged liver and spleen; chest X-ray showed scattered, speckled, high-density miliary shadows with blurred margins in the middle and inner zone of both lungs. Acute miliary tuberculosis was considered. He was treated with anti-inflammatory, anti-tuberculosis, and hormonal therapy, but his symptoms recurred, so he was transferred to our hospital.

> **Thinking prompts:** In this case, the symptoms recurred even after two weeks of anti-tuberculosis treatment, so we need to consider the following: ① Whether the diagnosis of tuberculosis was correct? ② Was there a possibility of drug resistance? ③ In addition to fever and cough, the patient's chest X-ray showed more scattered, speckled, high-density miliary shadows with blurred margins in the middle and inner zone of both lungs, suggesting other lung diseases.

II. Physical examination and auxiliary examination on admission

1. Physical examination

T 38.5°C, P 100 times/min, BP 120/60 mmHg; clear consciousness, acute facial features, no rash or scab anywhere on the body; superficial lymph nodes not enlarged; both pupils equal in size and roundness, responding to light. The patient's neck was soft, the breath sounds of both lungs were coarse, and no dry and moist rales were heard. Heart sounds were strong and rhythmic. The abdomen was soft, and the liver was palpable 1.5 cm below the right costal margin.

2. Auxiliary examination

Routine blood tests: WBC 12.2×10^9/L, Hb 123 g/L, PLT 271×10^9/L, E 31.4%.

ESR 70 mm/h, CRP 143 mg/L.

ASO (anti-streptococcal O test): 321 IU/ml.

Liver and kidney functions were normal.

Rheumatology 11 (–), Weil-Felix test (–), Widal test (–), Hepatitis-B five tests (–), multiple PPD skin tests (–).

TB-Ab (+).

Chest CT: Diffuse distribution of small nodular shadows in both lungs, but uneven in size and distribution; some nodular shadows were blurred; no hilar or mediastinal lymph node enlargement was seen.

Blood culture + drug sensitivity: No bacterial growth.

Plasmodium was not detected.

III. Diagnosis and analysis

1. Acute miliary pulmonary tuberculosis: The patient presented with fever and cough as his predominant symptoms. A chest CT showed diffuse distribution of small nodular shadows in both lungs, but the size and distribution were not uniform; some of the nodular shadows were blurred, and no hilar or mediastinal lymph node enlargement was seen. It seemed to resemble pulmonary tuberculosis, but the patient had multiple PPD skin tests (–), no discomfort after the fever subsided, no anemia, and ineffective anti-inflammatory and anti-tuberculosis treatment; therefore, acute miliary tuberculosis was ruled out.

2. Diseases related to eosinophilia: Tests showed a significant increase in routine WBC and E. A significant increase in C-reactive protein suggested a condition related to eosinophilia.

(1) Parasitic infections: The most common cause of eosinophilia. Unicellular protozoan infections generally do not cause eosinophilia, while multicellular helminths and trematodes can cause it, the extent of which parallels the number and extent of tissue invasion by worms, especially larvae. Infections confined to the intestinal lumen (such as roundworms and tapeworms) generally do not cause eosinophilia. In clinical cases of unexplained eosinophilia, it is important to analyze the patient's living environment and dietary history and to examine the stool to detect eggs or larvae.

(2) Allergic reactive diseases: Allergic rhinitis, bronchial asthma, urticaria, and allergic reactions to drugs can present with eosinophilia. This patient had no previous relevant medical history.

(3) Pulmonary eosinophilic infiltrates: Clinical features are cough, chest tightness, shortness of breath, and increased blood eosinophilia. X-ray examination (scattered or wandering infiltrative foci in the lungs in the form of cloudy patches) and lung tissue biopsy (showing eosinophilia) are the main points of diagnosis. Simple pulmonary eosinophilic infiltrates may be a transient alveolar allergic reaction caused by parasitic infection or drugs. The symptoms are mild, and usually do not require treatment, often resolving spontaneously within a month. Asthmatic pulmonary eosinophilic infiltrates, starting at the age of 40–60 years, characterized by recurrent cough and asthma, were not considered for this patient.

(4) Neoplasm: Eosinophilic leukemia is rare. As well as fever, anemia, hepatosplenomegaly, and lymph node enlargement common in leukemia, heart, lung, nervous system, and skin infiltration are prominent. Two out of three patients have leukocytes above 50×10^9/L, of which eosinophils account for 60%–85%.

3. Diagnosis and treatment: Based on the above analysis, a bone marrow examination was conducted, and showed eosinophilia and negative tumor markers. Detailed medical history was taken, and it was discovered that the patient had lived in a schistosome infected area for a long time, and had swum in a small river in his hometown two months earlier. We sent his blood specimen to the city's epidemic prevention station for a schistosome antibody test and a schistosome ring egg precipitation test, and the test results were positive. A total of 120 mg/kg of praziquantel was given for six days, along with symptomatic support treatment.

IV. Condition at discharge (twentieth day after admission)

The fever subsided on the fourth day of praziquantel, which the patient continued to take for another two days (a total of six days). On the nineteenth day after admission, blood was drawn and examined; C-reactive protein and sedimentation had decreased significantly, peripheral blood leukocytes and classification were normal; fecal hatching turned negative.

V. Follow-up

Three months after discharge, the patient's body temperature was normal, C-reactive protein and blood sedimentation were normal, fecal hatching was negative, and the chest X-ray lesion was completely absorbed at six months of re-examination.

VI. Lessons learned

Schistosomiasis is an infection caused by contact of the human skin mucosa with contaminated water containing cercaria. Schistosomes are mainly parasitic in the portal system, and their eggs are deposited in the submucosa of the intestinal wall, causing corresponding pathological damage. The lesions are most significant in the liver and colon. The pulmonary form of schistosomiasis is characterized by ectopic deposition of eggs, causing allergic alveolitis, granulomatous, and interstitial lung lesions. Clinical manifestations include fever, anorexia, abdominal pain, usually mild respiratory symptoms, occasional coughing, little sputum, vague chest pain, and inconspicuous pulmonary signs; a chest X-ray may show diffuse, cloudy, punctate, miliary infiltrative shadows with uneven distribution, variable size, and fuzzy margins; blood eosinophils are significantly increased; praziquantel treatment is effective.

This case was characterized by fever and a miliary infiltrative shadow on a chest X-ray. The main reason for clinical misdiagnosis was that the clinical manifestations were not very specific, so there was a lack of positive signs to support the diagnosis. In addition, ectopic schistosomiasis is rare in non-epidemic areas, which makes it very easy to misdiagnose. Clinicians are advised to do the following:

(1) Take and analyze a thorough medical history, particularly epidemiological data, especially contact with contaminated water infected areas; establish a precise diagnostic idea

(2) Perform a detailed physical examination with all of the necessary medical and technical examinations in a timely manner, such as eosinophil count, a schistosome antibody test, and a schistosome ring egg precipitation test

(3) Confirm the diagnosis with the medical history promptly, and note differential diagnosis, so that treatment can begin as quickly as possible

(Sheng Jifang)

Persistent fever, headache, and drowsiness for three days; unconsciousness for one day

I. Medical history

Patient: Male, seven years old, from Guangdong Province. He was hospitalized between 13 and 25 July 2004 with persistent fever, headache, drowsiness for three days and unconsciousness for one day.

The patient presented with fever (temperature usually around 39°C) three days earlier accompanied by significant headache, nausea, and projectile vomiting several times, with the vomitus being gastric contents. He had diarrhea three times – thin, yellow stools without mucus and pus and blood, and no tenesmus. He took self-administered aspirin at home to reduce fever, which was not effective. He had a poor appetite and spirit, and drowsiness. One day earlier, he fell unconscious, and did not respond to calls, suffering one convulsion of the limbs.

The patient had previously been healthy and denied any history of dizziness or headaches, allergies to medication or food, or exposure to contaminated water. He went to Beijing on a trip with his family from Guangdong in the last month. He denied any family history of hereditary disease, and there were no similar infections in the surrounding area.

> **Thinking prompts:** There are many diseases that can cause fever in children. Because they may be inarticulate when complaining of symptoms (this patient was already in a coma at the time of admission), understanding the course of the illness may be difficult. Therefore, it was necessary to ask the parents for a detailed medical history, as well as performing a thorough physical examination and other relevant examinations. There may be a process of supplementary medical history or review.
>
> The history should provide a detailed account of the sequence of symptoms and the progression of the disease, including conditions that may guide the current diagnosis or choice of treatment, as well as helping to identify and rule out certain diagnoses. Symptoms of diarrhea help to differentiate and exclude gastrointestinal diseases as in this case. The child's fever, headache, projectile vomiting, and impaired consciousness suggest the possibility of intracranial infection, and the focus should be on neurologic examination.

II. Physical examination and auxiliary examination on admission

1. Physical examination:

T: 39.5°C, BP 90/60 mmHg, HR: 97 times/min, unconscious, no response to calls. Respiratory rhythm regular, superficial lymph nodes not enlarged, and there was no rash. His pupils were equally large and round, and responded to light. There was neck stiffness, increased muscle strength, and hyper-reflexes of the knees and Achilles tendons. Pathological signs were negative. His abdomen was soft, and the liver and spleen were not palpable below the costal margin; shifting dullness was negative. No positive cardiopulmonary signs were seen.

> **Thinking prompts:** Routine blood tests, blood cultures, C-reactive protein, and ESR tests should be performed on the basis of a complete history and physical examination to indicate bacterial, viral, or non-viral infections, and PPD tests and Mycobacterium tuberculosis tests to exclude Mycobacterium tuberculosis infections. Cerebrospinal fluid examination is essential for the clarification of meningoencephalitis. Routine urine and stool tests and cultures should be performed to exclude urinary tract or intestinal infections. With fever, if septic, local infections (migratory lesions) are often present, and chest radiograph and abdominal ultrasound are the most routine tests. In summer, unexplained coma and cholera should not be forgotten or excluded, and motility and immobilization tests for Vibrio cholerae are very necessary.

2. Auxiliary examination

Routine blood: WBC 16.7×10^9/L, N 89.6%, L 9.1%, RBC 3.41×10^{12}/L, Hb 10^9 g/L, PLT 280×10^9/L.

Cerebrospinal fluid examination: Suggested increased pressure, slightly turbid appearance, WBC 318×10^6/L, N 78%, normal sugar and chloride.

Urine and stool routines normal.

Immobilization test negative.

Chest X-ray and abdominal ultrasound normal.

III. Diagnosis and treatment process

1. Preliminary diagnosis

The patient had an acute onset, and quickly fell into a coma with high fever, headache, vomiting, impaired consciousness, and positive meningeal stimulation signs. Meningoencephalitis was suspected initially, but the cause was still unclear. The possibility of infection from other sites spilling over into the skull should also be noted.

> **Thinking prompts:** There are various causes of meningoencephalitis. The most common are bacterial, viral, and tubercule bacillus, and all three are possible in school-aged children. In addition, unexplained coma in children in summer

should be considered as a possible result of toxic bacillary dysentery. However, the onset of toxic bacillary dysentery is rapid, often accompanied by high fever, convulsions, and coma within 24 hours, and toxic shock, usually without signs of meningeal irritation and normal cerebrospinal fluid. A stool test can help with diagnosis. This patient had a slow onset compared to toxic bacillary dysentery. There were no signs of shock nor obvious signs of meningeal irritation, and most importantly, normal stool routine and culture, so toxic bacillary dysentery could be ruled out. Cholera could also be ruled out because the patient had no obvious signs of dehydration, and the motility and immobilization tests for Vibrio cholera were negative. Therefore, clinicians should focus on the diagnosis and differentiation of meningoencephalitis.

2. Differential analysis

(1) Purulent meningitis: Meningococcus is a common pathogen causing purulent meningitis, which occurs mostly in winter and spring, with petechiae often appearing on the skin mucosa and coma occurring within 1–2 days of onset. The primary lesion can mostly be found in those caused by purulent bacteria. Cerebrospinal fluid shows bacterial meningitis changes. Petechiae or cerebrospinal fluid smear staining or culture may reveal bacteria. In this case, purulent meningitis was not considered.

(2) Tuberculous meningitis: Tuberculous meningitis is not seasonal; it has a slow onset and long course, and is dominated by meningeal irritation signs. There is often a history of tuberculosis. The levels of chloride and sugar in cerebrospinal fluid decreased, and the levels of protein increased obviously. Cerebrospinal fluid culture can detect tuberculosis bacilli, and a chest X-ray can mostly find tuberculosis lesions. Therefore, tuberculous meningitis was ruled out in this case.

(3) Epidemic encephalitis B (Japanese encephalitis): This is mostly distinctly seasonal (summer and autumn) and is common in children under ten years of age. The onset is rapid, with symptoms such as high fever, headache, vomiting, impaired consciousness, and convulsions. Typical signs are meningeal irritation signs, often with positive pathological reflexes. Laboratory tests show increased peripheral blood leukocytes and neutrophils, and cerebrospinal fluid examination is consistent with aseptic meningitis changes. Serological tests may help to confirm the diagnosis. Combined with the clinical manifestations of this patient, a diagnosis of Japanese encephalitis can be established. It is important to note that some patients do not necessarily have the typical symptoms described above, such as in this case, and do not elicit pathological reflexes, but a correct diagnosis can be made on the basis of the other manifestations. Diagnosis can be confirmed by further serum specific IgM antibody assay, a complement fixation test, a hemagglutination inhibition test, and a neutralization test, which can detect the specific corresponding antibodies. According to

the clinical symptoms of Japanese encephalitis, it can be classified as mild, moderate, severe, or critical. This patient had a fever of 39°C–40°C, shallow coma, occasional convulsions, negative pathological signs, and obvious signs of meningeal irritation, so was considered as having the moderate type.

> **Thinking prompts:** Japanese encephalitis is caused by viral infection, so culturing body fluids does not help to identify it. However, specific IgM antibody measurement can be performed to assist in the diagnosis. Generally, it can be detected 3–4 days after the onset, or as early as the second day of the disease course in the cerebrospinal fluid. The peak can be reached in two weeks, which can be useful for early diagnosis. The detection rate is high in patients with mild and moderate Japanese encephalitis, and low in severe and critical cases. There are no specific antiviral drugs for the treatment of this disease, but ribavirin and interferon can be used. Active symptomatic treatment and care should be provided, with emphasis on dealing with hyperthermia and convulsions and being alert to the occurrence of respiratory failure.

3. Ward-round analysis on the seventh day after admission

After admission, multiple blood cultures showed no growth of pathogenic bacteria. Urine and stool cultures were normal, the PPD test was negative, and the tubercule bacillus test was negative. The B encephalitis-specific IgM antibody was positive, and the hemagglutination inhibition test was positive.

Immediately after admission, intensive care was given to monitor vital signs. The patient's oral and skin cleanliness was maintained, and he was regularly turned over and patted on his back to prevent oral, skin, and lung infections. Ice packs and alcohol baths were given for physical cooling from high fever, supplemented by indomethacin medication to lower his temperature. Fluid replacement was administered to correct dehydration, acidosis, and electrolyte abnormalities. Nasal feeding was administered to ensure nutritional intake. On the second day after admission, the patient's body temperature began to drop, and on the fifth day it returned to normal. His mental state began to clear. His mental and psychiatric recovery was normal, without limb movement disorder. His general condition was good.

IV. Condition at discharge (twelfth day after admission)

The patient's body temperature was completely normal, his mental state was better, and his diet and sleep had improved. Limb movements were normal. On the twelfth day after admission, blood was drawn and re-checked for B encephalitis-specific IgM antibodies, which were higher than the first time. The routine blood test and classification returned to normal.

V. Follow-up

After discharge, the patient continued to take medication, and gradually resumed normal life. His body temperature continued to be normal. One month after discharge, his blood test was normal. At six months, he reported that he was going to school and living his life as usual without any discomfort, and his body temperature was normal.

VI. Lessons learned

This is a relatively typical case of Japanese encephalitis. Children visiting Beijing for the first time in summer and autumn are a high-risk group, and should be closely observed. The initial diagnostic idea should be analyzed according to the various characteristics of meningoencephalitis caused by specific pathogens. The disease can be quickly identified by ruling them all out. In this case, the treatment was effective and did not leave any sequelae. It should be noted that meningoencephalitis is not the only disease that causes fever and coma in children, because young physicians tend to limit their thinking to it. Although toxic bacillary dysentery and cholera were ruled out in this case, identification of the two is essential, because limiting diagnostic thinking to a single system will largely increase the chances of misdiagnosis.

(Hou Wei & Meng Qinghua)

High fever and irritability for two days; recurrent convulsions and unconsciousness for one day

I. Medical history

Patient: Female, three years old, from the suburbs of Beijing. She was hospitalized between 17 August and 5 September 2005 with high fever, irritability for two days, and recurrent convulsions and unconsciousness for one day.

Two days ago, the patient presented with a fever of about 40°C, accompanied by significant irritability, crying, hitting herself on the head, and vomiting her stomach contents several times. There was no diarrhea, and she suffered from a poor diet and nighttime sleep. She was seen at a local clinic and diagnosed with a bacterial infection through laboratory tests, WBC 18.3 × 10^9/L, N 86.7%, L 8.2%. She was given ceftriaxone sodium intravenously for two days and aspirin-dl-lysine antipyretic treatment, but the effect was poor. There was a short decrease in body temperature with antipyretics, but it quickly rose again. One day ago, the patient had recurrent limb convulsions, then stopped crying, became unconscious, and did not respond to calls. She was quickly transferred to our hospital.

The patient was previously healthy, delivered at full term, with normal growth and development, and completed vaccinations on schedule. She had no history of drug or food allergy, and had not come into contact with contaminated water in an infectious area. She had no family history of hereditary disease, and there was no recent occurrence of similar diseases in the surrounding area.

Thinking prompts: The pediatric patient was too young to express herself accurately, and her rapid descent into coma made taking medical history very difficult. Therefore, a careful physical examination and related tests are particularly important. Parents should be questioned in detail about the sequence of symptoms, the progression of the disease, the growth and development history of the pediatric patient, and the family history, which may play a guiding role in the diagnosis and differential exclusion of the disease and the choice of treatment. Since this pediatric patient had been treated with third-generation cephalosporins for two days at the local hospital with poor results, her illness cannot be put down to a simple bacterial infection, and other causes should be investigated.

II. Physical examination and auxiliary examination on admission

1. Physical examination

T 40.1°C, BP 105/65 mmHg, H 100 beats/min. The patient was unconscious and did not respond to calls. Her heart rhythm was uniform. Respiration was superficial with a regular rhythm. The respiratory sounds of both lungs were clear, and no dry and moist rales were heard. There was no enlargement of the superficial lymph nodes throughout the body, and no rash. Her pupils were equally large and rounded bilaterally. She had a slow light reflex, and the bulbar conjunctival edema was obvious. Stiff neck and resistance were obvious. Both deep and superficial reflexes were absent, and the pathological signs were positive. Positive signs were seen in the abdomen.

> **Thinking prompts:** Routine blood test, blood culture, CRP to suggest bacterial or viral infection, blood gas analysis, biochemistry, glucose, and electrolytes were performed based on a complete history and physical examination to help assess the current vital status. Cerebrospinal fluid examination was necessary because of obvious positive signs in the nervous system. Routine urine and stool and culture, chest radiograph, and abdominal ultrasound were helpful in finding the primary foci of infection. A PPD test and Mycobacterium tuberculosis test were performed to rule out tuberculosis infection. Motility and immobilization tests of Vibrio cholerae can rule out cholera.

2. Auxiliary examination

Routine blood: WBC 13.2 × 10^9/L, N 79.8%, L 8.6%, RBC 3.55 × 10^{12}/L, Hb 112 g/L, PLT 257 × 10^9/L.

Routine urine and stool were normal.

Blood gas analysis suggested respiratory acidosis combined with metabolic acidosis.

Biochemical, liver, and kidney functions were basically normal.

Blood glucose was 3.1 mmol/L and electrolytes suggested sodium 135 mmol/L.

Cerebrospinal fluid examination suggested increased pressure, clear appearance, WBC 120 × 10^6/L, N 75%, normal sugar and chloride, and protein 0.45 g/L.

Motility and immobilization tests for Vibrio cholerae were negative.

Chest X-ray and abdominal ultrasound were normal.

III. Ward-round analysis after admission

1. Preliminary diagnosis

The patient had an acute onset, with high fever, convulsions, impaired consciousness, and positive meningeal stimulation signs. The main causes of coma with positive meningeal irritation signs are meningitis or meningoencephalitis caused by various bacteria, viruses, and fungi; pseudo-meningitis caused by systemic infection; blood entering the subarachnoid space from cerebral hemorrhage and traumatic brain injury; and a brain tumor or brain abscess invading the subarachnoid space. This patient had no history of head trauma before the onset of the disease, so traumatic brain injury could be ruled out. Brain hemorrhages and brain tumors are common in middle-aged and elderly people. They rarely occur in children, and do not have high fever as the first symptom. Therefore, the initial diagnosis was meningoencephalitis, but the etiology was not completely clear. The possibility of pseudo-meningitis and a brain abscess caused by systemic infection should also be noted.

Thinking prompts: There are various causes of meningoencephalitis, namely bacteria, viruses, tubercle bacillus, and fungi, all of which are possible in preschool children. There is also pseudo-meningitis due to systemic infections such as toxic bacillary dysentery, which is common in children during the summer. However, the onset of toxic bacillary dysentery is more rapid, often with high fever, convulsions, and coma within 24 hours, and toxic shock, usually without signs of meningeal irritation. Cerebrospinal fluid is more normal, and stool examination can help with diagnosis. This pediatric patient had a slow onset compared to toxic bacillary dysentery, with no signs of shock, obvious signs of meningeal irritation, and a marked increase in peripheral blood leukocytes. However, antibiotic treatment was not effective, and did not support bacterial infection. Most importantly, the routine stool was normal, so toxic bacillary dysentery could be ruled out.

Cholera could also be ruled out because the patient had no obvious signs of dehydration, and the Motility and immobilization tests for Vibrio cholerae were negative.

Meningitis-type leptospirosis and cerebral malaria are also systemic infectious diseases that can cause neurological symptoms. Leptospirosis mostly occurs after contact with contaminated water, and has symptoms such as fatigue, gastrocnemius pain, conjunctival congestion, axillary or inguinal lymph node enlargement, and mild cerebrospinal fluid changes. The fever pattern of cerebral malaria is more irregular, with chills, fever, and sweating at the onset followed by cerebral symptoms, splenomegaly, and anemia. This patient lacked the specific above-mentioned symptoms, so a diagnosis was unlikely, but specific serum antibodies and blood smear could be checked for Plasmodium to help confirm the diagnosis.

Brain abscesses can also present with high fever, convulsions, and neurological symptoms, and the primary focus can often be found elsewhere in the body. Antibiotic treatment can be effective, and a further cranial CT scan can be performed to assist in confirming the diagnosis.

Finally, the focus in this case was on the diagnosis and differentiation of meningoencephalitis.

2. Differential analysis

(1) Purulent meningitis can be ruled out: See "Differential analysis" in Case 61.

(2) Tuberculous meningitis can be ruled out: See "Differential analysis" in Case 61.

(3) Mumps, poliomyelitis, coxsackie, and echovirus infections of the central nervous system: The cerebrospinal fluid leukocytes in this type of disease can range from (0.05 to 0.5) × 10^9/L, but the classification is predominantly lymphocytic. Some patients with mumps may first present with symptoms of meningoencephalitis and later develop swelling of the parotid gland, and any exposure to mumps should be noted when differentiating. A small number of patients with JE may have flaccid paralysis, which can be misdiagnosed as poliomyelitis, but the latter does not have impaired consciousness. Coxsackie virus, echovirus, herpes simplex virus, and varicella virus can also cause similar symptoms. The patient lacked appropriate epidemiological evidence and clinical features, and routine blood tests were not supportive. These types of diseases can be ruled out by serological examination.

(4) Fungal meningitis: Cryptococcus Neoformans Meningitis is the most common intracranial fungal infection. It occurs in patients who are extremely immunocompromised, often the elderly and frail, in patients with tumors, or in those who have been heavily using broad-spectrum antibiotics or hormones and immunosuppressive agents for a long time. The diagnosis can be confirmed by finding Cryptococcus neoformans on an ink smear of cerebrospinal fluid. This patient was previously healthy, had normal growth and development, and denied a history of the above-mentioned drug use, so this diagnosis could be ruled out.

(5) Epidemic encephalitis B (Japanese encephalitis): See "Differential analysis" in Case 61. Considering the patient's clinical manifestations, a diagnosis of B encephalitis can be established. According to the clinical symptoms of B encephalitis, it can be classified as mild, moderate, severe, or critical. This patient had a fever of more than 40°C, coma, repeated convulsions, loss of both deep and superficial reflexes, positive pathological signs, and obvious signs of meningeal irritation, so she was considered to be a critical case.

> **Thinking prompts:** Japanese encephalitis is caused by viral infection, so a culture of bodily fluids does not help to identify it. However, specific IgM antibody measurement can be done to assist in the diagnosis. Generally, it can be detected 3–4 days after the onset, and can be detected as early as the second day of the disease course in the cerebrospinal fluid. The peak can be reached in two weeks, which can be used for early diagnosis. The detection rate is high in patients with mild and moderate JE, and low in severe and critical cases. There are no specific antiviral drugs for the treatment of this disease, but ribavirin and interferon can be used. Active symptomatic treatment and care should be provided, with an emphasis on dealing with hyperthermia and convulsions, and being alert to the occurrence of respiratory failure.

IV. Ward-round analysis on the fifth day after admission

After admission, multiple blood cultures showed no growth of pathogenic bacteria. The urine and stool cultures were normal, the PPD test was negative, and the tubercule bacillus test was negative. Leptospira-specific serum antibodies were negative, a blood smear was negative for Plasmodium, and a cerebrospinal fluid smear with ink stain was negative for Cryptococcus. Encephalitis B-specific IgM antibodies were positive, and a hemagglutination inhibition test was positive. The cranial CT was normal.

Immediately after admission, intensive care was given to monitor vital signs, noting oral and skin cleanliness, and regularly turning the patient over and patting her back to prevent oral, skin, and lung infections. For high fever, ice packs and alcohol baths were given for physical cooling, supplemented with indomethacin medication to lower her temperature. Fluid replacement to correct dehydration, acidosis, and electrolyte abnormalities was administered. Nasal feeding was administered to ensure nutritional intake. The patient had repeated convulsions and significant bulbar conjunctival edema, so intracranial hypertension was considered. 20% mannitol and furosemide were given for dehydration, together with glucocorticoids. Comatose patients with more respiratory secretions can be given sputum suction and nebulized inhalation to keep their airways clear.

On the fifth day of admission, the patient's temperature began to drop. She was still in a coma, but her deep reflex could be elicited. Her pupils were equal in size and round, and a light reflex could be elicited. The number of convulsions gradually decreased to 1–2 times per day. The routine blood test was repeated with WBC 9.1×10^9/L, N 75%, L 6.9%. Blood gas analysis, blood glucose, and electrolytes results returned to normal.

V. Ward-round analysis on the tenth day after admission

The patient's body temperature gradually returned to normal. Her vital signs were stable, her consciousness became clear, but her reactions were slow. She had weakness in both lower limbs, and had difficulty moving on her own. No further convulsions occurred after she regained consciousness. The patient's blood count and cell classification returned to normal.

VI. Condition at discharge (nineteenth day after admission)

The patient's body temperature was completely normal. Her consciousness was clear but her reactions were still slow. Her mental state was better, and her diet and sleep were normal. Both lower limbs were still weak; muscle strength was grade 3, muscle tone was normal, and there were difficulties in spontaneous activities. On the fourteenth day after admission, blood was drawn and retested for a fourfold increase in encephalitis B-specific IgM antibodies compared with the first time, and the routine blood and cell classification were normal.

VII. Follow-up

After discharge from the hospital, no further medication was administered, and the patient's body temperature remained normal. Her reactions were still slow at the three and six-month follow-ups after discharge, with weakness in both lower limbs and no significant recovery of muscle strength. With the help of her parents, she can barely walk a few steps; no speech issues, and no more convulsions or muscle spasms.

VIII. Lessons learned

This case was classified as a severe form of JE, and the epidemiology, clinical symptoms, and specific ancillary tests all supported the diagnosis. The diagnosis was based on fever, coma, and meningeal irritation signs as the entry point. Systemic infectious diseases, cerebral hemorrhage, brain abscess, and trauma were ruled out, and then analyzed according to the various characteristics of meningoencephalitis caused by different pathogenic bacteria. Finally, encephalitis-B was considered. Due to the severity of the patient's condition, although there was no respiratory failure, there was parenchymal brain damage, and there were still obvious sequelae six months after discharge.

(Hou Wei & Meng Qinghua)

Fever and fatigue for more than ten days with chills, weakness, and dizziness

I. Medical history

Patient: Male, 32 years old, a middle school teacher from Jiangxi. He was hospitalized between 9 March and 11 May 2005 with fever and fatigue for more than ten days, accompanied by chills, weakness, and dizziness.

The patient developed a persistent fever with no obvious inducement more than ten days ago, with a temperature as high as 39.6°C, accompanied by chills, weakness, and dizziness, which disappeared when the fever subsided. No headache, no cough and expectoration, no chest tightness, shortness of breath, no sore throat, no blurred vision. He went to his local hospital for medical treatment, but no diagnosis was made. He was treated with ceftriaxone sodium and ribavirin, but his body temperature still fluctuated around 38.5°C, so he was referred to our hospital for further treatment.

> **Thinking prompts:** Fever is a common symptom of many diseases. Medical records should describe the conditions at the onset and at the time of the turn of events in detail, while concomitant symptoms can often provide clues to local organ damage. The treatment aspects that will guide the subsequent treatment plan should also be described in detail as concisely as possible, such as the use of antibiotics for febrile diseases. For example, whether the dose and course of antibiotics are adequate can be summarized by the standard application.

This patient was found to be positive for hepatitis B five years ago, and started taking lamivudine in 2001 (100 mg daily). He decided to stop taking it after two years of treatment due to a fever. He began to feel weak and lost his appetite. Last year he was diagnosed with hepatitis and liver cirrhosis at the local hospital, and was hospitalized for six months, but his symptoms were not significantly relieved and his abnormal liver function did not improve. He resumed oral administration of lamivudine in January 2005, but his liver function was not reviewed regularly. He denied eating unclean food, had no contact with contaminated water, and did not breed or slaughter pigeons. The patient's mother had a history of hepatitis B.

Thinking prompts: When the patient was questioned, it was clear that he had a history of hepatitis cirrhosis, which is most likely to be complicated by infections, especially of the abdomen. This history of cirrhosis also suggested that the patient was immunocompromised and prone to complications from infection by conditionally pathogenic bacteria. Based on a detailed physical examination of his whole body, focused attention was given to abdominal signs. The patient had been treated with antibiotics for more than ten days, and signs of secondary infections, such as oral leukoplakia, should be noted.

II. Physical examination and auxiliary examination

1. Physical examination

T 39°C, P 90 times/min, R 18 times/min, BP 111/70 mmHg. Fine mental state, skin sclera moderately yellow stained, no white spots in the oral cavity, soft neck, no liver palm, no spider nevus, no enlarged lymph nodes anywhere on the body, no abnormalities in the heart and lungs, soft abdomen, no pressure pain, no rebound pain; the liver was not palpable below the costal margin, and the spleen was palpable 1.5 cm below the ribs, shifting dullness (+), no edema in both lower limbs. Brudzinski's sign (−), Kernig's sign (−), pathological reflex (−); muscle strength and tension of the limbs were normal.

Thinking prompt: Auxiliary examinations focus on abnormalities of the liver function and manifestations of portal hypertension caused by cirrhosis, which can be checked by liver function tests and B ultrasound examination. As for fever, infection indicators such as C-reactive protein, blood count, and blood sedimentation can be checked, and ascites cell count and biochemical tests can often indicate the presence of intra-abdominal infection.

2. Auxiliary examinations on admission

Routine blood: WBC 4.7×10^9/L, N 72.0%, L 17.2%, Hb 83 g/L, RBC 2.16×10^{12}/L, PLT 45×10^9/L.

Liver function: A/G 23.1/36.6 g/L, ALT/AST 43/63 U/L, CHE (cholinesterase) 812 U/L, TB/CB 81/41 μmol/L, γ-GT 47 U/L, PT 26.4 seconds.

Routine ascites: WBC 83/μl, RBC 320/μl, Rivalta test weakly positive, yellow in appearance, clear, no bacterial growth in the ascites culture.

B-ultrasound: Cirrhosis, splenomegaly, ascites, no significant abnormalities in either kidney ureter and retroperitoneum.

PPD test: 1:2,000 (−), 1:10,000 (−).

Routine urine and stool were normal.

Urinary bilirubin (+).

ANA full set tests, ANCA, C-reactive protein, and anti-streptococcal O hemolysin were normal.

III. Preliminary diagnosis and differentiation
1. Preliminary diagnosis
The young adult male patient had chronic hepatitis B for five years and hepatitis cirrhosis for nearly one year; persistent fever for more than ten days with chills, weakness, and dizziness; examination revealed positive abdominal shifting dullness. Based on the above features, the preliminary diagnosis was hepatitis cirrhosis with spontaneous peritonitis.

Spontaneous peritonitis: This occurs in patients with decompensated cirrhosis combined with ascites, and is one of the most common complications of cirrhosis. It is often due to intestinal vascular stasis, with the intestinal tube immersed in ascites, which decreases intestinal barrier function and intestinal flora translocation, causing abdominal infection. Besides fever, the main clinical manifestations are abdominal distension and decreased urine output. Abdominal pressure pain and rebound pain can be insignificant or even absent. When cirrhotic ascites are combined with infection, routine and biochemical changes in ascites can be atypical, but the leukocyte count should exceed 300/μl. If it exceeds 200/μl, the diagnosis can be clarified with the clinical conditions. This patient's ascites leukocyte count was not high. This did not support infectious ascites, so it should be reviewed in the near future. The antibiotics chosen should be sensitive to intestinal flora, such as acylurea penicillin, aminoglycosides, third-generation cephalosporins, or carbapenems. Combined with the fact that this patient had used ceftriaxone sodium at his local hospital for a longer period, the causative organism is probably the intestinal flora that produces ultra-broad-spectrum β-lactamase, so a compound antibiotic or carbapenems needs to be chosen.

2. Differential analysis
The diagnosis needs to be differentiated from the following diseases:

(1) Biliary tract infections: The typical biliary tract infection features fever, abdominal pain, and jaundice. In the elderly or in patients without significant biliary obstruction, abdominal pain or even jaundice may not appear. However, there is often pressure pain in the right upper abdomen, and bilirubin in the blood is predominantly conjugated, (normally, conjugated bilirubin accounts for about 25% of total bilirubin. During an attack of hepatitis, hepatocytes can swell, and their ability to metabolize unconjugated bilirubin decreases; both conjugated and unconjugated bilirubin can increase. In this case, conjugated bilirubin can exceed 30% to 40%), urinary urobilinogen is reduced or absent, and glutamyl transpeptidase and alkaline phosphatase are often significantly increased in the blood. In this patient, the bilirubin increment was biphasic, the urobilinogen was increased, and the glutamyl transpeptidase and alkaline phosphatase were normal, so the increased blood bilirubin was considered to be of hepatocellular origin, not biliary origin. Moreover, the patient lacked abdominal signs and symptoms, which did not support biliary tract infection.

(2) Upper respiratory tract infection: This is mainly caused by rhinovirus. Clinical manifestations include catarrhal upper respiratory tract symptoms, such as nasal congestion, runny nose, sneezing, sore throat, and coughing and expectoration. Catarrhal symptoms

may not appear, but the duration of fever is usually 3–7 days and rarely exceeds 14 days. The main treatment is rest, fluid intake, and symptomatic treatment. In case of combined bacterial infection, antibiotics should be prescribed, such as first-generation cephalosporin. However, this patient did not have the above symptoms, and the fever duration was relatively long, so it was not considered.

(3) Typhoid fever: Typhoid fever is characterized by persistent fever – a typical early step-like rise in body temperature, which may present as continued fever with a relatively long fever duration, as well as vagueness, hearing difficulties, abdominal distention, constipation, relatively slow pulse, leukopenia, and splenomegaly. S. typhi mainly invades the mononuclear phagocyte system and has a second bacteraemia. The first bacteraemia is not clinically manifested, and the second bacteraemia leads to the onset of clinical signs and symptoms. Culturing S. typhi in blood, bone marrow, and urine and stool is the criterion for confirmation of the diagnosis, but the probability of culturing the bacteria is low in patients who are already on antibiotics. Serological tests include the Widal reaction. Typhoid lipopolysaccharide antibodies are not very specific or sensitive, so they can only be used as an auxiliary diagnosis. However, if the serologic changes are dynamically observed, this will increase the value of the diagnosis. The main treatment options are quinolones and third-generation cephalosporin. Although this patient had a long febrile course, he had an acute onset and moderate degree of fever. He lacked other manifestations of typhoid fever, and denied eating unclean food, so typhoid fever was not considered for the time being.

(4) Pulmonary tuberculosis: Tuberculosis occurs in people with weakened immunity, mainly manifesting as low to moderate fever, night sweats, emaciation, coughing, and expectoration. If the lesion is in the periphery of the lung, the cough and expectoration may not be obvious, and densitometric changes can be found on chest radiography; there may be no change on the chest radiography in the early stage of miliary tuberculosis, but when it is repeated after 2–3 weeks, miliary foci can be found. In addition, patients with miliary tuberculosis usually have severe toxemia symptoms such as high fever and poor mental health. A positive PPD test is helpful for diagnosis but can be negative in immunocompromised patients or those with early tuberculosis (4–8 weeks). This patient had a fever for more than ten days, and was in the loss compensation period of liver cirrhosis, so the possibility of tuberculosis should be noted. However, the chest X-ray and PPD test did not support tuberculosis, so it was not considered. However, the presence of extrapulmonary tuberculosis should be noted, especially in sites that are more difficult to detect, such as liver tuberculosis and intracranial tuberculosis. Therefore, the condition and the efficacy of antibiotics should be observed, and appropriate tests should be performed if necessary.

(5) Urinary tract infection: Of the upper or lower urinary tract. In the former, bladder irritation signs (frequency, urgency, and painful urination) may not be obvious, but there are often systemic symptoms, such as fever and lower back pain. The latter is the opposite. This patient had no bladder irritation signs. No anatomical channel changes such as stones were detected by B-ultrasound of the urinary system, and a routine urine test was normal. Therefore, a urinary tract infection was not considered.

(6) Pelvic infection: The pelvic cavity is closed in men, so pelvic inflammatory disease is rare. However, rectal lesions should be noted, such as sinus tracts and fistulas causing infection of the rectal bladder fossa, which are not easily detected in their deep anatomical location. Often there is a history of anal fissures, with clinical manifestations such as fever, increased frequency of stools, tenesmus, and anal pain. This patient lacked a history of local diseases and local symptoms, so pelvic infection was not considered.

(7) Secondary infection: The patient had been on antibiotics for a long time at his local hospital. Decompensation of cirrhosis resulted in relatively low immunity, so we should note the possibility of secondary infection. Secondary infections occur in the oral respiratory tract, with Candida albicans as the most common pathogen. The patient's oral cavity did not show white spots, and he lacked respiratory manifestations, so it was not considered for the time being. However, it should be noted that the prolongation of antibiotic treatment increases the possibility of secondary infection, so it is important to observe the oral cavity and give antifungal treatment if necessary.

IV. Ward-round analysis on the ninth day after admission

The patient was treated with compound antibiotics (piperacillin-tazobactam) for seven days, but his body temperature still fluctuated around 38.5°C. He had no significant appetite, but the amount of food eaten was acceptable. There was no relief for his fatigue, and his mental status was fair. During the checkup, white spots were found in his oral cavity, and the results of the ascites review did not suggest an infection. Considering that his persistent fever was caused by a secondary infection (Candida albicans infection), fluconazole (Diflucan) 0.2 g was administered intravenously once daily, first dose doubling, and oral care was strengthened.

V. Ward-round analysis on the forty-third day after admission

The patient's temperature gradually decreased the day after fluconazole was added to his treatment on the ninth day of admission, and normalized on the third day of treatment. When the fever subsided, fluconazole was continued for two days and all antibiotics were stopped. Blood bilirubin also decreased during the treatment with fluconazole, and abdominal distension was relieved. Normal body temperature was maintained for 19 days. However, nine days ago, his temperature rose again, fluctuating around 38.5°C. Blood bilirubin rose again on re-examination, and the abdominal distension returned. No headache, no vomiting. No new positive signs were found on physical examination. Ultrasound revealed that ascites had recently increased again, and a CT examination of the lungs was normal. Since cirrhosis combined with abdominal infection was the most frequent, the treatment was still targeted at abdominal infection. After seven days of cefoperazone and sulbactam, the patient's body temperature still did not regulate, reaching over 39.0°C (Figure 63-1). Therefore, antibiotics were discontinued, and he was observed for two days. His temperature remained unchanged. Since this fever, his abdominal distension had increased, his urine output had decreased, and his liver function suggested further increments of blood bilirubin. The prothrombin time was prolonged.

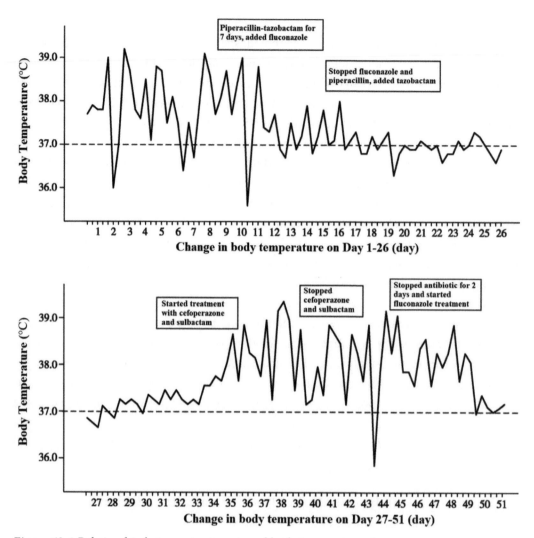

Figure 63-1 Relationship between treatments and body temperature changes

The patient had a renewed fever with a persistent temperature, a recurrence of abdominal distension, and a concomitant increase in blood bilirubin. What was the reason for the ineffective treatment with a broad-spectrum combination of antibiotics? Can the cause of the two fevers be explained by monism or dichotomy? Were they infectious fevers or non-infectious fevers? If they were infectious, what pathogens were they and where was the site of infection? The patient's current hospitalization data was the most direct, specific, and definitive, so the relationship between the change in temperature, treatment measures, and efficacy of the patient's two successive fevers since admission was analyzed retrospectively, and the differential analysis is as follows:

1. Drug fever: Drug fever is one of the more common causes of non-infectious febrile diseases. Drug fever caused by antibiotics is the most common, and can appear after four days of medication, usually 7–8 days, often caused by drug-induced allergic reactions. The fever subsides 24 to 48 hours after stopping the medication. This patient stopped taking antibiotics

for two days and still showed no signs of temperature reduction, so it was not considered.

2. Tumor fever: There are two main causes of fever caused by parenchymal tumors, namely tumor necrosis and release of a pyrogen. No mass was found in the patient during routine examination, so it was not considered. However, there are some tumors that are difficult to find through conventional examination, such as small intestine tumors. They were not considered because the intestinal lumen of the small intestine is small, and can often cause obstructions. Certain hematologic tumors, such as lymphoma (especially extranodal lymphoma, which is likely to occur in patients with relatively low immunity), may manifest as periodic fever, and lymph node and bone marrow biopsies may be helpful for diagnosis. The rate of positive bone marrow biopsies for extranodal lymphoma is only 15% to 20%, so it is sometimes difficult to determine clinically. However, the most frequent cause of fever is infection. This should be ruled out first before diagnosing a tumor, so it was not considered for the time being.

3. Opportunistic infections: One type of opportunistic infection has already been mentioned in the first clinical analysis, namely double infection. The patient was admitted to hospital with an initial fever, and his temperature decreased the next day after the addition of fluconazole treatment, supporting the diagnosis of Candida albicans secondary infection. The renewed fever, again with the ineffective application of broad-spectrum antibiotics, triggered the following thoughts and reasoning:

(1) Could it be that the course of the fluconazole treatment was not sufficient to control the fungus completely, so it caused another fever? However, deep fungal infections caused by Candida albicans are usually manifested in the respiratory system. The patient's lung CT was normal, and transient Candida albicans sepsis is rare, so a diagnosis of Candida albicans infection was not supported.

(2) The therapeutic efficacy of fluconazole and the temperature drop are not associated, so are they just coincidental? No clinical information should be overlooked. If it is not a coincidence, then the efficacy of fluconazole treatment and fever remission must be related. Using monism to explain the two fevers, the first consideration is an opportunistic fungal infection of the same non-Candida albicans.

(3) If it is a fungal fever, where is the site of infection? The medical history, clinical manifestations, and auxiliary examinations failed to identify one, so could it be a systemic infection? However, the course of the disease is almost one and a half months, so it is unlikely to be a systemic infection. Then could it be a fungal infection in a site that is not easily detected, or is overlooked by general clinical examination and auxiliary tests, such as an intracranial fungal infection? Therefore, cryptococcal meningitis can be considered.

4. Cryptococcal meningitis: This is a relatively common form of deep fungal infection, often in immunocompromised patients. Cryptococcus is found in the feces of birds such as pigeons. The patient's relatively slow onset and sensitivity to fluconazole support the diagnosis of the disease. Headaches tend to be more intense because of the marked increase in intracranial pressure. However, if the cryptococcal pathogenicity is weak, the symptoms of increased intracranial pressure and signs of meningeal irritation can be insignificant, which can lead to

clinical misdiagnosis and missed diagnosis. Once a central infection is considered, cerebrospinal fluid examination should be performed as early as possible in order to clarify the kind of pathogenic infection and to carry out targeted treatment. This is of great clinical importance because the earlier the treatment of pathogens is carried out, the better the curative effect and the fewer the sequelae. A cranial magnetic resonance imaging (MRI) scan and enhancement can also be performed to detect any changes in the meninges and brain parenchyma.

VI. Ward-round analysis on the forty-fourth day after admission
1. Differential diagnosis
Yesterday's cerebrospinal fluid examination report (Table 63-1): Colorless appearance, clear, leukocytes 40/μl, neutrophils 68%, lymphocytes 30%, no cryptococcus found, chloride 118 mmol/L (reference value 119–129 mmol/L), glucose 0.8 mmol/L (reference value 2.5–4.4 mmol/L), protein 0.99 g/L (reference value 0.20–0.45 g/L). Cerebrospinal fluid was sent for culture. See the report for the results.

Table 63-1 Routine cerebrospinal fluid test

Date	Appearance	Clarity	Pandy's reaction	Leukocytes (pcs/μl)	Neutro-phils %	Lympho-cytes %	Look for Cryptococcus
2005.4.20	Colorless	Clear	+	40	68	30	−
2005.5.5	Colorless	Clear	+	20	10	90	−
2005.5.24	Colorless	Clear	−	1			−

A routine cerebrospinal fluid test indicates the presence of a central infection. The four common types of pathogens are bacterial, viral, tubercular, and fungal. Clinical manifestations include fever, headache, vomiting, convulsions or decreased muscle strength, neck resistance, Brudzinski's sign, positive Kernig's sign, or positive pathological reflexes. However, each of the four types of central changes has its own characteristics, which are analyzed as follows:

(1) Common bacterial central infections: Bacterial central infections generally have an acute mode of onset, such as epidemic meningoencephalitis, often with subcutaneous hemorrhagic spots, cloudy cerebrospinal fluid, significant increment of white blood cells, predominantly increased neutrophils, decreased chloride and glucose, significantly increased protein, and bacteria being found in cerebrospinal fluid pictures and cultures. This was not considered.

(2) Viral central infection: Viral central infection is generally more acute in onset, often with more prominent damage to the brain parenchyma, manifested as convulsions, muscle strength, and respiratory changes. Cerebrospinal fluid is colorless and clear in appearance, with mild to moderate increment of white blood cells, predominantly lymphocytes (can be predominantly neutrophils early on), mild to moderate increment of protein, chloride, and glucose changes are generally not obvious, and the pathogen cannot be found. If the meningeal damage is not obvious, the cerebrospinal fluid can be completely normal. This was not considered.

(3) Tuberculosis and cryptococcal central infections: These are often secondary in patients with immune deficiency, and both may have pulmonary manifestations first. Sometimes the central manifestations can be obscure, and the appearance of the cerebrospinal fluid is typically ground-glass opacity in the former. Both can be colorless, pale yellow, clear or slightly mixed, with mild to moderate increment of white blood cells. Both can be predominantly lymphocytic and sometimes neutrophilic, with decreased chloride and glucose and increased protein. However, tuberculous meningitis is difficult to find in Mycobacterium tuberculosis, while cryptococcal meningitis is found in more than 80% to 90% of cases (which must be stained with ink and looked for under a microscope by an experienced physician). If the number of cerebrospinal fluid examinations is increased, the probability of finding cryptococci increases to almost 100%. Sometimes it is difficult to distinguish between the two. However, when all indicators of the cerebrospinal fluid are analyzed, especially the biochemical reports, the decrease in chloride in tuberculous meningitis is often more pronounced than the other biochemical changes in the cerebrospinal fluid. In contrast, the decrease in glucose was more prominent in cryptococcal meningitis. The biochemical alterations of the cerebrospinal fluid in this case were marked by a decrease in glucose. Looking back at the positive response to fluconazole treatment on admission, all were consistent with the diagnosis of cryptococcal meningitis. It is recommended to look for cryptococci again and if still not found, and wait for the results of cerebrospinal fluid culture. In the meantime, multiple lumbar punctures and cerebrospinal fluid examinations should be performed over a short period of time to improve the detection rate of cryptococci.

Some ten minutes later, the bacteriology laboratory verbally reported that Cryptococcus had been found, and thus the diagnosis of cryptococcal meningitis was clear. Anti-cryptococcal treatment was administered immediately.

2. Drug therapy

Currently available drugs include amphotericin B, fluconazole, and 5-fluorocytosine.

(1) Amphotericin B: A bactericidal agent, and the drug of choice for cryptococcal meningitis. However, it is the most toxic, and may cause chills and fever, along with gastrointestinal reactions such as nausea and vomiting. It can also lead to hypokalemia, and myocardial, liver, and kidney damage. Treatment must start with small doses, gradually increasing to 30–35 mg daily, generally not exceeding 40 mg. Previously, the daily dosage was as high as 50 mg, but it was difficult for patients to tolerate and could not be applied for a long duration. Such a high dose is not recommended in the current literature. Because of the poor compensatory capacity of liver function and active hepatitis in this case, it is estimated that amphotericin B will not be tolerated, so it is not selected for the time being. Amphotericin B does not cross the blood-brain barrier easily, so intrathecal injection is sometimes chosen along with systemic administration. During an intrathecal injection, the drugs are diluted with cerebrospinal fluid. It is advisable to inject slowly. However, the efficacy is not certain. Sometimes it can cause damage to the cauda equina nerve, which can lead to paraplegia in severe cases. Therefore, intrathecal injections are currently controversial. Whether it was

chosen for this patient was determined by his sensitivity to subsequent antifungal treatment.

(2) Fluconazole: A triazole antifungal drug that is an antibacterial agent. It has a certain degree of hepatotoxicity, and crosses the blood-brain barrier easily. In the treatment of cryptococcal meningitis, the dose requirement is large – 0.4–0.8 g per day intravenously during the intensive treatment phase and 0.2 g per day during the maintenance phase. Due to the patient's poor hepatic compensation ability and good response to the first application of fluconazole, a daily dose of 0.4 g was recommended for intensive treatment and 0.2 g for maintenance treatment.

(3) 5-fluorocytosine: An inexpensive antibacterial agent with a short half-life. It often causes drug resistance, so it is generally not applied alone. Combined with other antifungal drugs, it can produce synergistic effects. However, there are side effects such as bone marrow suppression and liver function damage, so it was not used in this case.

VII. Condition at discharge

A daily treatment regimen of 0.4 g fluconazole was selected. After eight days of intensive treatment by intravenous drip, it was changed to 0.2 g daily. The patient's body temperature gradually returned to normal after three days of fluconazole. After one week of treatment, the pre-treatment cerebrospinal fluid culture was reported (Table 63-2): Cryptococcus neoformans, sensitive to fluconazole, 5-fluorocytosine, and amphotericin B. Fluconazole treatment was continued in hospital for 34 days. The cerebrospinal fluid cell count, protein, chloride, and glucose returned to normal, and the patient was discharged.

Table 63-2 Cerebrospinal fluid biochemistry and culture

Date	Chloride mmol/L	Glucose mmol/L	Protein g/L	Incubation
2005.4.20	118	0.8	0.99	Cryptococcus neoformans: fluconazole/5-fluorocytosine/amphotericin B are sensitive
2005.5.5	120	1.6	0.51	–
2005.5.24	120	3.1	0.33	–

VIII. Follow-up

1. After discharge, maintenance treatment of 0.2 g fluconazole was continued for 65 days, and the cerebrospinal fluid was rechecked several times. All indicators were normal, and no cryptococcus was found.
2. Three years after discharge, the cerebrospinal fluid was normal and no cryptococcus was found in the culture. Liver function was basically normal.

IX. Lessons learned

1. The choice of antibiotics should be clearly targeted until the cause of fever is clear. Simultaneous application of antibiotics against different species of pathogens such as bacteria and fungi should be avoided as far as possible. Observations based on therapeutic measures and efficacy can provide clues for diagnosis.

2. The most common cause of fever is infection, and infection is caused by common pathogens, which should not be forgotten in clinical practice.

3. When clinical symptoms, signs, and auxiliary examinations fail to provide any clues, particular attention should be paid to clinically difficult to reach and easily ignored sites of infection.

(He Jianqin & Li Lanjuan)

Sore throat for more than ten days; arthralgia, fever, and hypotension for one day

I. Medical history

Patient: Female, 19 years old, a freshman at a local college. She was admitted to hospital with a sore throat for more than ten days, and arthralgia, fever, and hypotension for one day.

The patient visited her college health facility 11 days ago with a sore throat and fatigue. She was diagnosed with infectious mononucleosis after testing positive for heterophilic agglutination and negative on a group A streptococcal rapid screen. The results of laboratory tests are shown in Table 64-1. One week prior to admission, the patient developed nasal congestion and oral ulcers, and was followed up at the college health facility. Physical examination revealed oral ulcers, and enlarged anterior cervical lymph nodes with tenderness. Lidocaine and pseudoephedrine were given. Four days prior to admission, she experienced worsening sore throat and otalgia with dysphagia, bilateral tonsillar erythema, nasal mucosa congestion, and enlarged anterior cervical lymph nodes. She revisited the college health facility, where she was given 60 mg of prednisone orally for five days. Her symptoms progressed on the second day after the visit. Within 24 hours prior to admission, the patient presented for follow-up with additional symptoms of nausea, vomiting, chills, and lower abdominal pain. On physical examination, the symptoms were obvious, with a temperature of 37.6°C, heart rate of 129 beats/min, and blood pressure of 86/64 mmHg in the supine position, and a standing pulse rate of 144 beats/min and blood pressure of 100/72 mmHg. Her tonsils were enlarged but not accompanied by purulent exudate, and the degree of redness and swelling was relieved compared to before. Laboratory findings are shown in Table 64-1. Symptomatic treatment (antipyretic acetaminophen and antiemetic ondansetron) did not relieve the symptoms.

Thinking prompts: The patient – a college student – presented with a sore throat, enlarged lymph nodes in the neck, and fatigue. The possibility of a diagnosis of infectious mononucleosis should be considered initially, and can be confirmed by the classic heterophilic agglutination test, especially if the symptoms have persisted for more than one week. However, mononucleosis is not an easily treatable disease, and patients often revisit the clinic because of worsening symptoms. The key to the diagnosis in this case is to identify which symptoms are caused by EBV infection and which are not.

The patient returned to the clinic with nasal congestion and oral ulcers four days after being diagnosed with infectious mononucleosis. Common infectious causes of oral ulcers include the herpes simplex virus (HSV), coxsackievirus, and acute human immunodeficiency virus (HIV) infection, while non-infectious factors include neutropenia, iron deficiency, and Behcet's syndrome. Ulcers caused by HSV tend to appear in the anterior part of the mouth, including the gums and lips, whereas ulcers caused by the coxsackievirus often occur in the posterior part of the mouth and may also appear as lesions on the palms of the hands and the soles of the feet. Typical aphthous stomatitis is characterized by a fine yellow border at the back of the throat and painful swallowing, which may be secondary to other pathogenic infections, such as HSV or HIV, or may be idiopathic. However, aphthous stomatitis is not usually associated with EBV infection.

The patient came back for another follow-up three days later with a sore throat, otalgia, dysphagia, enlarged tonsils, and enlarged lymph nodes in her neck. These symptoms were consistent with those of mononucleosis, with the otalgia probably caused by a blockage of the Eustachian tube due to swelling of the pharynx. Doctors at primary hospitals are often torn about whether to give hormone therapy to patients with such severe sore throats. In this case, the patient received it. The results of previous clinical studies do not prove the benefit of hormone therapy, but the use of hormones is indicated when patients with mononucleosis present with severe complications, such as acute airway obstruction due to tonsillar enlargement.

The patient revisited the clinic one day after receiving hormone therapy, with symptoms of nausea, vomiting, chills, lower abdominal pain, and dehydration. Although toxic hepatitis (a common complication of mononucleosis) could explain the patient's GI symptoms, her serum transaminase level was only mildly elevated on a transient basis, so the diagnosis of toxic hepatitis was not established.

Until this point, the patient's symptoms could be explained by infectious mononucleosis. However, on the day of hospitalization, a dramatic change in her condition occurred with the development of fever, hypotension, muscle pain, arthralgia, and abdominal pain (see next page).

Table 64-1 Laboratory test results

Items	Reference normal value range	11 days before admission	Two days before admission	Before admission (clinic at college)	Before admission (first hospital)	On admission
Hematocrit (%)	36.0–46.0 (Female)	48.9	41.7	41.4	37.6	30.2
Hemoglobin (g/l)	120–160 (Female)	165	134	138	124	105
White blood cell count (× 10^9/L)	4.5–11	9.3	20.9	23.2	20.4	22.2
Leukocyte Sorted Count (%) Neutral leukocytes	40–70	36	86	79	74	
Banded (nucleated) type				6	6	
Lymphocytes	22–44	41	6	7	11	
Atypical lymphocytes		19	3	3	6	
Monocytes	4–11	4	5	5	3	
Platelet count (× 10^9/L)	150–350	146	296	334		247
Mean blood cell volume (fl)	80–100			90	89.6	88
Blood sedimentation (mm/hr)	0–20				62	36
Prothrombin time (seconds)	11.1–13.1					12.8
Activated partial thromboplastin time (seconds)	22.1–35.1					21.7
Sugar (mg/dl)	4.2–6.4				5.3	7.2
Sodium (mmol/L)	136–145				141	136
Potassium (mmol/L)	3.5–5.0				3.5	2.8
Chloride (mmol/L)	98–106				104	111

Table 64-1 (*Continued*)

Items	Reference normal value range	11 days before admission	Two days before admission	Before admission (clinic at college)	Before admission (first hospital)	On admission
Urea nitrogen (mmol/L)	3.57–7.14				5.00	5.00
Creatinine (μmol/L)	< 133				71	80
Total bilirubin (μmol/L)	5.1–17.1		10.3		5.1	5.1
Direct bilirubin (μmol/L)	1.7–5.1		5.1			1.7
Total protein (g/l)	55–80		69		70	54
Albumin (g/l)	35–55		37		38	24
Globulin (g/l)	20–35		32			30
Phosphorus (mmol/l)	0.8–1.5					0.29
Magnesium (mmol/l)	1.8–3.0					1.1
Calcium (mmol/l)	9.0–10.5				2.4	1.7
Alkaline phosphatase (U/L)	30–120		107		101	72
Aspartate aminotransferase (U/L)			35 (Reference range 7–10)		16	16
Alanine aminotransferase (U/L)	0–31		80 (Reference range 5–40)		47	38
Lipase (U/dl)	0.0–160.0					2
Amylase (U/L)	60–180					16
C-reactive protein (mg/L)	0.02–8.00					51.1

On the day of hospitalization, the patient woke up from the pain in her right elbow and left ankle. She returned to the health facility. Physical examination showed a temperature of 37.4°C, pulse of 92 beats/min, blood pressure of 104/64 mmHg, and significant tenderness in the right elbow and left ankle. Deep abdominal palpation showed tenderness in the mid and right lower abdomen. No rash was found anywhere on her body. A Group A streptococcal rapid screening test was negative; other laboratory findings are shown in Table 64-1. The patient was taken to another hospital by ambulance.

Upon arrival, the patient's complaints included headache, cough, generalized weakness, sore throat that was aggravated again from the previous day, diffuse myalgia, right elbow pain, left calf to ankle pain, and a pain severity score (1 to 10) of 10, but the patient had no history of injury. Physical examination revealed a temperature of 38.3°C, pulse of 108 beats/min, respiration of 22 breaths/min, blood pressure of 109/71 mmHg; her neck was soft, and there was tenderness in the right lymph node, swelling and pain in the right elbow, and tenderness in the left Achilles tendon. Laboratory findings are shown in Table 64-1. Oxygen saturation was 100%. A lumbar puncture examination of her cerebrospinal fluid was clear and colorless, with protein 0.17 g/L (reference value 0.20–0.45 g/L) and sugar 4.38 mmol/L (reference value 2.5–4.5 mmol/L), and smear staining did not reveal pathogens or leukocytes. A chest radiograph and elbow plain radiograph did not reveal any abnormality.

Two hours after presentation, the patient had a temperature of 38.6°C, a heart rate of 108 beats/min, and a blood pressure of 76/38 mmHg. Routine urinalysis was negative except for a trace of protein. Urine was sent for culture at the same time. She was given 1 g intravenous ceftriaxone sodium. Ten minutes later, generalized pruritus started, and urticaria was found on her neck and back. 25 mg of Benadryl and 125 mg of methylprednisolone were given intravenously immediately. An electrocardiogram showed sinus tachycardia. Her blood pressure dropped to 61/39 mmHg despite 3 L of saline infusion, so continuous dobutamine hydrochloride was given through a peripheral vein, followed by 1 g vancomycin intravenously and nasal cannula oxygen. After infusion of 4 L of saline, the patient was taken to our emergency center in an ambulance.

The patient was previously healthy. She lived in a dormitory, had one regular sexual partner, and always used condoms. She had received a meningococcal vaccine before entering college at the age of 18. The only oral medication she took was oral contraceptive pills. Azithromycin had caused nausea and vomiting in the patient, and meclozine had caused dyspnea and altered sanity. The patient had a history of alcohol consumption but not smoking, and no history of intravenous drug addiction. She was physically active and had been camping in Maryland two months earlier; she had traveled to the United States, Cuba, and the Mediterranean several years earlier. The patient had no family history of immunodeficiency.

II. Physical examination

Body temperature was 37.1°C, pulse rate was 105 beats/min, respiration was 14 breaths/min, and blood pressure was 84/48 mmHg. The patient was conscious and had no obvious discomfort. She was treated with 5 μg/(kg-min) dopamine hydrochloride, and oxygen was administered by nasal cannula at 2 L/min with oxygen saturation of 98%. Examination revealed ulceration of the left oral mucosa, petechiae in the posterior oropharynx and isthmus mucosa, tenderness of the cervical lymph nodes, and mild cervical resistance, but meningismus could be excluded. There was pressure pain in the right upper abdomen, and the liver margin was palpable below the costal margin. The patient's right elbow was painful with passive movement, swelling was evident, and pus was flowing. No erythema was seen at the joints. Urticaria could be found on the arms, chest, and thighs. The rest of the examination (including a gynecologic examination) revealed no abnormalities. Laboratory findings are shown in Table 64-1. The chest radiograph was normal and a urine pregnancy test was negative.

III. Diagnosis and treatment after admission

After admission, a rapid drip of saline and supplemental potassium chloride via a jugular vein catheter was administered, and vital signs began to stabilize. The patient underwent a right elbow arthrocentesis in the emergency room, and orange fluid was sucked out. Routine examination showed 17,250/ml leukocytes, 94% of which were polymorphonuclear cells, 2% lymphocytes, and 4% monocytes, and no pathogenic microorganisms were detected by Gram staining. Blood specimens were sent for detection of antibodies to EBV and Lyme disease. Cultures of synovial fluid and blood, nasal, cervical, rectal, and urethral secretions were also performed. The patient was taken to the intensive care unit for treatment.

> **Thinking prompts:** Is it possible to explain these symptoms as uncommon complications of mononucleosis? Acute monoarthritis due to EBV has rarely been reported in the literature, and EBV has been isolated in synovial fluid in only one case. Infectious mononucleosis can cause hemodynamic changes, but they tend to be seen in cases of splenic rupture. This patient did not show signs of splenic rupture.

1. Ward-round analysis on admission

The following possible causes of arthralgia should be considered in this case: infection or inflammation of the joint capsule (arthritis), infection or inflammation of the periarticular tissues (tenosynovitis), or inflammation of the skeletal tendon attachment points (inflammation of the tendon bone anchor point). The differential diagnosis of acute onset mono- or oligoarthritis includes bacterial infections (e.g., Staphylococcus aureus and Streptococcus pneumoniae), reactive arthritis, nodular disease, injury, hemarthrosis, gout, pseudogout, and rheumatoid arthritis of a single joint. On the other hand, the differential diagnosis of polyarthritis should take into account endocarditis, serum sickness, acute HBV infection, HIV infection, microvirus infection, rheumatic fever, rheumatoid arthritis, and systemic lupus erythematosus. Arthritis due to Lyme disease can be oligoarticular or polyarticular, but is often not dominated by pain but by joint stiffness. In this case, the patient presented with oligoarticular arthritis without other concomitant symptoms, and the differential diagnosis could be narrowed to septic arthritis and reactive arthritis.

(1) Reactive arthritis: An acute asymmetric arthritis, often secondary to urethral mycoplasma infection or infectious gastroenteritis within six weeks, which mainly affects the joints of the legs, especially the knee, ankle, and foot. Inflammation of the tendon bone junction in the Achilles tendon is characteristic, and was also present in this patient. However, she lacked evidence of infectious gastroenteritis (nausea and vomiting without diarrhea), and had no signs of urethritis (although female patients can present with asymptomatic urethral mycoplasma inflammation). Her illness involved the elbow joint and, more importantly, had hemodynamic changes that could be explained by septic arthritis. Usually, a diagnosis of reactive arthritis can only be clarified when septic arthritis has been excluded.

(2) Septic arthritis: The most common pathogens in young patients are Neisseria gonorrhoeae and Staphylococcus aureus, while others such as pneumococci, Gram-negative bacilli, and Candida are very rare.

1) Staphylococcus aureus arthritis: The pathogen can be detected by Gram stain, and in 90% of cases the joint fluid culture is positive, with a large number of neutrophils (count over 100,000/ml) in the joint fluid. The patient in this case had only 17,000/ml of neutrophils in the joint fluid and a negative Gram stain smear, which was not consistent with the typical presentation of S. aureus arthritis.

2) Septic arthritis due to Neisseria gonorrhoeae: Neisseria gonorrhoeae – the causative agent of disseminated gonococcal infection – can cause two types of septic arthritis, namely limited septic arthritis and arthritis-dermatitis syndrome, which manifest as arthralgia, skin damage, and tonsillitis. Limited septic arthritis is rarely accompanied by bacteremia; dermatitis syndrome has positive blood cultures and characteristic skin lesions that appear as petechiae, ecchymosis, and small suppurative herpes. Neisseria gonorrhoeae causing disseminated infection can be differentiated from strains causing urinary tract infection by biochemical methods. Disseminated gonococcal infection is commonly seen in women. Menstruation may be an important factor in the dissemination of the bacteria, as most cases occur within one week of a menstrual period. Therefore, it is necessary to gather detailed information about a patient's menstrual history.

The diagnosis of disseminated gonococcal infection is confirmed based on cultures of blood and cervical, urethral, rectal, pharyngeal, and synovial fluid. Treatment is usually simple, the preferred option being intravenous ceftriaxone sodium. However, in this case, the treatment was somewhat problematic. The patient developed a severe allergic reaction to ceftriaxone sodium when administered in the emergency room. For patients with cephalosporin allergy, the alternative is usually a quinolone, ideally ciprofloxacin. However, the CDC recommends avoiding the abuse of fluoroquinolones because of the epidemic of drug-resistant bacteria that has emerged in the United States.

In conclusion, the most likely diagnosis of this disease is septicemic arthritis due to disseminated gonococcal infection accompanied by EBV-associated infectious mononucleosis.

2. Post-admission condition

On the day following admission, the patient's temperature dropped to 37.3°C. Her pulse and blood pressure returned to normal, her rash subsided, her right elbow pain was relieved, her liver was palpable 3 cm below the rib cage, and the tip of her spleen was palpable. The rest of the physical examination was no different from the previous day. Tests for adenovirus, influenza A and B viruses, parainfluenza virus types 1, 2, and 3, and respiratory syncytial virus antigen (direct fluorescent antibody method) were negative.

On the same day, all four blood culture specimens previously retained at the first hospital were found to have Gram-negative diplococcus growth. Since the patient was allergic to cephalosporins, 400 mg of ciprofloxacin was given intravenously twice daily. The following day, the Gram-negative cocci were identified as Neisseria meningitidis. The pathogen was further identified by the state laboratory and was confirmed as Neisseria meningitidis group B. In contrast, blood, synovial fluid, and pharyngeal, cervical, and urethral cultures obtained at the current hospital were negative and positive for EBV-specific antibodies, suggesting that the patient had a combination of acute mononucleosis.

The patient received desensitization with cephalosporins followed by 1 g/d ceftriaxone intravenously for two weeks. As a prophylaxis, all people with whom she had recent close contact received a single oral dose of ciprofloxacin. All of the patient's symptoms were quickly relieved and did not recur after discontinuation of the drug, with no sequelae such as joint deformity (see Table 64-1 for the patient's laboratory results above).

IV. Lessons learned

Invasive meningococcal infections often occur in the unvaccinated adolescent population. College freshmen are particularly susceptible because they live in an environment (group dormitories) where the pathogenic organisms can be easily isolated. In this case, the patient was previously immunized and may have developed the infection secondary to an upper respiratory tract infection or influenza when the respiratory tract was in a susceptible phase. Winter is a susceptible period, and it is relevant that this patient developed the disease in spring. She did not have the typical manifestations of invasive meningococcal infection such as meningitis, fulminant sepsis, and petechiae and ecchymosis of the skin. Chronic meningococcal bacteremia is a rare complication that manifests as characteristic skin lesions that may worsen abruptly if hormones are applied. This patient did receive hormonal therapy for a short period of time before the onset of the disease.

Septic arthritis is not a common complication of meningococcal infection, but it has been reported. In this case, the patient was infected with a strain of meningococcal bacteria that is not commonly covered by vaccines, and the susceptibility of the upper respiratory tract due to EBV infection and the use of hormones for the treatment of mononucleosis may have transformed an otherwise asymptomatic bacteremia into symptomatic septic arthritis. Refractory hypotension, which is only partially corrected by dilation and use of antihypertensive agents, is a clinical manifestation suggesting that the patient may be infected with meningococcal sepsis.

Infectious mononucleosis is not uncommon in clinical settings, but its under-diagnosis rate is quite high due to the haphazard application of antibiotics to patients with upper respiratory tract infections and the self-limiting nature of infectious mononucleosis, coupled with the fact that there is still a large gap between the laboratory diagnosis of viral infectious diseases in China and developed countries. In practice, hospitals often make only a suspected diagnosis of infectious mononucleosis due to the lack of sensitive EBV PCR test kits and rapid serum antibody test kits certified by national standards, so it is very difficult to confirm a diagnosis.

Case 64 shows that in adolescent patients with complaints of fever and sore throat, EBV infection should be considered, and it is advisable to take appropriate laboratory tests, if available, to aid diagnosis. It also reminds us that although one diagnosis (monism) should be applied to a disease as much as possible, the progression and complications of the disease should also be taken into account to avoid delaying treatment.

(Wang Xinyu & Shi Guangfeng)

Fever for two weeks
with weakness and weight loss

I. Medical history

Patient: Female, 20 years old, a college student. She presented to the hospital with fever for two weeks with weakness and weight loss. She had occasional headaches without neck stiffness or photophobia, shortness of breath, and occasional nausea.

The patient had a clear previous history of Holt-Oram syndrome, which is an autosomal dominant disorder characterized by malformations of the heart and upper extremities. Pulmonary venous malformation reflux, ventricular septal defect, and patent ductus arteriosus were surgically repaired when the patient was two months old. She had been in good health since then. She was recently diagnosed with primary EBV infection by examining for positive EBV serology and a positive PCR test. The infection led to a decrease in her whole blood cells. Due to the undetermined diagnosis, the patient underwent a bone marrow biopsy. The blood count returned to normal on re-examination, and a second EBV PCR test was performed two months prior to admission, but the results were negative.

The patient had no history of recurrent infection, no history of sexual activity, no addiction to cigarettes or alcohol, and no use of prohibited drugs. She had no recent history of travel or tick bites. Her mother and brother both had Holt-Oram syndrome.

> **Thinking prompts:** The patient came to the hospital with a two-week-long fever. The chief complaint here was relatively clear but not specific. In patients with FUO (fever of unknown origin), it is difficult to clarify the etiology from the chief complaint. This patient had a headache but no neck stiffness, which allowed us to rule out an acute CNS infection.
>
> The patient's previous history was unique, with a relatively rare syndrome, but this syndrome was not a key factor in this case. EBV infection is relatively common, but there is a lack of standard testing in China. The internationally accepted test is still serology and PCR, and once the EBV PCR amplification is positive, it is clear that the patient is presenting with the infection. The patient's condition was self-relieved before admission. Her life history can help rule out some conditions like

HIV and rickettsial infection. In addition, Holt-Oram syndrome is a dominant inherited disease.

II. Physical examination

The patient's body temperature was 38.5°C, heart rate 96 beats/min, and blood pressure 106/65 mmHg. She had a look of acute illness, and her neck was soft. On cardiovascular examination, a grade 3/6 systolic murmur could be heard at the left upper sternal border, which did not change from the physical examination in the previous medical history. Both upper extremities were shorter than normal due to a congenital syndrome, and she was missing her index fingers. No rash was found anywhere on her body. No hepatosplenomegaly or lymph node enlargement was found. The rest of the physical examination was negative.

> **Thinking prompts:** The physical examination on admission did not reveal too many positive signs. Both cardiovascular and upper extremity problems were related to Holt-Oram syndrome.

III. Laboratory tests

Total WBC count was 0.5×10^9/L, of which 40% were banded nucleated cells, 16% were neutrophils, 40% were lymphocytes, and 4% were monocytes, orthocytic anemia (erythrocyte count 25%) and thrombocytopenia (platelet count 102×10^9/L).

The international normalized ratio (INR) and activated partial thromboplastin kinase time (APTT) rates were within normal limits.

Lactate dehydrogenase (LDH) of 575 IU/L, alanine aminotransferase, aspartate aminotransferase, bilirubin, and haptoglobin levels were normal.

Multiple blood, urine, and fecal bacterial cultures, and Mycobacterium tuberculosis and fungal cultures were negative.

Serological tests were negative for HIV-1, HIV-2, hepatitis B and C viruses, cytomegalovirus, microviruses spp., and Ehrlichia spp.

Positive IgG but negative IgM antibodies to Toxoplasma gondii were consistent with previous infection.

Serum Cryptococcus antigen test and urinary Histoplasma antigen test were negative.

EBV capsid IgG antibody and EBV nuclear antigen were both negative. However, the EBV serum PCR test was 36,800 copies/ml [using the RealArt EBV PCR kit, Artus (San Francisco, CA, USA), with a lower limit of detection of 300 copies/ml].

A post-admission bone marrow biopsy showed that all cell lines were dysplastic with some fibrosis, but cytogenesis was normal.

> **Thinking prompts:** In Case 64 we learned about infectious mononucleosis typically caused by EBV infection. Although sepsis ensued later, the diagnosis was not too difficult from the point of view of infectious mononucleosis, and the patient

was diagnosed at the university hospital. However, in this case, since the patient presented with whole blood cytopenia after EBV infection, rather than the common mononucleosis, what could the cause be?

IV. Ward-round analysis on admission

Laboratory tests have a significant role in diagnosing patients with fever. The patient had pancytopenia (trilineage decline), which can be caused by hematologic tumors (lymphoma), systemic lupus erythematosus, and severe infections. However, her general condition was fair and therefore no signs of serious infection were found for the time being. Elevated LDH suggested that tumors, especially lymphomas, could not be ruled out. The patient was later screened for possible pathogens, but unfortunately many of these tests are not currently available in China, so diagnosing these diseases lacks a confirmatory laboratory tool. Bone marrow biopsy can be helpful in the diagnosis of patients with pancytopenia, and it is recommended that it be performed along with bone marrow aspiration to avoid delays.

V. Progress of the disease after admission

The patient started on ceftazidime (2 g intravenously three times daily) because of neutropenia with fever. Due to EBV infection, she received valacyclovir (1 g three times a day), followed by intravenous acyclovir and one dose of cidofovir (5 mg/kg intravenously). Non-steroidal anti-inflammatory drugs and cortical hormone were also used to relieve the fever. The patient received several blood transfusions and different doses of granulocyte-macrophage colony-stimulating factor (GM-CSF) to treat the pancytopenia. However, her fever persisted with a maximum temperature of 40.6°C. The patient went on to develop hepatosplenomegaly and extensive lymph node enlargement with tenderness.

> **Thinking prompts:** Here we can see how to standardize the application of antibiotics, and in particular the circumstances under which empirical antibiotics should be initiated. The patient started empirical anti-infective treatment only because of granulocyte deficiency with fever. Medical staff chose ceftazidime, a third-generation cephalosporin, for anti-infective treatment. As the disease progressed, it became clearer that it was multi-organ invasive, and the invasion of the immune system was more pronounced.

On day 10 of hospitalization, a CT scan of the lungs revealed three nodules in the lungs along with hepatosplenomegaly and cervical glandular enlargement. Bronchoscopy and lavage revealed active hemorrhage; stain examination was negative for pneumocystis, fungi, mycobacteria, cytomegalovirus, and herpes simplex virus (HSV). Pulmonary nodule biopsy revealed organizing acute pneumonia, which suggested a possible viral cause due to the discovery of nuclear fragments. However, immunoperoxidase staining for cytomegalovirus, HSV, and adenovirus, as well as EBV and fungal staining were all negative. A transjugular vein liver tissue biopsy showed central stem cell degeneration as well as sinusoidal histiocyte destruction of the hepatic blood, and all stained pathogens remained negative.

> **Thinking prompts:** By day 10, the disease had progressed further and nodules were found in the lungs, at which point it was determined that these nodules should be related to the patient's disease. So a lung biopsy was performed, which also supported the diagnosis of viral infection. Further staining did not help much in the diagnosis.

On the fifteenth day of hospitalization, the patient developed shortness of breath, which progressed to altered consciousness and multiple organ failure. The minimum white blood cell count was 0.5/µl. Blood creatinine rose to 283 µmol/L and required hemodialysis. Aspartate transferase and total bilirubin levels rose to 2,132 IU/L and 270 µmol/L, respectively. Ferritin rose to 4,800 ng/ml and triglycerides to 381 mg/dl. The patient developed disseminated intravascular coagulation (D dimer 4,456 ng/ml, INR 8.3, APTT 152 seconds, and fibrinogen below 60 mg/dl). EBV PCR revealed a progressive rise in the virus, from 443,000 copies/ml to 974,000 copies/ml.

> **Thinking prompts:** On the fifteenth day of hospitalization, the patient's condition deteriorated further, as seen in the manifestation of multiple organ failure. Meanwhile, the EBV PCR increased along with the progression of the disease, indicating that the virus was still in the process of replication.

The patient was treated with high doses of hormones to control the disease. The patient was admitted to the intensive care unit and given maximum support, but died on the nineteenth day of hospitalization. An autopsy revealed proliferating macrophages and hemophagocytes in the bone marrow, lymph nodes, and spleen, and EBV immunohistochemistry was positive. The patient met the diagnostic criteria for EBV-associated hemophagocytic syndrome, including persistent fever, splenomegaly, severe pancytopenia, abnormal liver function, and elevated ferritin. Additional diagnostic markers missing in this patient included genetic mutation testing, natural killer (NK) cytotoxicity assessment, and soluble CD25 levels, none of which had been tested prior to her death.

> **Thinking prompts:** The patient eventually died, and the pathological autopsy finally clarified that the etiology was indeed EBV-related hemophagocytic syndrome. The clinical presentation of the patient was found to be typical according to the diagnostic criteria.

VI. Analysis of the fatality

Hemophagocytic syndrome, or hemophagocytic lymphohistiocytosis, is a life-threatening clinical manifestation characterized by an imbalance or dysfunctional NK cells or cytotoxic body cells. This imbalance results in uncontrolled and ineffective immune activation, which in turn leads to cell destruction and multiple organ failure, as well as proliferative activation of the reticuloendothelial system and macrophages becoming hemophagocytic, resulting in pancytopenia, hepatosplenomegaly, and lymph node enlargement.

The concept of hemophagocytic syndrome was first floated in 1939 by Scott and Robb-Smith. The disease can be primary or congenital hemophagocytic syndrome, and secondary or reactive hemophagocytic syndrome. Historically, this distinction helped to differentiate between cases of hemophagocytic syndrome – one with an infantile onset and a high mortality rate (defined as primary hemophagocytic syndrome), and one with an adult onset due to other etiological triggers, often with a better prognosis (secondary hemophagocytic syndrome). However, this distinction is artificial and has inadequacies. The first is that primary hemophagocytic syndrome may develop at any age, not only in infants and young children. Secondly, only 40% of patients with primary hemophagocytic syndrome can be found with a definite genetic mutation. Again, both primary and secondary syndromes may develop from infection. Finally, some secondary cases of hemophagocytic syndrome have a higher case fatality rate than primary hemophagocytic syndrome.

VII. Lessons learned

The patient was diagnosed with EBV-associated hemophagocytic syndrome, for which there is currently a lack of effective diagnostic tools in China. Therefore, making a diagnosis is relatively difficult, and the consequence is often the death of the patient. Moreover, EBV-associated hemophagocytic syndrome is currently seen to have the highest mortality rate among the various hemophagocytic syndromes. In terms of treatment, the early use of etoposide-based chemotherapy regimens is currently clinically recommended to improve the survival rate. The lack of effective EBV-specific antiviral drugs means that current iterations such as acyclovir do not help much in the overall treatment of the condition. In addition, there is evidence that the use of granulocyte-macrophage colony-stimulating factor in patients with hemophagocytic syndrome may instead accelerate the progression of the disease, and therefore its application is not advocated.

This case is arguably not a typical case of infectious mononucleosis. However, it was purposefully selected because EBV infections tend to be mild in general presentation and are self-healing. However, if they progress to become a hemophagocytic syndrome, the case fatality rate is very high. The author has encountered several cases of hemophagocytosis at the hospital. Only a few survived, and some of the surviving cases later relapsed and ended up dying. In this case, although EBV infection was diagnosed early, the disease continued to progress and did not respond to treatment. It would be a breakthrough to find an effective drug that could improve the survival rate for this type of case by even 10%.

(Wang Xinyu & Shi Guangfeng)

Case	1	SARS
Case	2	Amoebiasis
Case	3	AIDS
Case	4	AIDS
Case	5	Diphtheria
Case	6	Septicemia
Case	7	Septicemia
Case	8	Echinococcosis
Case	9	Viral hepatitis
Case	10	Brucellosis
Case	11	Brucellosis (chronic phase)
Case	12	Enterovirus infection
Case	13	Infectious mononucleosis
Case	14	Dengue fever
Case	15	Pulmonary aspergillosis
Case	16	Lung fluke disease
Case	17	Liver fluke disease
Case	18	Toxoplasmosis
Case	19	Toxoplasmosis
Case	20	Leptospirosis
Case	21	Relapsing fever
Case	22	Cholera
Case	23	Tuberculous meningitis
Case	24	Mixed meningitis (cryptococcal, tuberculosis mixed infection)
Case	25	AIDS combined with Pneumocystis carinii pneumonia
Case	26	Rabies
Case	27	Rabies
Case	28	Lyme disease
Case	29	Bacterial dysentery
Case	30	Bacterial dysentery
Case	31	Shock-type toxic bacillary dysentery
Case	32	Epidemic cerebrospinal meningitis Influenza
Case	33	Epidemic typhus
Case	34	Endemic typhus
Case	35	Influenza
Case	36	Mumps complicated by pancreatitis
Case	37	Mumps complicated by meningitis

ABOUT THE EDITOR-IN-CHIEF

LI LANJUAN is a member of the Chinese Academy of Engineering, a professor, a chief physician, and a doctoral supervisor. Renowned in China for her expertise on infectious diseases, she has been engaged in clinical and scientific research and education on this topic for more than 30 years. As the pioneer of the artificial liver in China, she made a major breakthrough in creating a unique and effective support system for the treatment of heavy hepatitis. She proposed the theory of using infection microecology to examine the occurrence, development, and outcome of infection, providing a new idea for the prevention and treatment of infection.

Professor Li has presided over ten national projects, including the 863 Program, the 973 Program, the tenth Five-year National Key Scientific and Technological Project, and key projects for the National Natural Science Foundation of China. She has published more than 200 papers, more than 30 of which are SCI-indexed, and has authorized eight patents. She has won two National Science and Technology Progress Awards, four first prizes for Progress in Science and Technology in Zhejiang Province, and a second prize for Popularization and Application in Colleges and Universities granted by the Ministry of Education. She is now the director of the Key State Laboratory for the Diagnosis of Infectious Diseases, the leader of the Key State Discipline Department of Internal Medicine (Infectious Diseases), the academic leader of the Key National Discipline of Infectious Diseases for Project 211, the chair of the Zhejiang Association for Science and Technology, and the director of the Zhejiang Key Laboratory of Infectious Diseases.

She also serves as Vice President of the Chinese Medical Association, Vice President of the Chinese Health Information Society, Associate Board Chair of the Chinese Society of Biomedical Engineering, Chief of the Infectious Diseases Division at the China Medical Association, Leader of Liver Failure and the Artificial Liver Group in the Infectious Diseases Division of the China Medical Association, Director of the National Artificial Liver Training Center, President of the Infectious Diseases Doctors' Branch of the Chinese Medical Doctor Association, Associate Division Chief of the Microecology Branch of the China Preventive Medicine Association, Director of the International Society for Blood Purification, and Chair of the Science and Technology Association in Zhejiang. She serves as Editor-in-chief of the *Chinese Journal of Clinical Infectious Diseases*, the *Chinese Journal of Microecology*, and the *Zhejiang Medical Journal*. She is also the Vice Editor-in-Chief of the *Chinese Journal of Infectious Diseases* and the *International Journal of Epidemiology and Infectious Disease*. She has edited and published 15 monographs, including the first edition of *Artificial Liver and Infectious Microecology of China*, and has planned teaching materials on infectious diseases for the Ministry of Education.

In recent years, she has been an advocate for the Face-to-Face Action Plan for Health, and as the General Director of the National Science and Technology Support Program, she has worked on the National Digital Health Key Technology and Regional Demonstration and Application Research Project, which aims for the realization of digital health in China. She has also served as a technical officer for the expert group of the 11th Five-Year Plan for major scientific and technological projects on the prevention and control of major infectious diseases, as well as the expert team leader for the Integrated Prevention and Control Demonstration Area and Field Study, and the head of the clinical diagnosis and treatment group of the National Influenza A (H1N1) Expert Committee, making significant contributions to the diagnosis and treatment of infectious diseases in China.